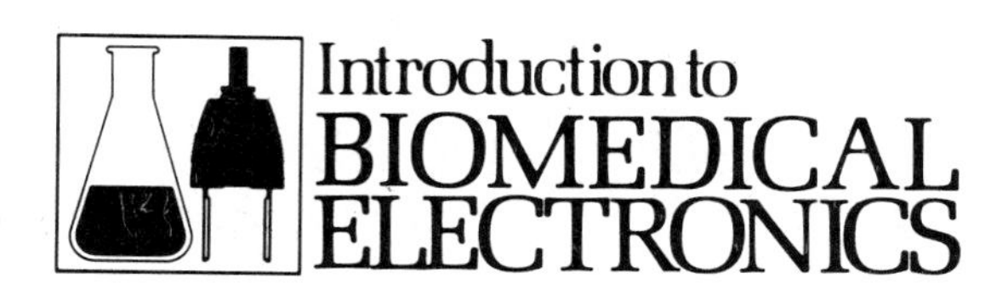
Introduction to
BIOMEDICAL
ELECTRONICS

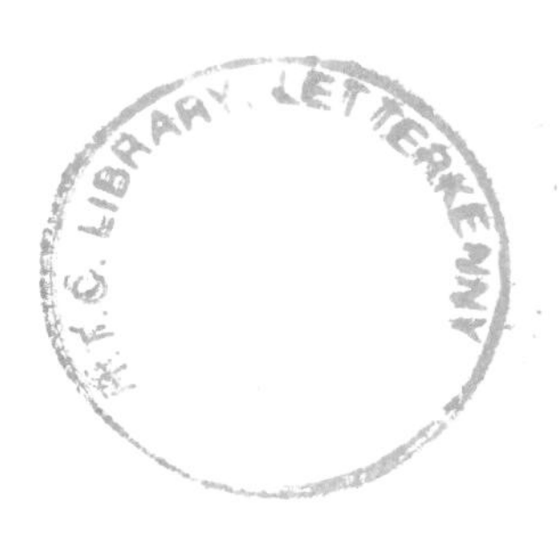
R.T.C. LIBRARY, LETTERKENNY

About the Author

Joseph DuBovy has been a biomedical consultant for Philadelphia General Hospital. He has been a biomedical engineer at Burke Rehabilitation Center in White Plains, New York. He has also been an instructor in biofeedback at the State University of New York at New Paltz, and has been an electronics instructor at Technical Careers Institute in New York. In addition, he has served as publisher and editor of the *Journal of Medical Electronics*.

Joseph DuBovy
Biomedical Consultant

Introduction to BIOMEDICAL ELECTRONICS

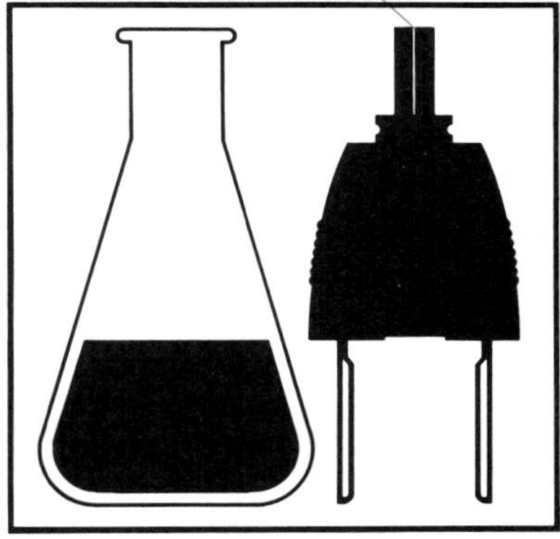

Gregg Division
McGraw-Hill Book Company

New York
St. Louis
Dallas
San Francisco
Auckland
Bogotá
Düsseldorf
Johannesburg
London
Madrid
Mexico
Montreal
New Delhi
Panama
Paris
São Paulo
Singapore
Sydney
Tokyo
Toronto

Library of Congress Cataloging in Publication Data

DuBovy, Joseph.
Introduction to biomedical electronics.

Includes index.
1. Medical electronics. I. Title.
R856.D7 610'.28 77-17920
ISBN 0-07-017895-X

INTRODUCTION TO BIOMEDICAL ELECTRONICS

2 3 4 5 6 7 8 9 0 DODO 7 8 5 4 3 2 1 0 9 8

The editors for this book were George J. Horesta and Alice V. Manning, the designer was Charles A. Carson, the cover designer was Jackie Merri Meyer, the art supervisor was George T. Resch, and the production supervisors were Kathleen Morrissey and May Konopka. It was set in Melior by Progressive Typographers.
Printed and bound by R. R. Donnelley & Sons Company.

To my father, whose life might have been prolonged had progress in biomedical electronics arrived earlier, and to my mother, whose loving thoughts have eased my way

CONTENTS

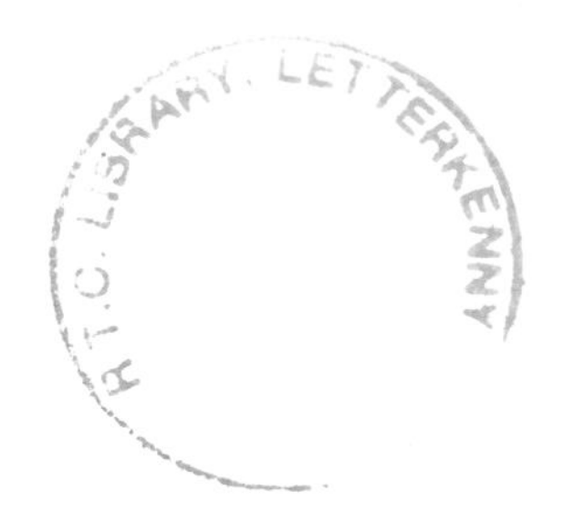

PREFACE

When one thinks of an electric generator, the generator a power company uses to produce electricity comes to mind. It is a miracle of modern technology, whose magic is only exceeded by another far more complex electric generator—the human body.

There are some 425 muscles that would never move if internal and external electric signals did not bid them to. The brain has been compared to a computer of some advanced age. It receives data and is programmed by the senses. It can store over 6 billion bits of information. All 6 billion bits can be evoked by proper stimulation. In sleep, in a coma, or in any other state, the brain generates electrical activity. When this activity ceases, life ceases with it. In fact, this activity has become the definition of life itself, indicating the dividing line between life and death. The pacemaker inside the wall of the right atrium emits a series of pulses which cause the heart to pump blood through the arteries. Without electric signals sensing a lateral pressure differential within our head, we would find our sense of balance impaired. Everything we sense must be converted into electrical activity before the brain will respond to it. A well-regulated feedback loop consisting of electric signals functions through the autonomic nervous system to regulate heart rate and other organs. As a source of electrical activity, the human body is far more sophisticated than anything humans have invented.

Of all the revolutions that have taken place in history, by far the most radical is the revolution in medical electronic technology. Yet the biomedical engineering revolution is in its infancy. The best is yet to come. At present we can monitor physiological data or use it for diagnosis. In the future, physiological electrical activity will become an automatic extension of the nervous system itself, with the results completely programmable. In the past, medicine has treated disease and organic dysfunction after they have occurred. Computerized tabulations of norms in physiological data are making preventive medicine a reality through mass population screening. Electronics can reveal advance clues to every known disease and malfunction. The flights of the astronauts dramatized the fact that human physiological data can be telemetered around the world at the speed of light. By combining advanced telemetering technique with satellite communications technology, the most renowned medical specialist could be at the bedside of any patient anywhere on the face of the earth.

The revolution in medical electronics technology has created one problem. That is the desperate need for biomedical engineering technicians (BMETs) with the following qualifications:

1. A thorough understanding of the concepts involved in the application of biomedical instrumentation and systems
2. An ability to maintain equipment in good operating condition even when only second-rate test equipment is available
3. A talent for communicating effectively with physicians, describing both the capabilities and the limitations of the hardware, to help physicians make the most of their electronic tools

This text begins with a basic exploration of the biomedical frequency spectrum and its physiochemical origins, then continues with a discussion of how physiological data are changed into electric signals or amplified. Once the electric signals are ready to be processed, we had better make certain that no unwanted or nonmedical data are included. Therefore, Chapter 4 explores interference and instability. Second only to interference as a problem is maintaining biomedical fidelity in the readout device. That is covered in Chapter 5. It would be impossible for a text of this type to contain every circuit to be found in biomedical instrumentation. Instead, this text explores in detail only those circuits which are most commonly found in various types of medical instrumentation.

Chapters 8 to 10 explore the troubleshooting of solid-state devices, integrated circuits, and the entire system. Readers familiar with TTL and CMOS concepts will find in those chapters a review of what they already know. However, an attempt has been made to relate this material specifically to medical instrumentation. In addition, preventive maintenance is constantly emphasized. Equipment failure at a critical time can cost the patient's life. The pages devoted to calibration are specifically for the BMET who must meet high standards of reliability, often with a limited or nonexistent test-equipment budget.

The population explosion and the expansion of rural medical facilities point to an increasing reliance upon medical electronic tools. In some of the larger hospitals in the country, the single BMET has already been updated by a team of biomedical technicians. The trend in this direction will accelerate as the rapid influx of new electronic instruments into hospitals continues.

As biomedical instrument systems become more and more complex, performing an increasing number of functions, the BMET will be obliged to continue to study beyond the material presented in this text. This material has been written to serve as a general reference to facilitate subsequent in-depth study in a particular area.

The problem-solving material after each chapter will test the reader's comprehension of the various concepts discussed. The questions do not belabor specific numbers and details, as these are soon forgotten. Instead, the questions are geared to determine the extent of the reader's overall understanding of that chapter.

Joseph DuBovy

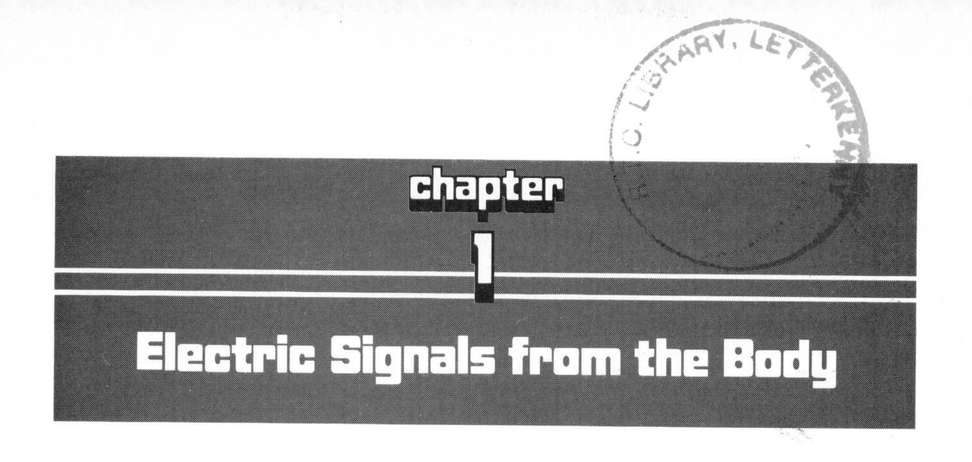

PART 1: ELECTRICAL ACTIVITY OF CELLS, TISSUE, MUSCLE, AND THE NERVOUS SYSTEM

1-1 GENESIS

In 1775 Austrian mystic and physician Franz Mesmer announced that he had discovered a force he called "animal magnetism," which permeated the universe. Mesmer's concept of a mysterious force at work within animals and humans was ridiculed by his fellow physicians. He soon was forced to give up his flourishing medical practice.

However, only 16 years later, in 1791, physiologist Luigi Galvani made a startling observation. An electric suture had accidently touched the dissected legs of a frog and the legs twitched violently. Galvani declared that there was indeed a mysterious force at work within animals and humans as Mesmer had proclaimed. Galvani called this force "animal electricity." The process through which animal electricity functioned became known as *galvanism* or a *galvanic reaction.* Several years later Galvani's friend Alessandro Volta placed dissimilar metal pieces on both sides of his tongue and noticed a strong, unpleasant taste. He had discovered more evidence of Galvani's animal electricity. Only this time it applied to humans. With the invention of the galvanometer, this new force could be measured.

As technology advanced, the vacuum tube finally permitted bioelectric potentials of very small magnitudes to be observed, classified, and analyzed. Bioengineering became a discipline that revolutionized medical science, and thus far we have only seen its early stages.

1-2 MOLECULES

Galvani's animal electricity, or bioelectric potential, exists in all living nerves, muscles, tissues, and cells. Its origin can be traced as far back as the molecule that combines to make up the cell. Even the molecule is subject to the laws that govern the atom itself. However, once the electrochemical energy of the atoms has bound them into a molecule, the smallest unit in existence with its own chemical properties has been created. A molecule may have identical atoms, as does hydrogen (H_2), or it may have dissimilar atoms, as does water (H_2O). Molecules of rare gases and hydrocarbons are highly volatile and easily evaporate (obtain enough energy to leave the liquid and enter the surrounding atmosphere). They are one extreme of the nonpolar family of molecules. At the other extreme are the nonpolar ionized (charged) molecules, such as sodium chloride (table salt). These ions move about in all directions in a uniform electric field and exert intense electrostatic energy on their neighboring molecules.

A polar molecule, on the other hand, does not develop into an ion capable of moving about freely in a uniform electric field. The polarized molecule will quickly orient itself whenever it encounters an electric field. All polar molecules (like the nonpolar ion) will exert a powerful attractive force on their neighbors. Polar molecules are less volatile than nonpolar molecules, boiling at a much higher temperature. Most of the organic compounds (alcohols, amines, esters, ketones, and nitriles) except for the hydrocarbons are polar molecules. Their electrostatic force or electric moment is stronger than that of nonpolar molecules.

1-3
IONS IN SOLUTION

Ionized molecules such as sodium chloride (NaCl) move about in all directions in a uniform electric field and exert a strong electrostatic force on neighboring molecules. In liquid solutions these ions migrate and thus conduct electric energy. These ions have become charge carriers. In living tissue, it is ions that conduct the charge. In tissue or solutions there are majority and minority carriers. A majority carrier may be sodium or chlorine ions or intercellular potassium. Such ions occur in large concentrations and are extremely mobile. When current flows, they carry most of the charge. Minority ions exist in low concentrations and carry very little charge. For example, in a battery, ions move about between electrolytes and thus are able to supply a substantial amount of current. To a far lesser degree this "battery effect" occurs in living tissue. In the living cell, if the concentration of ions is low on one side of a barrier and high on the other side, pressure builds up for an equalization to take place, that is, for the high concentration to move over to the low concentration. In other words, nature attempts to balance the concentration gradient.

Each ion can also be considered a charge carrier. Inside an electric field, an electron (close to zero mass) is a charged particle influenced by the surrounding field. Ions in solutions seek to equalize their concentrations across barriers as electrons move in accordance with the surrounding field. An electric potential has thus been created. The thrust to equalize the concentration gradient is counterbalanced by the electric charge. For example, in a pH glass electrode, only hydrogen ions pass in a solution with pH below 7. This is called a *hydrogen-ion concentration*. The voltage (electric potential) is determined by the concentration of hydrogen ions outside the electrode.

The pH electrode, like the living cell, is selective as to the ions that can pass through it. The pH electrode permits us to measure ion concentrations because a calibrated buffer (whose ion concentration is known) is compared to the test solution outside (where the concentration is unknown).

1-4 CELLS

The cell is the smallest system having all the characteristics that we associate with life. The cell will reproduce itself. The offspring of this reproductive process will be affected by material within the parent cell and the surrounding environment. As the new cell is formed, it will collect data from the parent cell and store these data in nucleic acid polymers. This storage takes place according to a specific code, and the new cells contain functioning protein corresponding to that code. The genetic code only serves as a foundation. The environment then becomes the leading influence on the future of the genetically coded data. The building block of the genetic data is adenosine triphosphate (ATP). Bioengineering as a discipline allows the researcher to plot the cell's growth and determine its future pattern.

1-5 THE CELL'S ELECTRICAL ACTIVITY

Electric potentials in living tissue begins with the chemical reaction within each cell. In this process, oxygen (O_2) is brought to the cell and waste is eliminated. Osmosis is the key to this process. Its function depends on the body-water concentration remaining within narrow limits. When the lower moisture limit is approached, osmoreceptors inform the brain by causing the secretion of ADH, an antidiuretic hormone. ADH is carried to the kidneys, slowing the removal of water from the body. Chemoreceptors monitor the carbon dioxide (CO_2) and oxygen (O_2) levels and the pH of the blood. When the CO_2 level increases, the inspiratory center is commanded to breathe more, bringing more air into the lungs and sending more O_2 to the tissues.

The proper chemical balance within cells and tissue both depends on and determines their electrical activity. Every cell has a similar resting electrical property. The outside of the cell has a potential of 65 millivolts (mV) compared to the inside of the cell. Potassium ions are concentrated inside the cell [155 milliequivalents per liter (mEq/L)] and sodium ions are concentrated outside the cell (145 mEq/L). There is also a concentration of chloride ions outside the cell (105 mEq/L). The cell has an electric resistance of 1000 to 10,000 ohms per centimeter (Ω/cm), a capacitance of 1 microfarad (μF), a dielectric constant of 5, and a phase angle of 75°. DNA and RNA in the cell's nucleus carry the information that determines how the cell will grow. The cell's energy plant, mitochondria, is found in the cytoplasm surrounding the cell's nucleus. Glycogen (a form of glucose) is stored in the chemical generator of the cell consisting of small canals. Enzymes in these canals change glucose to glycogen for storage. When energy is needed, glycogen is changed back into glucose.

In biomedical engineering we take advantage of the fact that a collection of living cells always has properties of resistance, displacement, capacitance, and impedance. Transducers can be designed to convert any of these parameters into electric signals. The cell's power plant (mitochondria) manufactures ATP (adenosine triphosphate) by the reaction of O_2 with nutrients supplied by cellular cytoplasm. CO_2 (a product of this reaction) is carried to the lungs, where it is eliminated and new O_2 is received. This cycle as well as all other bodily cycles is governed by the body's electric signals. An intricate feedback loop is the result. As each part of the body measures its own critical parameters, it sends signals in response to those measurements to maintain cyclical balance. Every time a muscle is moved, synapses in the spinal chord respond to action potential pulses. Body regulators maintain a fixed level for whatever variables they are responsible for, such as the regulation of body temperature, blood composition, or blood pressure. However, for these functions to maintain their balance, the entire electric system must be working properly, from the giant potentials of large muscles down to the tiny voltages across the membrane of each cell.

1-6 MEMBRANE POTENTIAL

The skin that covers a sausage might be compared to the membrane that surrounds the protoplasm of a living cell. A positive charge exists on the outside of the cell, while a negative charge exists on the inside. When the cell is stable or at rest, there is a 70-mV potential between the inside and outside of the cell. The human muscle can be compared to thousands of individual biological batteries or fibers lined up in parallel. The nerve is draped across this bundle of fibers, as shown in Fig. 1-1*b*. When a nerve carries an electric impulse to the muscle, it sets in motion a series of processes in which the membrane potential (70 mV) disappears in the individual muscle fibers. The result is the contraction of the muscle. After the collapse of the membrane potential, tissue cells immediately recharge to reestablish the membrane potential. This charging time can be as high as a thousandth of a second, or a millisecond. Both nerve and muscle tissue oxidize oxygen to maintain their charge potential and their ability to quickly recharge. It was this charge-and-discharge cycle in the frog's leg which startled Galvani into his discovery of animal electricity. Sixty years later (1848) Hermann von Helmholtz applied electric shocks to frog muscles at two different locations. Then he measured the time between the nerve shock and the muscle's contraction, first at one location, then at another. Helmholtz measured 0.0013 second (s) between the two locations. He then was able to conclude that the impulse travels down the nerve at the rate of 30 meters/second (m/s), or 65 miles/hour (mi/h). Since those early experiments it has been discovered that electric impulses travel faster down larger-diameter nerve fibers and slower through narrower nerve fibers. A fiber about 1 micrometer (μm) wide, such as the nerves telling your eyelids to blink, will conduct at approximately 1 m/s. However, nerve fibers causing your thigh muscle to contract (25 μm in diameter) can conduct up to 100 m/s. Nerve-fiber temperature also determines how fast electric signals can propagate, since nerve-conduction velocity in-

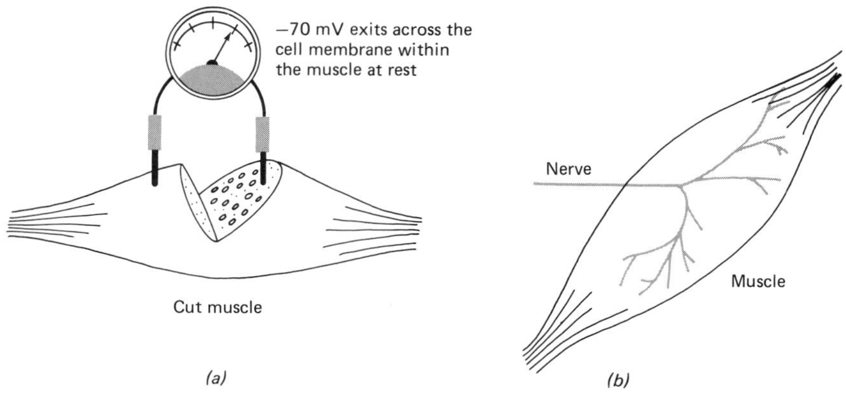

Fig. 1-1 (*a*) Voltmeter leads are attached to a section of cut muscle. A muscle can be compared to thousands of individual batteries or fibers connected in parallel. Thus the voltage difference between the surface and the interior will reflect the voltage across the cell membrane. The voltmeter reads the voltage, which is −70 mV. (*b*) The nerve is draped across a bundle of muscle fibers.

creases with temperature. This explains why you shiver when its cold and why excessive heat is so painful. Unlike humans, frogs, snakes, and fish possess poor temperature regulators. Their body temperature and nerve-fiber temperature respond to the seasons. Winter slows their nerve-conduction velocity to the point where they become sluggish or completely inactive.

Muscle and nerve fibers have only two alternative conditions: at rest or fully activated. Up to a critical or threshold level, the nerve fiber will not respond. But upon reaching a critical point, the nerve fiber is triggered into total response. This *all-or-nothing* situation affects fibers closer to the nerve cable (covering) than to the nerve's center. Figure 1-2 shows the fibers responding to various levels of stimulation. In the submaximal area the fibers are not yet excited. Maximal response corresponds to the fiber being turned on.

In the 1920s researchers Erlanger and Bishop introduced the cathode-ray oscilloscope to biological studies. The application of this sensitive instrument enabled these researchers to view precise variations in the waveshape as the fiber entered the supermaximal region (see Fig. 1-2) and how the waveshape appeared when the stimulation dropped below the threshold level.

The membrane effect can be compared to ions trying to pass through a plastic sheet with microscopic holes. The smaller ions will pass but not the larger ions. The result will be smaller ions of one type deposited on one side of the plastic sheet and larger ions of opposite polarity left behind on the other side of the plastic sheet. As the different-sized ions

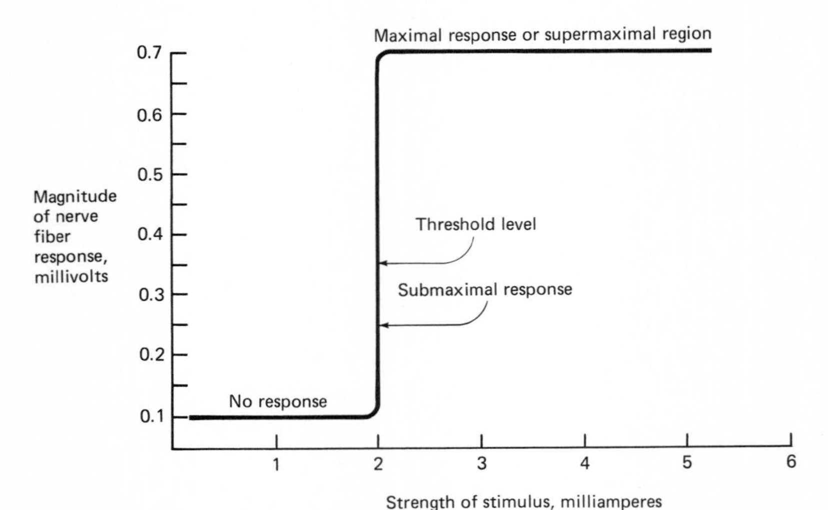

Fig. 1-2 Muscle response to gradually increasing electric stimulation.

have different charges, the result will be a voltage or charge across the plastic sheet. The physicist Nernst has given us an equation to calculate the voltage which exists across the cell membrane:

$$\text{Voltage across membrane} = K \times \log \frac{\text{concentration of ions inside membrane}}{\text{concentration of ions outside membrane}}$$

where K = constant indicating temperature of the solution and charge on the ions

There are approximately 20 potassium ions (K+) inside the cell to every one outside the cell. As with our plastic-sheet illustration, the cell boundary is selectively permeable to potassium ions and sodium ions (Na+). This is the essential reason for electric conductivity of nerves and the contraction of muscles. Sodium ions remain for the most part outside the cell. Thus we have potassium ions on the inside and sodium ions on the outside. In even numbers the approximate rations would appear this way.

	Inside the Membrane	Outside the Resting Cell
K+	400	20
Na+	40	400
Cl	20	280

1-7 THE ACTIVE CELL

When nerve or muscle activity reaches maximal value, sodium ions outside enter the cell. The concentration gradient of the resting cell disappears. At the same time the potassium ions pour out of the cell. When the sodium ions have reached their peak (inside the cell), potassium ions exit. However, after 0.0005 s a reversal of this process occurs, with potassium ions again entering the cell. After a second reversal, or a total time interval of 1 millisecond (ms), the cell is once again at rest. This sequence of cellular activity would appear on an oscilloscope as seen in Fig. 1-3. The significant fact for all living creatures is that as these events occur in one cell they spread like a prairie fire to all surrounding cells in nerves and muscles. The electric current generated in this way then travels to the farthest cells. Its speed is determined by the

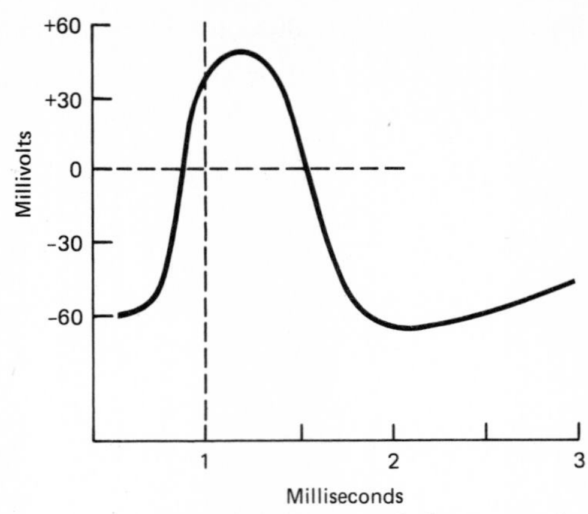

Fig. 1-3 Ion reversals create potential changes with time.

nerve diameter, with the fastest rates occurring in heavy fibers protected by a myelin sheath. This fatty sheath is an electrical insulator. It keeps the current inside the nerve cells so that leakage or a short circuit does not occur. Every few millimeters there are tiny breaks in the myelin where ions can move in and out and sodium and potassium interchange again takes place. These new interchanges further amplify the passing current. Thus the traveling impulse does not fade out. For example, if you step on a tack, sodium ions will pour into the cells at the sensory-nerve endings in the area of the tack. This sodium flow will repeat itself millions of times until the message reaches your brain. As we shall learn in Chap. 2, the brain generates its own sodium-in, potassium-out sequence. In this case, the brain acts like a radio relay station. It receives impulses from the sensory nerves, then transmits a responding set of impulses down through your motor nerves to your leg. The message is a command to your leg muscles to contract and pull away from the offending tack.

1-8 THE AUTONOMIC NERVOUS SYSTEM

For the responding message from your brain to quickly reach your leg, it had to travel along a very efficient route. This might be compared to a well-paved expressway. The multipolar, sympathetic nerve cells of the spinal cord act like a well-paved expressway for the traveling impulses. These cells are part of the autonomic nervous system that supplies cardiac muscles, pulmonary muscles, and the smooth muscles of the blood vessels and glands. Unless you practice meditation or trancelike rituals, you have no control over the autonomic nervous system, for autonomic means automatic (see Table 1-1). Let us suppose this were

Table 1-1 **How the Autonomic (Automatic) Nervous System Controls Bodily Functions**

Organ	Sympathetic Activity	Parasympathetic Activity
Heart	Change in rate and force	Decrease in rate and force
Blood vessels	Constriction	Dilation
Clot rate	Increases time	No effect
Glucose production	Increases	No effect
Pupil of eye	Some relaxation	Contraction
Tear, gastric, and pancreatic glands	Constriction	Stimulation
Sweat glands	Secretion	No effect
Reproductive glands	Ejaculation	Erection
Salivary glands	Slight secretion	Copious secretion
Gall bladder	Relaxation	Contraction

changed into a voluntary system. Then you would have to consciously command your lungs to expand, your heart to beat, your blood vessels to contract, and your glands to function. Obviously you would not survive this way. The specialized form of nerve pathway that enables this automatic function to occur exists in the brain and the spinal cord. Figure 1-4 is an illustration of this system. Nerve cells outside the central nervous system (CNS) are called *ganglion* cells. Within the CNS they are called a *nucleus*. The axons of ganglion cells terminate in cardiac muscle, smooth muscle, and gland cells. These impulse receivers are called *effectors*. The skeletal muscles supplied by motor-nerve fibers are the best-known examples of this system. These fibers start from motor cells in the brain or spinal cord and lead to the muscle fibers.

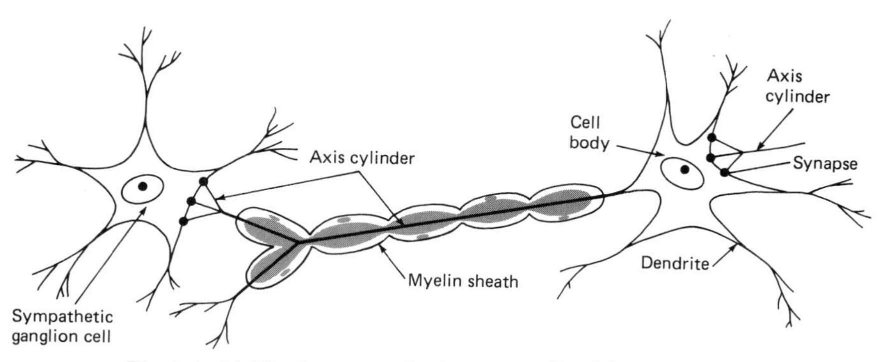

Fig. 1-4 Multipolar, sympathetic nerve cells of the spinal cord.

1-9 NERVE AND MUSCLE DISEASE

In healthy nerves no impulse will exist when no command is sent through the nervous system. Using an electromyograph, the neurologist or electromyographer will look for spurious electric potentials when no command is being sent through the nervous system. Fasciculation potentials of various sizes and shapes (irregular and less than three or four per second) when no command is being sent indicates a nervous-system abnormality in the dendrites, the cell body, the axon, or the terminal branchings. In motor-unit diseases, repetitive high-frequency discharges would indicate substantial atrophy.

Like the nerves, muscles should be electrically silent when at rest. The electromyographer will look for fibrillation potentials from a resting muscle. These potentials occur at a rate of 2 to 20 per second, and their amplitude can be as high as 200 μV with a 1-ms duration. They start with a positive phase, then become diphasic or triphasic. Fibrillation potentials reveal that the muscle-cell membrane is unstable. There may be several reasons for this membrane instability. A major one is denervation. In denervation, the nerve draped across the muscle fiber is not supplying the muscle properly. Consequently, the muscle compensates by becoming abnormally active electrically. Fibrillation potentials, indicating an unhealthy muscle, can also arise from spinal shock, an electrolyte unbalance, or an inflammatory process.

1-10 THE SYNAPSE

When muscles contract, it is due to the message from the nerve which has reached them through the synapse (Fig. 1-4). A single muscle fiber will receive only one nerve fiber, and the junction between them is called the *end plate.* The proper function of this end-plate region is a vital key in the workings of the nervous system. Its details can be seen in the reproduction of an electron microscope picture. Figure 1-5 shows that the nerve cell is separated from its surroundings by a tiny space measuring only about 200 angstroms (Å). In the brain as well as in the nerve, specialized cells called *glia* are concentrated in the vicinity of the nerve. These glia cells exist in heavy concentration; the junction between the nerve and muscle, however, contains nothing. The synaptic regions in the brain are very similar to the nerve-muscle junction of Fig. 1-5. Both contain a dense concentration of chemical substance required to pass impulses from one cell to the next one. Ion movement and the interchange of sodium and potassium ions occur as has previously been described. Curare, strychnine, and other deadly

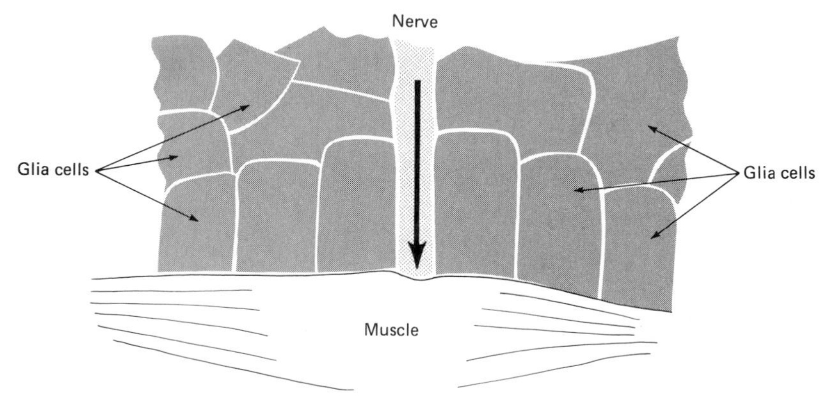

Fig. 1-5 The junction of a nerve with its muscle and the surrounding glia cells.

poisons are capable of interfering with the conduction of impulses across the synaptic regions. These poisons prevent the sodium ions outside the cell membrane from entering the cell, resulting in paralysis.

An electric eel is an example of a creature which can add its cell membrane potentials together to generate up to 600 volts (V) at 1 ampere (A). This large voltage is made possible by the fact that the tiny 70-mV potentials are all in phase or additive. When we explore the electrical activity of the brain, we will find out how phase relationships can produce waves of various frequencies. The brain contains highly specialized cells. As these cells relate to each other, the specific electrical activity associated with that organ is created. Another organ with specialized cells that interrelate to produce electrical activity is the heart.

PART 2: ELECTRIC SIGNALS FROM THE HEART AND BRAIN

1-11 THE HEART

All parts of the body depend on the blood supply for nourishment and cleansing. Thousands of miles of arteries, veins, and capillaries make up our circulatory system. Every day several tons of oxygenated blood are pumped through this system. Yet the powerful minipump, weighing less than a pound, that does all this work is capable of working over a hundred years without repair. The heart is made up of muscle fibers which continuously respond to electric and pneumatic signals. These muscle fibers are divided into four chambers. These

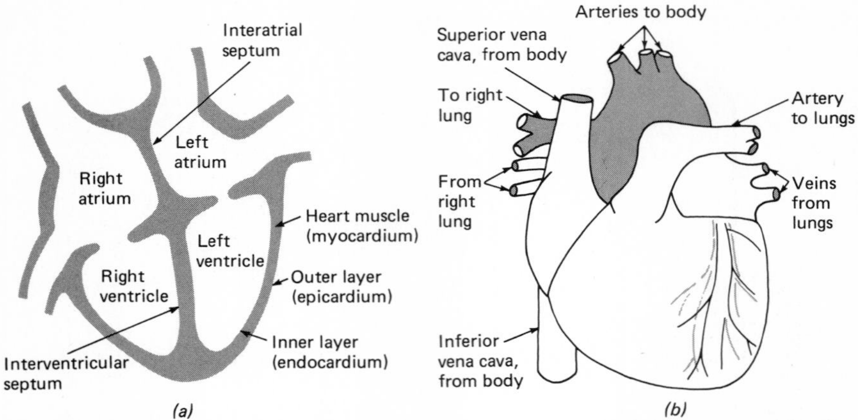

Fig. 1-6 (*a*) Simplified drawing of heart chambers; (*b*) actual heart. In (*a*) the four chambers of the minipump are shown. Their actual location can be seen in (*b*).

compartments fill with blood on expansion and are emptied on contraction. A simplified view of the heart is seen in Fig. 1-6.

Tired blood, having given up oxygen and acquired carbon dioxide or waste material, leaves the body and enters the right atrium. This blood is carried by large veins known as the *superior* and *inferior vena cava*. When the receiving chamber (right atrium) contracts, it forces blood down into the right ventricle. This chamber then contracts, squeezing the blood into the pulmonary artery. This large artery returns the blood to the lungs. Here, the carbon dioxide is removed and a new supply of oxygen is added. As we learned earlier, in Sec. 1-5, the potassium-sodium interchange in living cells cannot occur without oxygen. The oxygenated blood now enters the heart again through the left atrium. Upon the contraction of this chamber, blood is forced down into the left ventricle. When this chamber contracts, blood is squeezed into the massive aorta. Blood in the aorta begins its trip through the body to replenish the cells.

THE PACEMAKER

We have seen that the various heart chambers, during one phase of their cycle, undergo a contraction, forcing blood out. What causes these chamber walls of muscle tissue to contract? In the wall of the right atrium is a region of specialized tissue called the *sinoatrial* (SA) *node*. The SA node, acting as a pacemaker, generates electric pulses at a rate of from 60 to 80 per minute under normal conditions. Mystics, gurus, and some meditators are able to decrease this normal rate to as few as 10 pulses per minute. Hysteria and shock can create a condition called *brachycardia* where pacemaker pulses can increase up to 150 pulses

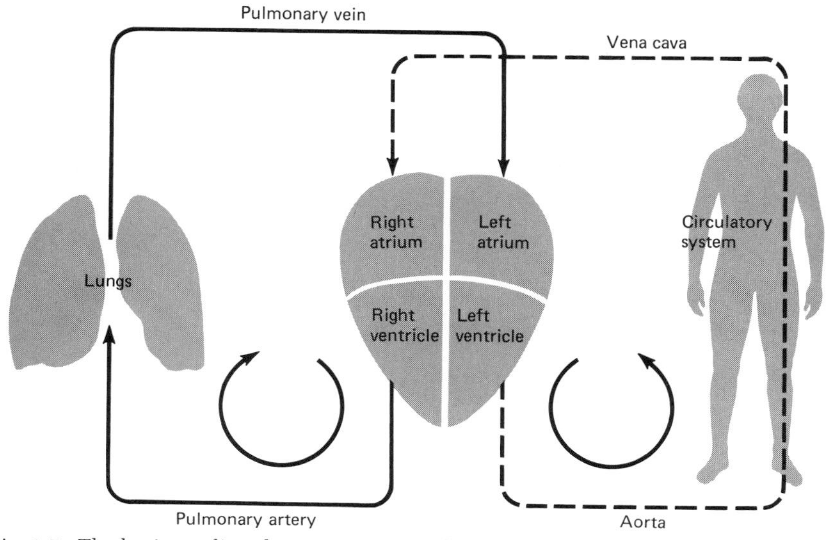

Fig. 1-7 The basic cardiopulmonary system. Blood begins its trip when the right atrium receives an electric shock from its pacemaker and contracts. This squeezes blood down into the right ventricle and into the lungs to be oxygenated. The blood then reenters the heart and is forced out through the aorta to replenish the body's cells.

per minute. These regulated pulses from the SA node spread through the atrial walls. From there they continue their journey to a region of specialized tissue called the *atrioventricular* (AV) *node*. The function of this node is to delay the trigger pulses so that the blood can get to the lower ventricles first. After reaching the AV node, the pulses enter an area known as the *bundle of His*. Once in this complex of tissue, the pulse causes both ventricular walls to contract, forcing blood out of the heart. In this manner, blood is forced both through to the body and into the lungs, as shown in Fig. 1-7. The pacemaker pulses can be picked up with an electrocardiogram (ECG). The shape of the ECG waveform depends on the placement of the pickup electrodes.

PHASES OF THE CARDIAC CYCLE

The first phase of the electric cycle causes the two atria to contract. Consequently, it is known as the *atrial depolarization phase* of the cardiac cycle. After the pacemaker pulses have passed through the AV node, they cause the ventricles to contract. The final phase in the cycle, called the *repolarization phase*, is the relaxation of heart muscle. Figure 1-8 shows a complete electric cardiac cycle.

Atrial depolarization or contraction of the two atria occurs at point P

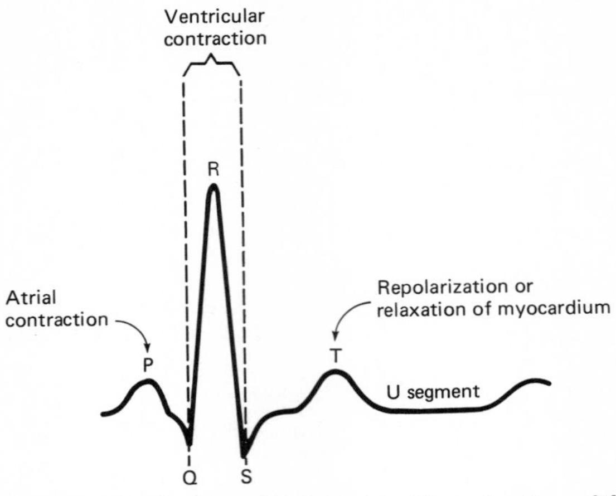

Fig. 1-8 A complete cardiac electric cycle. It starts with contraction of the two atria (the P wave). After the P-Q delay, the pacemaker pulse causes a sharp ventricular contraction (the QRS complex). The cardiac cycle ends with the T wave and the U segment, indicating cardiac-muscle relaxation.

(known as the *P wave*). After having been delayed by the AV node (this corresponds to the P-Q interval), the pulse then causes the sharp ventricular contraction. This is seen as the QRS complex. Finally, at the end of the cardiac cycle, repolarization or myocardium relaxation occurs. This is observed as the T wave. The U segment prior to the next P wave helps to indicate cardiac-muscle relazation. A depressed T wave with a depressed U segment usually indicates one or several abnormalities.

1-12 ABNORMALITIES

Should the initial pulses coming from the SA node be either slow or fast, then the cardiac rate will be either low or high. This type of abnormality is known as an *arrhythmia*. A prolonged P-Q interval would indicate that the pacemaker signal is having trouble reaching the lower chambers or the ventricular area. This would also be considered an arrhythmia. In Sec. 1-9 the denervation of muscle tissue was discussed. When denervated muscle is deprived of the minimum amplitude of voltage from the nerve (nerves) surrounding it, the muscle will compensate by generating its own impulses. These pulses are free-running; that is, they are not synchronized to other electrical events in the nervous system. During the cardiac cycle such pulses or ectopic beats may occur.

VENTRICULAR PREMATURE BEATS

The ventricular premature beat (VPB) is a ventricular contraction which occurs spontaneously. It is the best-defined sign of potentially lethal instability in the ischemic heart. The VPB is also known as the premature ventricular contraction (PVC) or extrasystole. On an ECG the VPB would be seen as shown in Fig. 1-9. VPBs can be readily recognized by the following characteristics:

1. *Prematurity*. The VPB occurs before (or at the same time) as the sinus-originated ventricular contraction.

2. *Compensatory pause*. Usually the VPB does not interfere with the normal sinus pacemaker. It ordinarily replaces one sinus-originated systole and has no effect on the succeeding beat. Thus the interval between the extrasystole and the next sinus beat is long by an amount exactly sufficient to compensate for the prematurity of the extrasystole.

3. *Bizarre morphology*. Since the extrasystole originates at some arbitrary location in the ventricles, its morphology is almost always quite different from the morphology of the normal systole. In practice, more often than not, it appears quite broad compared to a normal systole, as shown in Fig. 1-9.

To the cardiologist of the 1960s, today's electronic supersurveillance of VPBs would have seemed overdone. It was said at that time that VPBs, like gray hair, were a sign of advancing age. This is partially

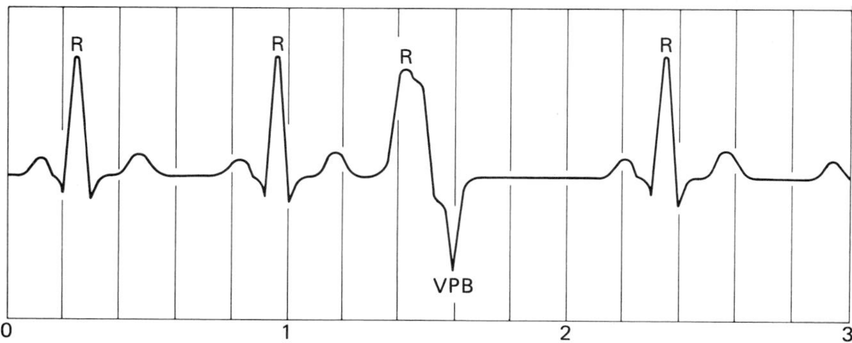

Fig. 1-9 The third R wave is a premature ventricular contraction replacing a normal systole. It is not generated by the sinus pacemaker but is instead spontaneously created by muscle irritability. As this offbeat pulse (R + VPB) originated in an arbitrary location in the ventricles, it usually is broad compared to a normal systole. VPBs have malignant potential and may precipitate fibrillation.

true. Computerized screening of large population segments has predicted likely candidates for coronary disease on the basis of VPB occurrence. While most VPBs may be benign, they have malignant potential when they appear together with ischemia. Experiments show that there is a critical zone of high vulnerability approximately 0.04 s before the apex of the T wave. During this time, extremely small electric shocks applied to the myocardium can precipitate fibrillation. Related experiments show that the threshold for free-running fibrillation monotonically decreases after sequential VPBs. Both the experiments and the clinical experience show that a single VPB during the vulnerable period can trigger ventricular fibrillation. The likelihood of fibrillation is multiplied when VPBs come paired, or in longer runs, called *ventricular tachycardia.*

Ventricular fibrillation is a nonsynchronized and rapid ventricular contraction. Its rate is up to 500 per minute. Actually, the ventricles are not contracting. Instead, they are quivering. Cardiac output (blood flow) drops almost to zero. This condition is fatal unless it is terminated within minutes. A similar condition caused by defective nerve impulses or irritable muscle tissue is known as *atrial flutter.* Its rate will range from 200 to 400 per minute. An occasional pulse may pass through the AV node to cause a ventricular contraction. Thus the ventricular rate may approach normal. However, atrial flutter waves can be seen on the ECG. Should these runaway atrial pulses slow down enough to cause contraction in the atrial wall, a premature atrial contraction would result.

In addition to the problem of irritable muscle tissue, there is the possibility of the pacemaker impulses being blocked. A *bundle branch block* is a conduction defect in the bundle of His. It can be a left bundle branch block (LBBB) or a right bundle branch block (RBBB). A conduction defect in the AV node would a complete block. A 2 to 1 or second-degree block means that every other impulse is able to pass from the atria to the ventricles. A 1 to 1 or first-degree block is when every pulse can pass but is delayed in the AV node. When the normal cardiac impulse has been blocked, biomedical electronic devices may have to provide an artificial pulse.

CARDIAC PACING

Galvani was stunned to see the frog's legs jump on contact with the electric suture. He thus became the first witness to the electric stimulation of living muscle. If the human heart is muscle tissue, could it not also be stimulated electrically? Indeed, artificial pacing of the heart has been one of the earliest examples of electronic techniques used for long-term treatment rather than merely diagnosis. In 1883 Gaskell discovered a bridging tissue between the atria and the ventricles. In 1907,

Keith described and named the sinoatrial (SA) node (the special tissue where the natural pacemaker originates). As early as 1819, Aldini had attempted electric stimulation of the hearts of decapitated criminals. Later, galvanic shocks became the treatment for cardiac standstill. In 1952, Zoll was able to restart an arrested human heart with electric stimulation through the chest wall. Sennings installed the first implanted pacemaker in 1958. It was powered by cells which were recharged from outside the body. A year later, Greatbatch developed a pacemaker which was powered by mercury cells implanted inside the body. Today some 280,000 people are using implanted pacemakers. The pacemaker is merely a solid-state pulse generator. Its rate can be either fixed or variable to compensate for increased activity on the part of the user. Section 8-7 will describe the two most commonly used pacemaker circuits.

1-13 PHONOCARDIOGRAPHY

Up until this point we have discussed the electrical activity of the heart. This electrical activity moves muscles and generates pneumatic activity. The pneumatic activity in turn moves the valves separating the various chambers. All this physical activity results in a great deal of noise or acoustic activity. The stethoscope is an acoustic amplifier. The application of electronics to acoustic amplification allows us to do more than merely listen to the sounds of the myocardial walls. We can hear the most detailed sound, reflecting even the smallest flutter of a heart valve. We can hear the blood flowing in and out of the chambers. Phonocardiography (PCG) sounds can be correlated with the heart's electrical activity and its pulse-pressure waveforms. In Sec. 1-14 we will see multichannel monitors that display these and other parameters together.

As shown in Fig. 1-10, PCG output is classified into four distinct sounds. The first and second sounds correspond to the lub-dub, lub-dub which is heard through the stethoscope. The second sound is shorter and higher in frequency than the first. The end of atrial contraction and the beginning of ventricular contraction is indicated by the first sound. The closure of the mitral and tricuspid valves (between the atria and the ventricles) is also heard in the first sound. In the second sound we hear the backflow of blood into the ventricles just preceding closure of the aortic and pulmonic valves. This sound splits into two parts. The first depicts inspiration and the next, expiration. Ventricular dysfunction, septal defects, or the stenosis or valves can cause failure of the second sound to split. A third sound may be heard with excellent recording equipment. This is the filling of the ventricles. An even more

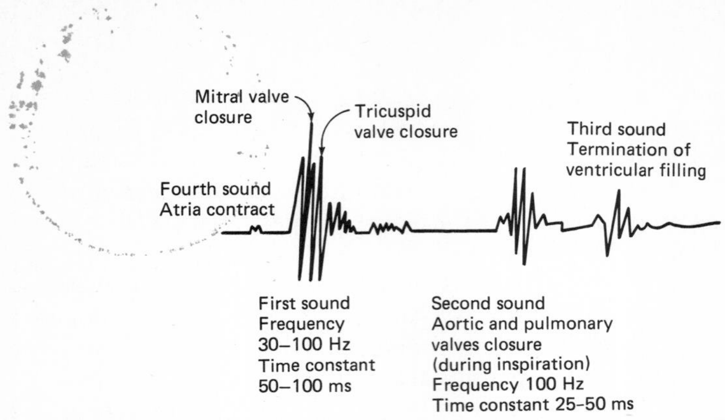

Fig. 1-10 The sequence of PCG acoustic activity. The first sound indicates closure of the mitral and tricuspid valves, respectively. During the second sound, the aortic and pulmonary valves close. The third, and weakest, sound is the completion of ventricular filling.

difficult sound to hear is the fourth, or the contraction of the atria. Heart murmurs usually have a higher-frequency component due to blood turbulence around obstructions when a valve fails to open or close. This can also be caused by a septal defect. The murmur can also occur during the systolic or diastolic period. Pulse waveforms are picked up by displacement transducers over the carotid artery, cardiac apex, or other pulse point. The PCG sounds are picked up by a microphone on the chest. Figure 1-11 shows the complete PCG data with ECG and pressure-pulse signals appearing in their proper time sequence. To develop this combination of data, the instrumentation shown in Fig. 1-12 would be required.

To the PCG specialist, the smallest acoustic activity offers significant information for diagnosis. A microphone on the chest may very well miss this minute activity. In this case, a microphone would be pushed into a heart chamber. This microphone is placed on the tip of a catheter, and the catheter is pushed through a peripheral blood vessel. This intracardiac technique has the advantage of eliminating sound artifacts caused by background noise.

1-14 SYSTOLIC TIME INTERVALS

Many cardiologists favor noninvasive techniques, where the patient's body is not "invaded." Today the well-known parameters of cardiovascular-system operation are being combined to detect heart problems noninvasively through a technique which allows measurement and analysis of the events during contraction, known as the *systolic time intervals* (STI).

The STI are derived from traces of the ECG, heart sounds, and the carotid arterial pulse, recorded simultaneously so that they appear in

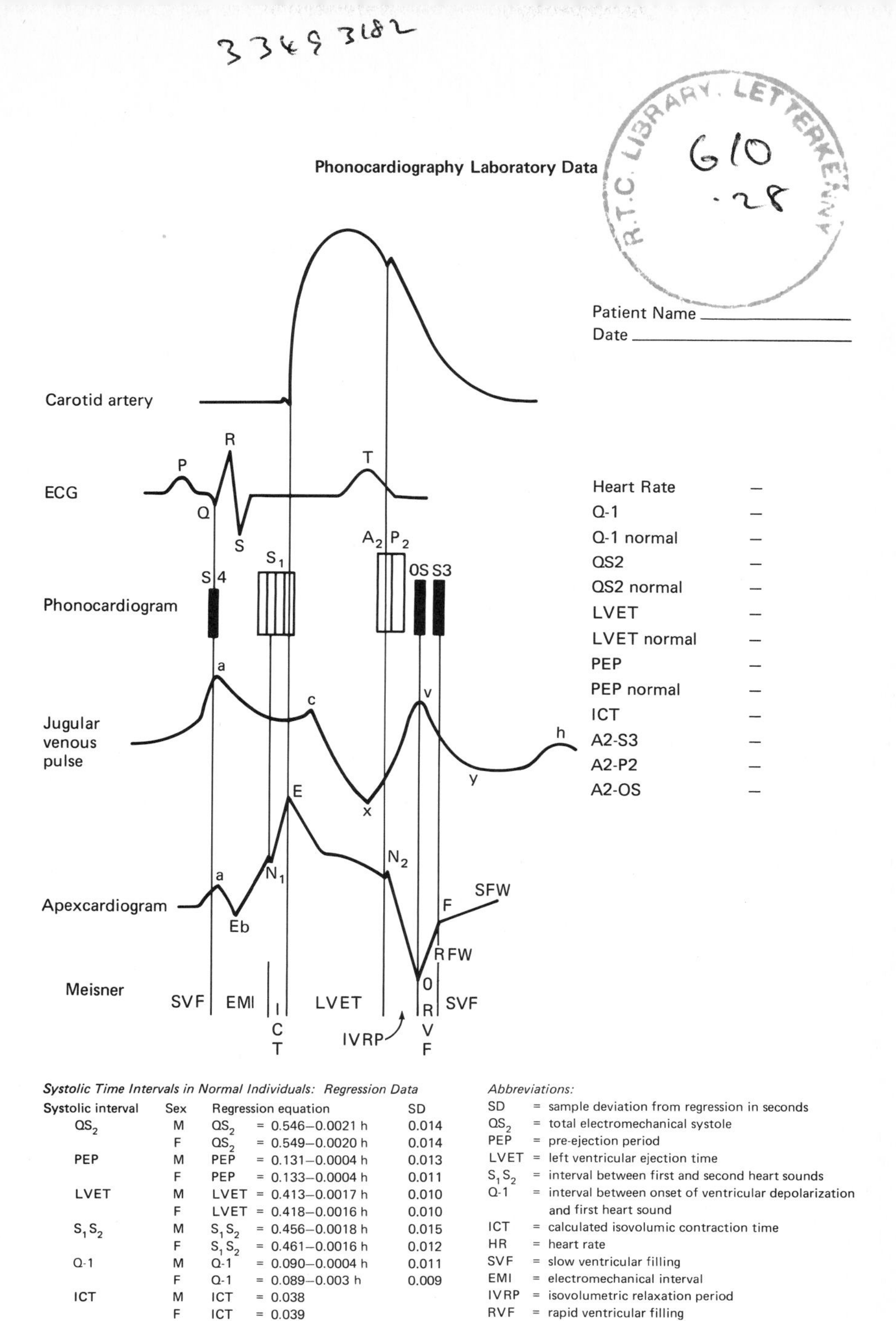

Systolic Time Intervals in Normal Individuals: Regression Data

Systolic interval	Sex	Regression equation	SD
QS_2	M	QS_2 = 0.546–0.0021 h	0.014
	F	QS_2 = 0.549–0.0020 h	0.014
PEP	M	PEP = 0.131–0.0004 h	0.013
	F	PEP = 0.133–0.0004 h	0.011
LVET	M	LVET = 0.413–0.0017 h	0.010
	F	LVET = 0.418–0.0016 h	0.010
S_1S_2	M	S_1S_2 = 0.456–0.0018 h	0.015
	F	S_1S_2 = 0.461–0.0016 h	0.012
Q-1	M	Q-1 = 0.090–0.0004 h	0.011
	F	Q-1 = 0.089–0.003 h	0.009
ICT	M	ICT = 0.038	
	F	ICT = 0.039	

(Taken from *Systolic Time Intervals in Heart Failure in Man*
A.M. Weissler, et al., Circ. 37:149, 1968)

Abbreviations:

SD	=	sample deviation from regression in seconds
QS_2	=	total electromechanical systole
PEP	=	pre-ejection period
LVET	=	left ventricular ejection time
S_1S_2	=	interval between first and second heart sounds
Q-1	=	interval between onset of ventricular depolarization and first heart sound
ICT	=	calculated isovolumic contraction time
HR	=	heart rate
SVF	=	slow ventricular filling
EMI	=	electromechanical interval
IVRP	=	isovolumetric relaxation period
RVF	=	rapid ventricular filling

Fig. 1-11 A typical PCG hospital data sheet. Specialists can note significant features of ECG, PCG, and pressure-pulse data. Time comparisons between the various types of data may be easily made using this data sheet.

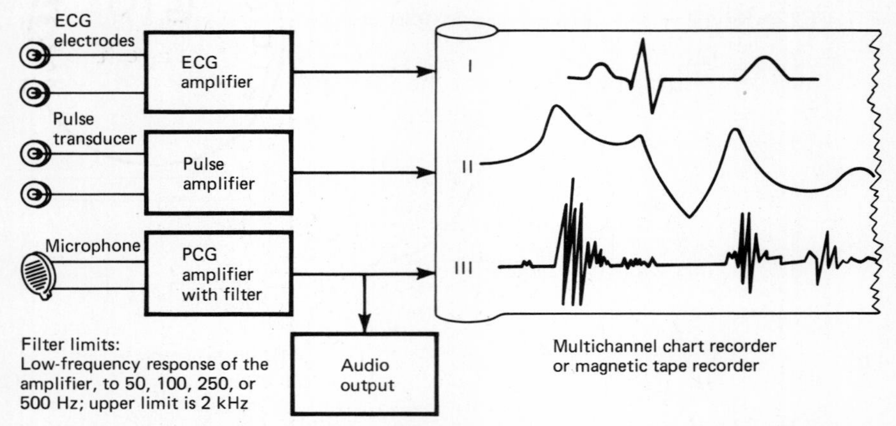

Fig. 1-12 Block diagram of a PCG system which might be used to generate the data in Fig. 1-11. ECG activity is amplified and appears as the first trace. Jugular venous pulse pressure is picked up by the pulse transducer and appears as the second trace. PCG data are filtered and amplified. They can be seen as the third trace and can also be heard.

their natural sequence relative to time, thus presenting a composite view of the heart in systole. Natural "landmarks" in the three tracings fix the beginnings and ends of the STI, which are illustrated in Fig. 1-13.

- **Total Electromechanical Systole (Q-S_2).** This interval spans the entire period of systole, from onset of the QRS complex on the ECG trace to closure by the aortic valve, as reflected by the second heart sound (S_2).

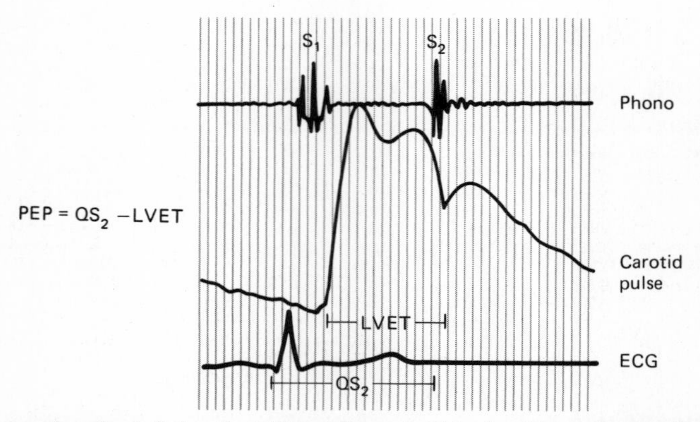

Fig. 1-13 Landmarks defining the STI are shown in this simultaneous record of a phonocardiogram, carotid pulse, and ECG, made with an Electronics for Medicine Simultrace Recorder. (Courtesy Electronics for Medicine Bulletin, Winter 1973–74, Volume 2, no. 4.)

- **Left Ventricular Ejection Time (LVET).** This interval spans the phase during which the left ventricle is ejecting its blood charge into the arterial system. The beginning of the interval is marked by the onset of the upstroke on the arterial pulse tracing, and its end occurs with the incisural notch.
- **Preejection Phase (PEP).** This phase delineates the interval between the onset of ventricular depolarization and the beginning of left ventricular ejection. PEP is obtained by subtracting LVET from the Q-S_2 interval. This eliminates the natural delay (typically 20 ms) in transmission of the arterial pulse from the proximal aorta to the point of measurement over the carotid artery. The timing of these events, as shown in Fig. 1-14, delineates the various phases of systole in the human left ventricle, as seen at catheterization.

The clinical significance of the STI stems from the fact that they, like the heart rate, cardiac output, and arterial pressure, are very well regulated under normal circumstances. Q-S_2, LVET, and PEP, appropriately corrected for sex and heart rate, fall into narrow ranges. Thus it is possible to measure these intervals in a large population of normal subjects and statistically arrive at a normal STI pattern. Abnormalities appearing in an STI measurement are readily detected because they fall

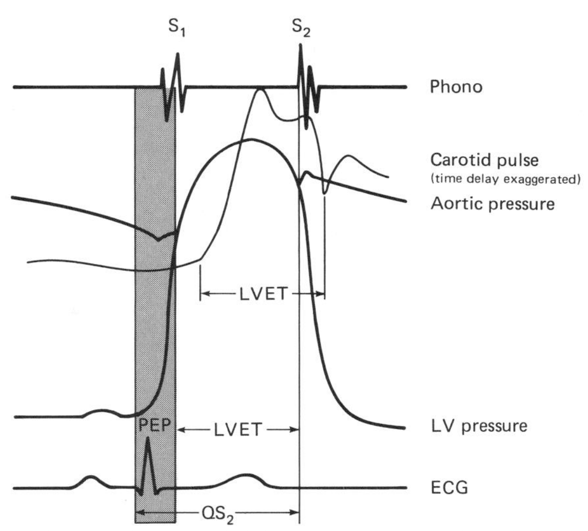

Fig. 1-14 The noninvasively derived STI are here compared to simultaneous pressures in the left ventricle and aorta. LVET measurable in the carotid pulse closely follows LVET measurable in the pressure tracing but is slightly delayed. This delay is canceled out when STI measurements are made from the same tracing. (Courtesy Electronics for Medicine Bulletin, Winter 1973–74, Volume 2, no. 4.)

outside the normal regulatory pattern. A distinct pattern of STI abnormalities accompanies chronic left ventricular failure: PEP lengthens, LVET shortens almost equivalently, while total systole Q-S_2 remains unchanged. This redistribution of the systolic intervals, in the presence of sinus rhythm and no intraventricular conduction defect, has been found to correlate with reduced cardiac output, stroke volume, and ejection fraction. The degree of alteration appears to correspond to the functional severity of the disease, suggesting that changes in the STI most probably reflect the functional state of the myocardium. Figure 1-15 illustrates a typical setup using an Electronics for Medicine Model VR-6. A phonocardiographic pickup is placed over the upper precordium, in a position optimal for recording the initial high-frequency vibrations of the first and second heart sounds (S_1 and S_2). Frequency limits of the phono amplifier are set to 100 and 500 hertz (Hz), respectively.

A Statham pressure transducer, air-coupled through a short polyethylene tube and small funnel placed firmly on the measurement site over the carotid artery, serves as an effective pickup for the low-frequency arterial pulsation. An Electronics for Medicine pressure amplifier processes the transducer signal and provides an arterial pulse trace of sufficiently large amplitude so that the points of upstroke onset can be clearly discerned. This technique, combined with other nonin-

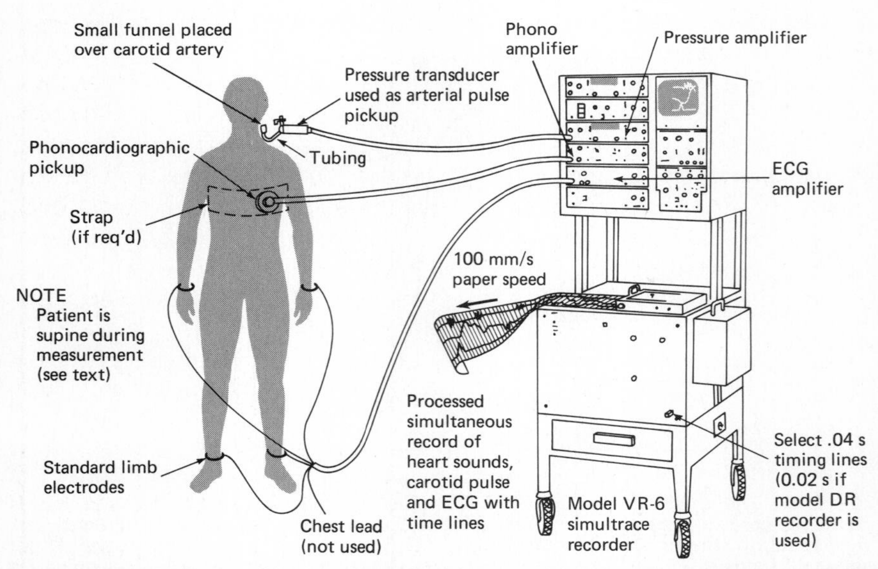

Fig. 1-15 Typical setup for recording simultaneous phonocardiogram, pulse, and ECG traces from which the STI are derived. Illustrated is a Model VR-6 Simultrace Recorder containing a pressure amplifier, phono amplifier, and ECG amplifier.

vasive procedures (echocardiography, scintiphotography, and radar kymography) can provide a "mosaic" of information regarding a patient's cardiovascular system. From this composite, the physician may gain sufficient knowledge of the patient's condition to conduct treatment without the need for catheterization.

1-15 THE BRAIN

All forms of life have some kind of nervous system; the mammal, however, has the most complex of all. This is primarily due to that most recently developed organ, the brain. The composition of this organ reveals the evolutionary status of the species. The various organisms have differing dominant brain spheres. Fish have dominant optic lobes; amphibians, a dominant smell center; and humans, a dominant cerebrum. The human cerebrum has grown over the other parts, forming wrinkled or convoluted gray matter. Whales, dolphins, and elephants have highly convoluted brains also, but the human brain has the most highly developed parietal region. This 3-lb organ (slightly less in the human female) approaches its full weight at about the seventh year of life. From that point its weight increases very slightly until the twentieth year, when it begins to decrease at the weight of a gram each year.

THE HEMISPHERES

The deep furrow separating the two hemispheres is called the *fissure of Rolando*. The hemispheres are bridged together by commissures or bundles of nerve fibers, the largest being the great cerebral commissure. Others include the posterior, anterior, hippocampal, and habenular commissures, the massa intermedia, and the optic chiasma. In humans, one hemisphere dominates, directing motor activity in the opposite side of the body, However, if one hemisphere has been injured, the opposite one can learn to do its job. Should any of the commissures be cut, no impulses will flow between the hemispheres.

Each hemisphere is capable of functioning independently. Normally, the left hemisphere dominates speech. The commissures can transmit visual or auditory patterns. Prefrontal areas control behavior. Oddly enough, the top of the brain controls the lower parts of the body, and the lower part of the brain controls the upper parts of the body.

THE CEREBRAL CORTEX

The cerebral cortex is close to the surface. It relates to motor control and to primary sensory response. Signals from the spinal cord pass through the reticular activating system (RAS) at the base of the brain. The RAS controls central nervous system (CNS) activity as well as wakefulness and attention. This system might be compared to the electric-power junction box in your home since both distribute electric energy. The RAS is dormant during sleep. However, almost any sensory signal, including pain from muscles or visual and auditory signals, can activate this system. Brain waves from the brain's surface relate to mental activity. Thinking produces asynchronous pulses in brain neurons. However, brain waves may originate from simultaneous firings of many neurons in the brain. Thus brain waves must be associated with a low level of thinking. Gurus who have spent most of their lives in meditation (a semitrancelike state where no thinking as we know it occurs) display much higher electroencephalogram (EEG) amplitudes than the average person.

THE HYPOTHALAMUS

This part of the brain (closest to the spinal cord) is called the *stem*. It is divided into a medial group and two lateral groups. Nuclei are also divisible, and several interconnections exist between hypothalamic nuclei and the hypothalamus. Tracts connect the hypothalamus and the spinal cord and the autonomic nervous system. Stimulation of the lateral nuclei in the hypothalamus will increase heart rate, raise blood pressure, increase sweating, inhibit the gastrointestinal tract, and cause secretion from the adrenal medulla.

Figure 1-16 shows an automatic control loop of the autonomic nervous system. As heat is radiated from the body and lost through evaporation and conduction (standing barefoot on a cold bathroom floor), more blood is brought to the body surface. Arterioles and capillaries close to the surface are opened wide and a large heat loss takes

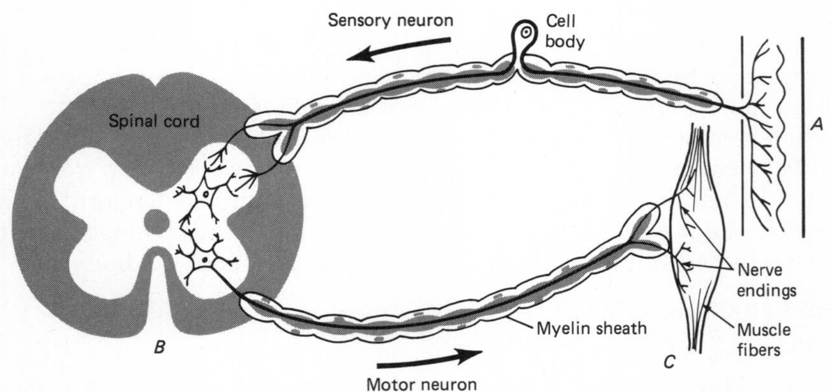

Fig. 1-16 A typical reflex pathway. Sensory fibers are stimulated at *A*, postsynaptic potentials are produced at *B*, and the impulses initiated in the motor neurons bring about a muscle response at *C*.

place. If blood is shunted away from the surface to the interior, the heat loss is minimal. Perspiration is another loss of heat. The hypothalamus functions as a thermostat and is sensitive to blood temperature, which it regulates. The hypothalmus is the center for anger, and its function is inhibited by the cortex. It also regulates food intake.

THE BRAIN'S MESSAGE CENTERS

The nerve cells which constitute the gray matter have two functions. They simultaneously transmit data over long distances and collect and compute data from different sources. The "wiring" system which facilitates data transmission is based on the axon. Axons branch out, making multiple connections. Each neuron or brain cell has its own axon, or transmitter. The remainder of the cell, the dendrites, receives data from other neurons. Dendrites are elongated continuations of the cell body. Their diameter narrows as they extend farther from the cell body. Figure 1-17 illustrates the basic composition of the highly specialized brain cell. As in the basic nervous system, the synapse sites are responsible for communication between nerve cells. When each axon branches, it does so through a synapse. Most synapses are found on the dendrites. Some are also found on the surface of the neuron body. Neurons direct data traffic. Each neuron can make a decision as to whether to pass data further along the axon. Each of the 50 billion (5×10^{10}) neurons may have up to 1000 synapses. Some cortical cells have 60,000 synapses. As with other nerve cells, the axon responds to electric stimuli in an all-or-nothing fashion. When the axon responds, it triggers the next one, and so on, like a set of falling dominoes. The voltage gradient across the axon is the same as in other cells: 70 mV. When a nerve impulse reaches the end of an axon, it triggers the release

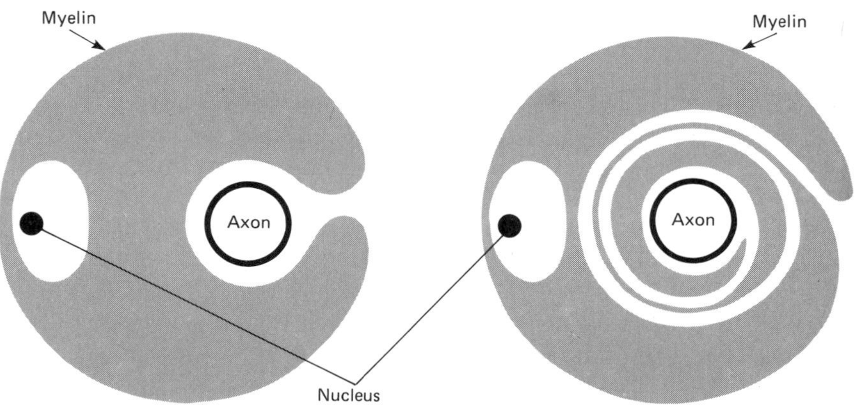

Fig. 1-17 Spiral layers of myelin surround the axon as seen through the electron microscope.

of a chemical transmitter which diffuses between the two neurons. Thus an electric charge is produced on the membrane of the next neuron.

1-16
THE ELECTROENCEPHALOGRAM

In 1929, Hans Berger first published his findings claiming that humans had brain waves. He had discovered a wave with an average duration of 90 ms (0.09 s) and a smaller wave with a duration of 35 ms (0.035 s). Berger called the larger wave the *alpha* wave. He found that the alpha wave underwent large variations in patients who suffered from epilepsy, multiple sclerosis, and other diseases of the central nervous system. The 8- to 11-cycle alpha waves can have amplitudes as high as 50 μV. They remain constant in frequency and have their highest amplitudes in the alert but relatively unoccupied brain. Berger found that the brain waves of retarded subjects were lower than those of normal subjects. He took an electroencephalogram (EEG) of a dying dog and found that as respiration ceased and the heart beat slowed, the brain waves increased in duration (decreased in frequency), with the amplitude slowly diminishing until death. During epileptic seizures, slow (3-Hz) waves with very high voltages predominate. Berger found artifacts from the eyes, as the retina is charged positively with respect to the cornea. *Beta* waves are associated with activity or states of tension. They have a frequency of 12 to 18 Hz. Cortical cells produce action potentials. When these potentials occur in the proper (additive) phase relationship, then summation results and voltage amplitude is created.

EEG specialists during World War II found that the alpha and beta rhythms had company. Another rhythm very evident in cats and rabbits was the *theta* rhythm. Traces of theta were found in children, monkeys, and some adults. Theta frequency is 4 to 7 Hz. It emanates from the temporal and adjacent parietal regions of the brain, midway between the front and rear of the head. These waves are strongest on the left side. Theta dominates among 2- to 5-year-old children. From ages 5 to 6 both theta and alpha are equal. From 6 up the theta diminishes. Theta seems to be associated with emotions, especially frustration. However, it increases with laughter as well as crying, hunger, and unpleasant stimuli. The slow *delta* waves seen in epileptic seizures were also seen in normal infants up to age 1 and in normal sleeping subjects. Delta is slower during light sleep, faster during deep sleep, and oscillates back and forth. During deep sleep there is a loss of muscle tone and rapid eye movement (REM) potential. Some specialists thought that the large, slow delta waves were protecting the brain, that when the neurons of the brain are in trouble (have difficulty in functioning) the delta waves are called upon to shut down the brain until order can be restored or until fatigue no longer exists. Such is the function of sleep when the neurons cannot do useful work. Sleep also allows a valuable mechanism, dreaming, to occur. Dreams have a cyclical nature, as shown in Fig. 1-18. Delta waves are often so large that they actually paralyze the cortex by electrocution. As a matter of fact, this may be their special function, just as pain is able to immobilize a muscle which is hurt or nonfunctional. At the opposite end of the EEG spectrum, *gamma* waves (low magnitudes) have been found in the high 35- to 50-Hz range. Also *lambda* waves were found to emanate from the back of the head. They occur at random times and have been asociated with vision. Another wave found only in a small percentage of subjects has been called the *mu* rhythm and was picked up from the central regions of either side of the head. Mu waves disappeared when the subject thought about moving limbs on the opposite side of the body. EEG investigators often find themselves strangled by their own raw data. This is why data reduction has become so valuable a tool in the EEG field. This will be discussed in greater detail in Chap. 5, The Readout.

During the years of EEG research, some unusual and interesting observations have come to light. Included among these are the following:

- Aspirin will cause an excess of slow waves.
- Two cups of coffee will stimulate the EEG.
- Abnormal EEGs are seen in persons who often have headaches.
- Marijuana produces slightly faster waves than normal.
- A convulsive EEG is observed at orgasm at the end of coitus.

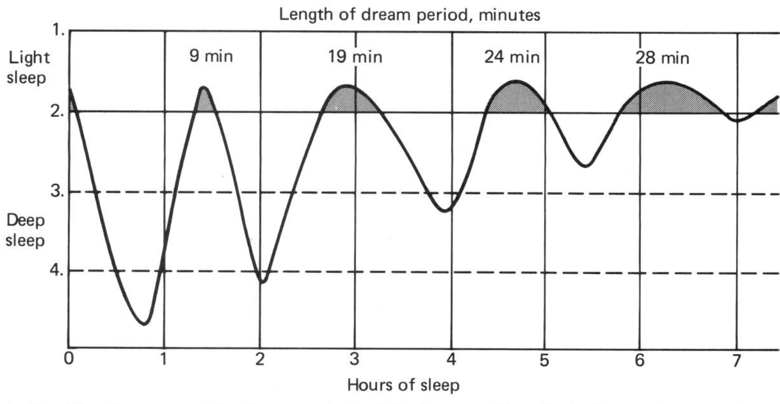

Fig. 1-18 We observe a 7-h sleep period with dreams (the shaded areas) occurring at cyclical intervals. Dreams occur only during light sleep. As sleep continues, each successive dream cycle becomes longer. The first dream period is only 9 min, and the last is 28 min.

- The EEG of an oppossum playing dead revealed a very alert animal.
- After a touchdown, a football player's alpha waves increased from 9 to 12 s.
- Yoga and Zen meditation increased the amplitude of alpha waves.

Researchers are in general agreement that the EEG as an index of cortical activity bears little relationship to the active discharge of individual cortical cells of the type which can be recorded with available microelectrodes. One hypothesis that has been offered suggests that brain waves might flow from membrane potentials in cortical cells. Such potentials would be changing synchronously. These oscillating potentials would not cause the cells to fire if they were below the threshold potential. A more recent theory suggests that EEG potentials originate within the dendrite material. Dendritic potentials are not spikelike pulses like those in the cells that fire. Dendritic potentials are more evenly graded, like EEG waves. According to this concept, the dendritic potentials are summed to produce the EEG rhythms. The basic concept is shown in Fig. 1-19.

Earlier we saw how the pacemaker pulse rate could control the heartbeat. This same concept can be carried over to the brain. Investigators are now at work on a pacemaker that would be located within the thalamus (seat of the brain). The pulses generated would then become a time base for the various brain waves.

Within the past decade, EEG researchers have shown a strong interest in the frequency analysis of EEG data. Many have thought that EEG amplitude analysis is closely related to the placement and type of elec-

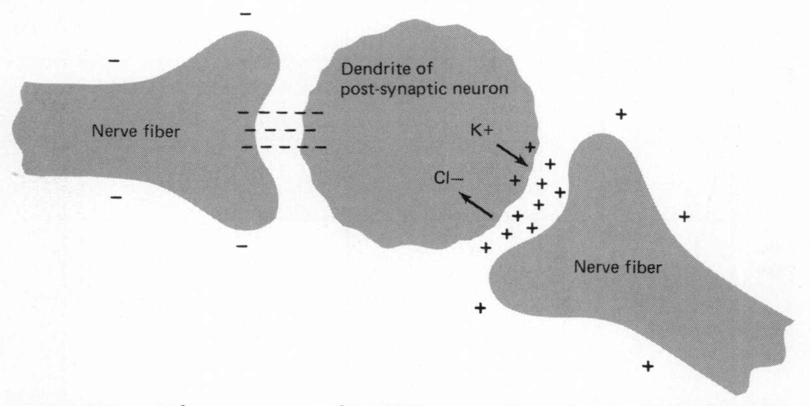

Fig. 1-19 A recent theory suggests that EEG potentials originate within dendritic material. These electric charges are transferred between one nerve fiber and the other through a dendrite of a postsynaptic neuron. A great number of these potentials are then summed to produce the EEG rhythms.

trodes as well as to the design of the electronic instrumentation itself. Because there are so many variables, it is possible to arrive at erroneous conclusions and results from the analysis of amplitude data. Frequency or phase data are referenced against time, and this makes possible repetitive experiments with the same standards and parameters over long periods of time.

When time data are being acquired, the frequency-analysis instrumentation periodically samples the input analog waveform. The Nyquist sampling theorem dictates that the sample frequency must be twice the highest frequency to be observed. This means the sample rate must be a function of the frequency range of the input data. This also influences sweep time. If the instrument is collecting 1024 data points per sweep, and the highest frequency to be observed is 25 Hz, then the sweep time would have to be 20.48 s. According to the Nyquist theorem, we would need a sample rate or frequency of 50 Hz (2 × 25 Hz). The time between samples would then equal 20 ms. If we need 20 ms for each point and we wish to collect 1024 data points per sweep, then

$$\frac{20\text{ ms}}{\text{point}} \times 1024\text{ points} = 20.48\text{ s}$$

If the EEG frequencies to be recorded are higher than the highest frequency setting of the spectrum analyzer, aliasing occurs. Aliasing is a distortion of the spectral picture, and consequently a false result. If the spectrum-analyzer frequency range is set far above the highest EEG frequency to be analyzed, then frequency is wasted and resolution is poor.

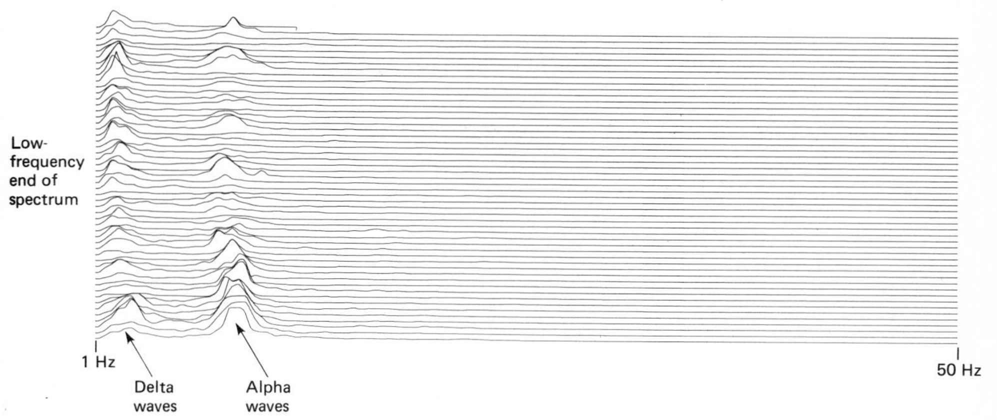

Fig. 1-20 Display of EEG spectrum on a Nicolet MED-80 analyzer. Useful data are packed on the left because the frequency range has been set too high.

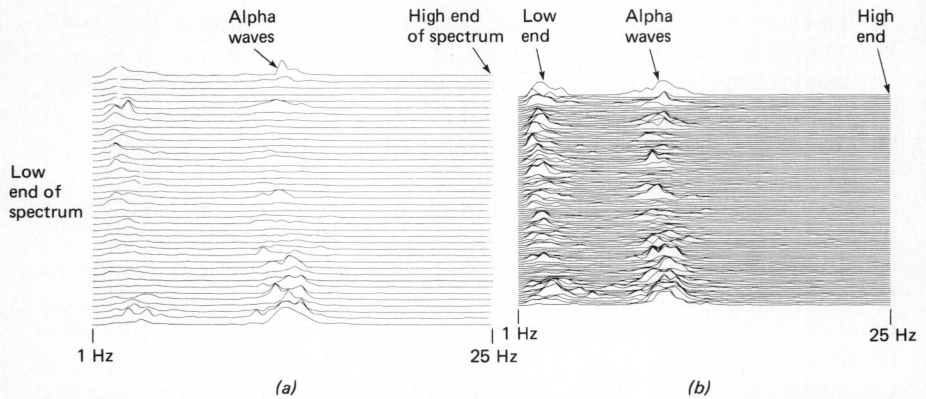

Fig. 1-21 Nicolet spectrum analyzer shows greater detail on the right, where there are twice as many blocks.

Figure 1-20 illustrates this situation. All the EEG data were known to be below 16 Hz, but the operator set the frequency-range control to 50 Hz. Most of the area to the right is seen to be wasted.

If we wished to observe two data channels at the same sweep rate, then we would only be able to look at each channel half the time. In the previous example we sampled 1024 points per sweep. Observing two data channels would allow us to sample 512 data points. If the channels were increased to four, we could only allow 256 points per channel. Increasing the number of channels for a given frequency range in turn reduces the resolution.

The number of blocks along with the number of sweeps and the sweep time determines the total analysis time required. The number of blocks is analogous to the number of plots which appears in the stack of plots. In Fig. 1-21*a* we see a stack of 50 blocks. In Fig. 1-21*b* we see much more detail of the EEG spectrum because there are 100 blocks of data. To observe EEG data from four distinct parts of the head, we would need four channels. In Fig. 1-22 we see a display of four data channels with good detail in each channel. This is so because the recording time was 6 hours (h).

1-17 LONG-TERM CYCLES OF THE AUTONOMIC NERVOUS SYSTEM

Chart recorders with extremely slow paper movement have revealed a very interesting aspect of the autonomic nervous system: It has a long-term cyclical pattern. Sleep, body temperature, urine excretion, and calcium and potassium output have a 25-h period. Surgeons have found hemorrhages during operations to be higher during the second

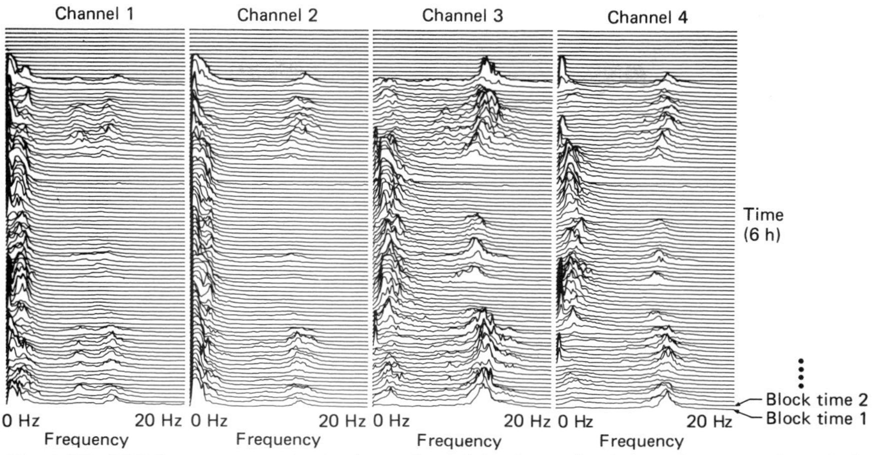

Fig. 1-22 EEG frequency analysis shows four data channels observed over a 6-h period. On the left-hand side of channel 4, changes in the delta, or sleep, wave can be observed. The theta, or activity, wave increases when the sleep wave has diminished in intensity.

quarter of a new moon. The insulin reaction also has its cycle. Diabetics are most sensitive to insulin at night. Even cockroaches have their biological clock. Setting their clocks out of phase with each other will lead to cancer and death. Researchers have data to indicate that there are cyclical diseases. Affected most are joints, bone marrow, lymph glands, stomach, salivary gland, kidneys, skin, and brains. Bile in the liver and glycogen production are also cyclical. There is an annual peak in human gonadal activity (November in the northern hemisphere) and an increased carbohydrate consumption in autumn.

1-18 THE ADRENAL CORTEX AND HOMEOSTASIS

The adrenal cortex produces two hormones. One of these, glucocorticoid, converts cholesterol into cortisol at a rate determined by corticosterone. Catalyzed by enzymes, this process is still only a minute part of a more complex system. Many glands interact to form the endocrine control systems that regulate our chemical constituents. The regulation of blood sugar is but on such control system. Constriction of the pupil is another control system; also our body temperature ignores the external environment.

This homeostasis (stability) is based on key variables being in or out of phase. For example, when blood sugar increases independently, insulin secretion is increased. However, when the insulin injection rate is increased, a different mechanism decreases blood sugar. Blood sugar is thus stabilized by in-phase and out-of-phase signals.

The electrical analogy is a closed-loop, negative-feedback system or a servosystem. A comparator (error signal) may be generated in the brain, where the algebraic subtraction of the key variables takes place. A disturbance in the equilibrium may generate a control medium to eliminate the effect of the disturbance. Thus the control system is stabilized by this self-generated correction signal. A circuit analogy might be current passing through a resistor R to charge capacitor C with a neon bulb across the capacitor. When the current through R allows the charging voltage across C to reach the neon firing potential, the neon bulb fires. The capacitor is discharged and the cycle starts again. Each cycle has the same time constant, depending on the hypothetical RC combination. This same circuit would apply to the long-term cyclical patterns. In the biological equivalent, the time constant (RC charging rate) depends on the body's electrochemical time constants.

1-19 THE RESPIRATORY SYSTEM

The spongelike material we call the lungs consists of five lobes, as shown in Fig. 1-23. Like the brain, the lungs are separated by fissures.

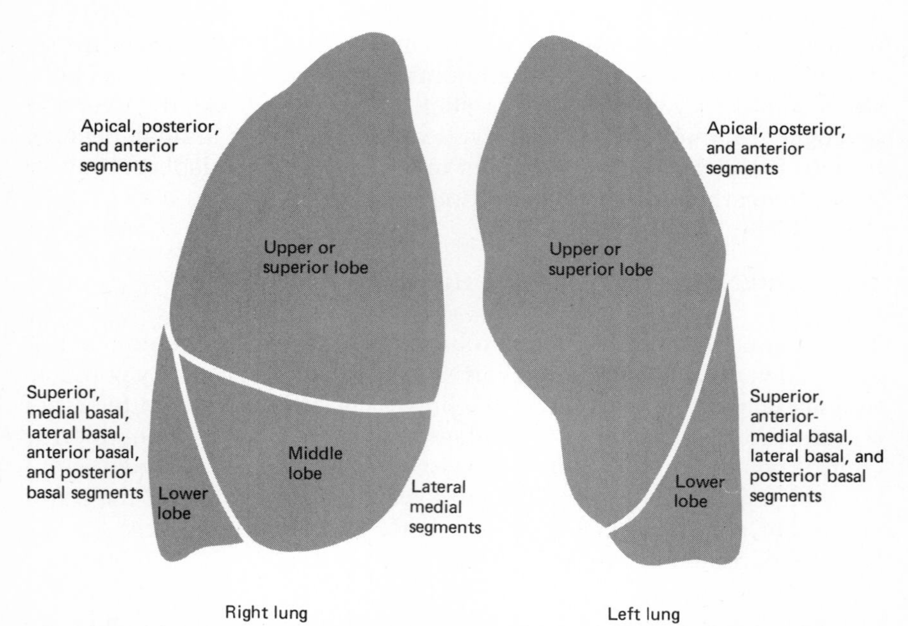

Fig. 1-23 The spongelike material we call the lungs consists of five lobes. The lobes are connected through fissures. Within each lobe are found several bronchopulmonary segments.

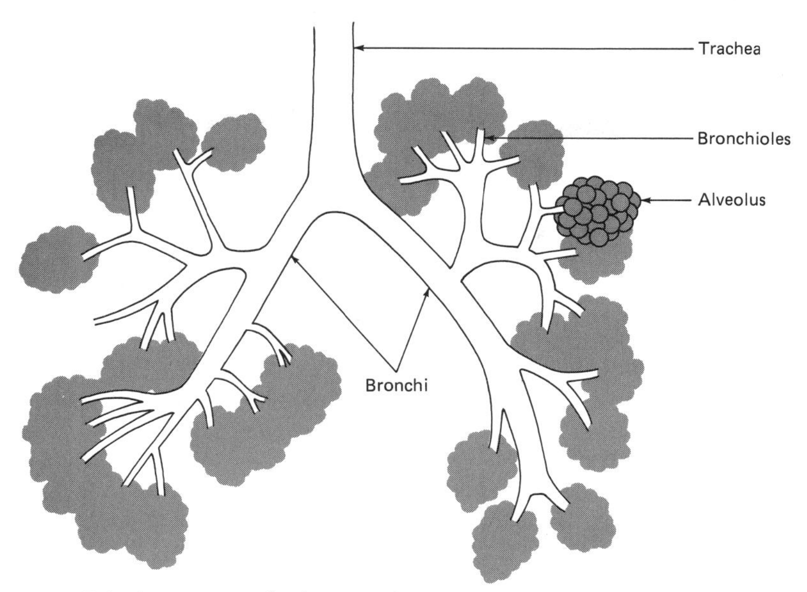

Fig. 1-24 Bringing air to and taking air from the lungs. The trachea has the greatest capacity in this air-conduction system. The bronchi lead to lesser tributaries known as the bronchioles.

Within each lobe are the various bronchopulmonary segments, as illustrated. Bringing oxygen to and taking CO_2 from the lungs is the air-conducting system. If we compare this system to the circulatory system, then the main artery would be the trachea. Branching out from the trachea are the bronchi, which in turn branch off into smaller bronchioles. The anatomy of this air-conducting system is shown in Fig. 1-24.

Just as the heart and the brain have specialized cells, so do the lungs. The three types of respiratory cells are the squamous, columnar, and goblet cells. Their anatomy can be seen in Fig. 1-25. The cilia (tiny hairs) lining the air passages are essential to the movement of air during the inhalation and expiration process. Many people have used commercial decongestants over a period of time, only to find that they have suppressed cilia activity, thus aggravating the original condition.

1-20 RESPIRATORY PARAMETERS

The BMET need only be concerned with the four key respiratory parameters. The first is *volume.* Volume is further broken down into its four components: tidal volume, expiratory reserve volume, inspiratory

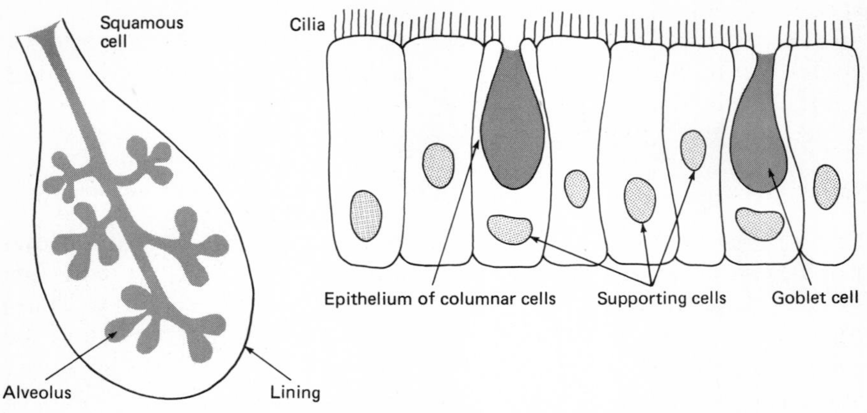

Fig. 1-25 Specialized cells in respiratory tissue.

reserve volume, and residual volume. According to how volume is calculated, we derive the second respiratory parameter, *lung capacity*. Capacity is divided into three components: total lung capacity, vital capacity, and functional residual capacity. A third parameter of importance is *ventilation*. This can be either dead space or alveolar ventilation. The *diffusion* of gas is another key parameter in respiratory studies.

VOLUME

We express the amount or volume of air in milliliters or liters. In the respiratory system we measure four types of volume. *Tidal volume* is the amount of air moved in or out per breath. *Expiratory reserve volume* is the additional amount of air which can be expired at the end of a normal expiration. *Inspiratory reserve volume* is the additional amount of air which can be inspired at the end of a normal inspiration. And last, the *residual volume* is the amount of air remaining in the lungs at the end of a forced expiration.

CAPACITY

By adding all four types of volume together, we get the *total lung capacity*. If we add only inspiratory reserve volume, tidal volume, and expiratory reserve volume, we get the *vital capacity*. If we add only the expiratory reserve volume and residual volume, we get *functional residual capacity*.

VENTILATION

Ventilation is the continuous process of moving air in and out of the lungs. Ventilation is usually expressed in volume per unit time, or liters per minute. Ventilation is either dead space or alveolar. *Dead-*

space ventilation is the amount of air moving in and out of the air-conduction system which is not directly involved in gas exchange. *Alveolar ventilation* is the amount of air moving in and out of the lungs which is directly involved in gas exchange. Alveolar volume is obtained by subtracting dead-space ventilation from tidal volume.

DIFFUSION

Diffusion is the movement of a gas from a high-pressure into a low-pressure area. Air is distributed to millions of alveoli or gas-exchange units. This alveolar air then encounters pulmonary membranes. These membranes separate the air from the blood in the capillary bed of the lungs. The membranes are made of endothelium and alveolar lining cells. Gas diffuses across the membrane, depending upon the pressure difference, gas solubility, and membrane thickness. When the oxygen finally reaches the blood, it attaches itself to hemoglobin. This explains why the hemoglobin count is so vital to good health—1.34 milliliters (mL) of oxygen combines with a gram of hemoglobin. In addition, carbon dioxide leaving the respiratory system is also attached to hemoglobin. Hemoglobin is the carrier that feeds the body's tissue (O_2) and removes waste (CO_2). This carrier contains iron molecules and thus has magnetic properties. Thus magnetic and electrostatic fields can affect blood flow. O_2 is more abundant in negatively ionized air than in positively ionized air. Negatively ionized molecules are small and easily give up their oxygen, whereas positive ions are larger and do not. Air pollution (heavy positive ionization) thus hinders oxygen distribution.

RESPIRATORY CONTROL

In the brain, the medulla and the pons initiate respiratory-control signals. Impulses from these centers are sent through the phrenic nerve to stimulate the inspiratory center and the inspiratory muscles, causing inhalation. Slightly more than 2 s later, delayed pulses are sent to the expiratory center to stimulate expiratory muscles. As soon as these pulses fade, the inspiratory pulses are repeated again. Respiratory pulse amplifiers are called *apneustic* and *pneumotax centers.* These centers also control ventilation according to the body's need. Nerve endings in the lungs are stimulated when the lungs are distended. Nerve impulses travel up the vagus nerve to the medulla. In response, the medulla transmits pulses which stop inhalation and start expiration. Overinflation of the lungs is prevented. This feedback loop regulates and controls the automatic rhythm of breathing.

Control is also affected by the amount of gas in the respiratory system. When oxygen is low, chemoreceptors are activated. Impulses are sent through the glossopharyngeal and vagus nerves to the medulla. This control center then sends pulses to increase alveolar ventilation. On the other hand, the respiratory center is also excited by carbon dioxide, Heavy concentrations of CO_2 can cause the breathing rate to increase 12 times above normal.

1-21 SPIROMETRY

The spirometer, once a mechanical instrument, now has electromechanical features. It can measure lung volume and lung capacity. Recordings can be made of vital volume, vital capacity, inspiratory and expiratory reserve volume, and maximum voluntary ventilation.

A common technique makes use of closed-circuit nitrogen dilution to investigate volume and gas distribution characteristics. Earlier pulmonary techniques used oxygen. Thus critical vacuum adjustments created difficulties. In the single-breath technique, the patient inhales from 700 to 1200 mL of nitrogen in a breath. A calibrated determination is made of the amount of expired nitrogen. Gas transducers responsive to nitrogen may be used. Time markers permit the evaluation of the key parameter vs. time. The key parameter may be forced vital capacity, flow volume, or voluntary ventilation. The electronic computation circuitry must have extremely low drift, a wide dynamic range, and good linearity. Older mechanical systems were severely limited in their sensitivity and dynamic range. They were unable to compare the key parameters in order to compute and integrate the results.

1-22 PLETHYSMOGRAPHY

This is a recent pulmonary technique. Using this system, lung or thoracic gas volume can be measured. In addition, the resistance to the passage of air, airway resistance (R_{AW}), can also be determined. In chronic respiratory disease, obstructions may impede the passage of air even though lung function is not impaired. The esophageal balloon technique is used to measure *lung compliance,* the lung's ability to follow voluntary expansion and contraction. A complete flow-volume loop of ventilation is measured with time markers spaced from 0.5 to 3 s for calibration of time.

A modern plethysmography system will have various readout devices. A split-screen oscilloscope may be included. Half the screen has a memory or storage cathode-ray tube (CRT) so that the physician can freeze valuable data. The other half of the display will continue to show live data as they are recorded. A Polaroid camera can be used to photograph a permanent record of a frozen image.

QUESTIONS

1. The smallest unit in existence with its own chemical property is the ___________.
2. True or false. A molecule must have identical atoms.
3. Hydrocarbon molecules combine readily with what substance?
4. Molecules that exert intense electrostatic energy on their neighbors are ___________ molecules.
5. Specify the primary electrical effect achieved by the ions in living tissue.
6. In a pH glass electrode where the solution has a pH below 7, what type of ions will pass?
7. How does the calibrated buffer in the pH electrode allow measurement of ion concentration?
8. What is the smallest arrangement with all the characteristics that we associate with being alive?
9. What is the key to the process in which the cell eliminates waste and absorbs oxygen?
10. Body-water concentration is critical to the cell's function. When a critical concentration is approached, an antiduretic hormone (ADH) is secreted. This secretion is controlled by ___________.
11. Chemoreceptors monitor the level of which chemicals in the body?
12. The resting potential of all cells is alike. What is the constant voltage difference between the inside and the outside of the cell?
13. ___________ ions are concentrated inside the resting cell. ___________ ions are concentrated outside the cell, and there is also a smaller concentration of ___________ ions outside the cell.
14. In the cytoplasm surrounding the cell's nucleus is the mitochondria. What is its function?
15. A(n) ___________ charge exists outside the resting cell, whereas a(n) ___________ charge exists inside the resting cell.
16. Explain the chemical interchange taking place when both nerve and muscle tissue maintain their charge potential and their ability to recharge quickly.
17. If nerve fibers are of larger diameter and relatively warm, how will this affect electric impulses traveling along the nerves?
18. What is the nerve's critical or threshold level?
19. What is the general name for nerve cells outside the central nervous system?
20. As an electromyographer, you see 12 fibrillation spikes per second being generated by a muscle at rest. This activity is observed on your medical oscilloscope. How would you analyze this electrical activity?

chapter 2

Patient Safety

INTRODUCTION

A biomedical instrument is designed to meet minimum safety requirements. When the equipment ages, protective components also age. When a safety fault develops, the equipment often becomes a hazard to the patient, the doctor, and the hospital staff. Increasingly, several instruments are combined to form a biomedical system. Safety precautions built into one instrument cannot provide complete safety for the overall instrument system. The BMET must be fully familiar with safety problems that will develop when instruments are used in combination.

Contrary to belief, higher currents passing through the body can sometimes be less lethal than lower currents. Also, the same amounts of current may produce different physiological effects, depending upon whether it is ac, dc, or high-frequency energy. Periodic testing and inspection of grounding systems is as vital to patient safety as regular inspection of the instruments themselves. Preventive maintenance must be performed faithfully to avoid predictable equipment hazards and to ensure that alarm circuits are functioning.

2-1 NATURAL PROTECTIVE MECHANISMS AGAINST ELECTRICITY

Under most circumstances, intact dry skin limits the flow of current through the body to safe levels. Furthermore, the natural withdrawal reaction to painful stimuli usually limits the duration of the shock to a very short period of time. If the current stimulates the flexor muscles, however, it may be impossible for one to let go of, or detach oneself from, the source of the shock. In any case, the application of current to the body surface usually results in distribution of that current in such a way that only a small fraction of it passes through the myocardium.

Medical procedures often defeat these natural safeguards. In the operating room, the patient's drapes frequently become soaked with blood and/or saline. In the cardiac-care unit, skin resistance is deliberately lowered with electrode jelly. Endoscopy may introduce current into the body through low-resistance mucous membranes rather than skin.

The anesthetized patient cannot react to painful sensations or withdraw from a current source. Cardiac monitoring involves the application of electrodes in the immediate vicinity of the heart, so that a fault current flowing through them might arrive at the myocardium with a high current density. In cardiac pacing, conductors are actually brought into direct contact with the heart. Cardiac catheterization is usually performed with nonconductive catheters, but during the procedure, they may be filled with conductive media such as angiographic dye or guidewires.

Hazardous sources of current are numerous. Direct contact with a live conductor is an obvious one. Any line-powered electric device may be a source of current if there is a connection between the power source and the metal case or some other accessible conductive part of the device. This connection can be by means of a direct short circuit, by conduction of current through relatively conductive substances such as dirt or biological fluids, by indirect coupling through capacitive or inductive effects, or by incorrect connections—improperly wired electrical outlets, probes plugged into the wrong jacks in a device, etc. Whether such a source is hazardous depends on the magnitude of the current available, on the intimacy of an individual's contact with the source and with the ground, and on the individual's physical condition.

Most electrically hazardous situations require simultaneous contact with a source of current and a ground pathway. The term *ground* here refers to any return path to the source of the current, whether or not it is connected to the earth. For current to flow, it must leave the source, pass through objects that are capable of conducting electricity, and return to the source. Such a system is called a *circuit*. In many circuits, the ground is earth, but it need not be. In an isolated system, such as an airplane, the ground may be the framework of the plane. In a building, anything connected to the building structure may possibly serve as a ground (return path), whether it is intended to do so or not.

2-2 ELECTRICAL HAZARDS

One milliampere (mA) of 60-Hz alternating current flowing in the intact body may produce a tingling sensation; 16 mA can cause "freezing" (inability to let go because of contraction of the flexor muscles); and at higher levels, tissue damage, respiratory arrest, and cardiac arrest can occur. Finally, current in excess of 80 mA applied to the body surface may cause ventricular fibrillation. It is interesting to note, however, that with currents greater than 100 mA, there is a tendency for muscular contraction to be so rapid and forceful that one is involuntarily jerked away from contact with the electrical source.

Such gross exposure of the body to currents of perceptible magnitude is referred to as *macroshock*. On the other hand, *microshock* occurs with exposure to minute electric currents well below the usual threshold of perception. When such imperceptible currents arrive at the myocardium with sufficient density, they can produce ventricular fibrillation. As little as 20 microamperes (μA), for example, leaking into a pacing catheter may constitute such a hazard. Currents of this magnitude are not regulated by ordinary electrical and building codes because they are not a threat to life except in certain unusual environments, such as the cardiac-care unit and the catheterization laboratory (Table 2-1). Currents in the microshock range are commonly encountered in kitchens and workshops by normal people who feel nothing and suffer no ill effects. Yet the same current flowing through a nurse and into a pacing catheter the nurse is adjusting may electrocute a patient.

Other electrical hazards are produced by misapplication of the therapeutic current. Examples include electric shock from a defibrillator, accidental burns by electrosurgical units, and ventricular fibrillation occurring when a pacemaker impulse coincides with the vulnerable period of the cardiac cycle.

Kouwenhoven has stated that static electricity may be a hazard. He reports an injury which resulted from an accident caused by a painful shock produced by static electricity. Walter states, but does not document, that static electricity can cause cardiac arrest if it is applied to a pacing catheter. This assertion is difficult to prove or disprove. The explosion hazard caused by static electricity in the presence of explosive gases is well known. Static electricity can also damage sensitive equipment.

DIRECT CURRENT

Direct current can sometimes cause injury even at very low amplitudes. Experimental application of direct current has been used to produce arterial thrombosis in animals, a principle applied clinically by Sawyer a decade ago. In a recent report, cutaneous burns in a patient exposed to a 14-V source of direct current during a surgical procedure were attributed to the electrolytic effect, with consequent production of caustic substances. Similar injuries have been reported at even 3 V. On the other hand, the fibrillation threshold for direct current is apparently somewhat higher than for alternating current.

HIGH-FREQUENCY ALTERNATING CURRENT

High-frequency alternating current, formerly thought to be relatively innocuous, has been reported to be capable of causing hemorrhagic lesions of the mitral valve. At very high density, it has also been known to induce ventricular fibrillation. High-frequency current may pass from point to point in unsuspected ways—transmitted by radiation, capacitive coupling, or inductive coupling—to produce effects at sites remote from the point of intended application.

Consideration must be given to the possibility of a startling (but ordinarily harmless) macroshock causing a *secondary accident* which results in injury or death.

Patients being treated with artificial pacemakers must be protected from exposure to certain types of electric and magnetic fields. Some of the sources include electric motors, automotive ignition systems, cautery, diathermy, microwave ovens, and a variety of other devices, some of which have yet to be identified. This is particularly true of demand pacemakers, for in some cases the external field is capable of turning off the pacemaker. But even fixed-rate pacemakers are not immune to dangerous interaction with electrically generated fields and magnetic fields.

Although the risk of interruption of electric power to life-support equipment is not a shock hazard, it is a vital design consideration. If a delay of over 10 s occurs before emergency power is brought into operation, the failure of a respirator, monitor, defibrillator, pacemaker, or other life-support equipment may be fatal. Power failure, whether caused by a blown fuse or a civil disturbance, must be considered in the planning of a power distribution system.

Finally, there is the well-known danger of explosive gases and vapors being ignited by static, direct, or alternating current, including current from therapeutic machines.

2-3 INSPECTION

Periodic testing and inspection of all ac receptacles and grounded surfaces is essential. It should be noted, however, that insertion of a polarity tester into an improperly wired receptacle can create a hazard by applying current to a grounding circuit. Tests should be made to determine both the resistance between ground points and the current that will flow through a resistor approximately equivalent to the impedance of the myocardium when it is connected to two separated ground

Table 2-1 **Potentially Hazardous Environments**

1. Most hazardous: Low-impedance conductor, insulated up to its tip, in contact with heart
   - Transvenous pacing catheter
   - Insulated transthoracic pacing wire
   - Pericardiocentesis with insulated needle
   - Nonconductive hollow catheter in heart with metal guidewire in place
   - Intravascular transducers (pressure, acoustic)
   - Intracardiac electrogram
   - Cardiac surgery
2. High-impedance direct path to myocardium
   - Hollow intracardiac catheter filled with conductive fluid (e.g., angiographic dye)
   - Cardiac surgery
3. Low-impedance path to heart which is not insulated to its tip and which passes through intervening tissue or blood vessel
   - Pericardiocentesis with uninsulated needle
   - Conductive intracardiac catheter
   - Intracardiac injections
   - Cardiac surgery
4. Potential inclusion of the heart in a low-resistance-current pathway entering and leaving at the body surface or via a body cavity remote from the heart

   Cardiology: Patient monitoring, taking an electrocardiogram, vectorcardiography, phonocardiography, echocardiography, telemetry, electronic stethoscope, esophageal electrode, blood-pressure monitoring, plethysmography

   Gastroenterology: Any endoscopic procedure, especially using line-operated equipment, constitutes a possible hazard. Even if the applied part of the instrument is nonconductive, it may become filled with a body fluid or an irrigating fluid, or a metal sucker or other instrument may be passed through it. These procedures are frequently performed on special tables, which are metal and are either electrically operated, grounded, or both. Cautery through an endoscope suggests additional hazards. The gastric camera and similar devices could also constitute a risk.

   Pulmonary diseases: Pulmonary physiology studies, oximetry, electric nebulizer, bronchoscopy

   Physical medicine: Diathermy, electromyography, nerve and muscle stimulators, hydrotherapy

   General surgery: Electrocautery, surgical drills, cryosurgery, body temperature probe (rectal or esophageal), aspirators (gastrointestinal, tracheal), blood-warming devices, surgical microscope, sitzbaths with electric heaters

   Otology: Operating equipment, line-powered examining instruments, electronystagmograph, audiometry

   Ophthalmology: Line-powered examining instruments, slit lamp, electroretinograph

   Psychiatry: Electroshock therapy

   Renology: Hemodialysis

   Dentistry: Dental drills and other diagnostic and therapeutic devices

   Miscellaneous: Intracorporeal television, electronarcosis, biogalvanic measurements (skin)

Table 2-1 **Potentially Hazardous Environments** (*Continued*)

5. Miscellaneous environments which are potentially hazardous because of exposure of the patient to wet or otherwise conductive bodies
   - Electric bed
   - Electric circle bed
   - Physiotherapy department
   - Medical emergency carts
   - Respirators
   - Operating tables
   - Operating chairs
   - Heating pads
   - Hypothermia apparatus
   - General surgical suite
   - Delivery room
   - Cast room
   - Nursery (isolettes, camera, etc.)
   - Hyperbaric chamber
   - Sterilizers
   - Dental units
   - Oscillating mattress
6. In addition, there may be hazards related to equipment not directly connected to the patient. Such remotely connected devices include slave monitors, digital readouts, and computers.

points. The polarity should be tested regularly, for a receptacle may have been improperly repaired between surveys. Contact tension should be tested. Broken or dead outlets should be repaired immediately.

SPECIAL CONSIDERATIONS

Because of the possible risk of ventricular fibrillation due to static electricity, carpeting is not recommended for patient-care areas where pacing catheters or similar instruments are in use. Methods intended to abolish static electricity are imperfect and necessitate grounding of the carpeting, thus creating an additional grounded surface and further complicating the problem of making the electrical environment safe.

Operating rooms require special design because of the risk of anesthetic explosions resulting from static discharges. The floor is deliberately made somewhat conductive and is grounded, and an isolation transformer is usually used to reduce the shock hazard to personnel. This additional ground path through the floor should not be forgotten when monitors, pacemakers, and defibrillators are brought into the operating room. Such devices should be properly connected to the power distribution system by appropriate plugs or adaptors. Defeating the system by means of extension cords leading to outside receptacles increases the shock hazard.

The fact that the electrically sensitive patient may be located anywhere in the hospital will eventually have to be considered. In other words, the entire hospital will have to be made electrically safe. The frequency with which certain procedures are currently performed determines which parts of the hospital are to be treated as electrically sensitive patient locations (Table 2-1) and to be designated by means of an approved sign.

PREVENTIVE MAINTENANCE

The purpose of preventive maintenance is to ensure:

1. That equipment is operating properly. The output of measuring instruments should have satisfactory fidelity and accuracy. Therapeutic instruments should deliver accurately and safely the therapeutic effect at the proper time.
2. That equipment and all accessories, cables, and power cords are safe.
3. That equipment is mechanically in good condition with no missing parts, loose switches or knobs, and no broken glass. Casters should be free and lubricated so that mobile equipment will not tip or make noise. Table 2-2 should be used as a general guide for maintenance schedules.

2-4 GROUNDING

The high-voltage energy from power generators is reduced to a lower voltage at substations. At the hospital these voltages are further reduced to 230 and 115 V. Receptacles are fed by conduit with a black wire (connects the shorter rectangular slot of the receptacle) to the 115-V transformer. This is the hot wire that runs through a circuit breaker located at the transformer or on a separate breaker panel.

Connected to the longer of the rectangular slots is a neutral white wire which goes to the joint terminal of two 115-V circuits. The white wire eventually goes to the transformer casing and to water pipes or a grounded metal stake. As the white (neutral) wire is grounded, the power voltage exists between the hot wire and any metallic object that is also grounded. All electronic apparatus gets its current from the hot wire, the return path being through the neutral wire. When wire insulation becomes defective, or grounding capacitors age, the instrument case is said to be "hot." With the neutral wire grounded, a current will pass through the body of a person if the person is touching the hot case and provides a ground path for the current.

This would never happen with an adequate ground; however,

Table 2-2 **Maintenance Schedules**

Parts of a maintenance schedule are offered here. While the listing has been made relatively detailed for some instruments, similar detail can be developed for each of the other sample devices. Many checks are common to all devices. Again the suggested frequency of testing and the personnel assigned to perform the tests are general guides, and specific schedules will depend greatly on the activity within and facilities of a given hospital. This table then *is not* a cookbook list which can be turned over to individuals untrained for responsibility with medical instrumentation. (Frequency is in months unless otherwise noted.)

In carrying out a device maintenance check, care must be exercised to protect patients during testing. In general, most tests should be performed *only* when the device is completely disconnected from a patient. An exception is the ECG monitor which can be spot-checked for correct operation using the built-in 1-mV step pulse while the device is attached to a patient.

	Maintenance	BME/ BMET	Nurse	Frequency
Monitors-ECGs				
1. Cable continuity (repair)	x			3
2. Strain relief (repair)	x			3
3. Leakage current and condition of power cord	x			1
4. Ground-wire continuity:				
Permanently installed	x			3
Portable units	x			1
5. Workability of knobs			x	weekly
6. CRT image			x	weekly
7. Alarm limits			x	weekly
8. Common-mode rejection ratio, input impedance, noise level, frequency response, maximum gain, sensitivity, linearity		x		6
9. Calibration marker	x	x		3
10. Sweep/paper speed	x	x		3
11. Rate meter	x	x		3
12. Interaction between controls		x		3
13. Transient leakage spikes		x		3
14. Internal component check		x		6
Defibrillators				
1. Strain relief	x			3
2. Continuity of cables	x			3
3. Ground integrity and power cord condition	x			3
4. Meter movement (needle should move smoothly)			x	after use
5. Paddle surface condition			x	after use
6. Charge and/or discharge relay operation			x	after use
7. Proper sterilization of internal paddles			x	after use

Table 2-2 (Continued)

	Main-tenance	BME/ BMET	Nurse	Frequency
8. Proper accessories on portable cart			x	daily and after use
9. Proper storage of defibrillator			x	daily and after use
10. Leakage current	x			1
11. Workability of control knobs			x	after use
12. Automatic discharge		x		3
13. Waveshape and energy		x		6
14. Storage capacitor leakage (for dc defibrillators)		x		3
15. Condition of internal discharge resistor		x		3
16. Deterioration of internal components due to age or otherwise		x		6
17. Capability of rapid, successive discharges		x		6
18. Synchronizing (or cardioverting)		x		6
19. Actual isolation of "isolated" paddles		x		6
20. Review of "emergency call" system performance		x		6
Pacemakers				
1. Pulse amplitude and rate		x		6
2. Amplitude control linearity		x		6

ground faults sometimes develop. For example, if the power plug is constantly pulled, the wire connecting the instrument to the grounding-pin third wire might break. Such a faulty ground connection on an electric bed would allow an ac voltage to exist on the bed frame as a result of capacitive coupling between the bed frame and the primary wiring in the bed. If a nurse unwittingly touched this bed frame and the patient's pacemaker wire, current from the bed frame would flow through the patient's body. Ground-fault alarms and interrupters are devices that will sense these abnormal conditions and either cut the power or give an alarm.

Whenever these protective devices are not available, routine checks with a low-resistance ohmmeter should be made to detect either a ground fault or a resistance between the instrument case and the power-cord ground pin.

LEAKAGE AND FAULT CURRENT

The user of equipment in special-care areas should know the leakage and fault currents that exist in all ac-connected instrumentation. Insu-

Table 2-2 (Continued)

	Estimated Workload*			
Instrument	**Quantity**	**Hours per Inspection**	**Inspection Period**	**Hours per Annum**
ECG	60	0.5	1 week	1560
Cardioverters and defibrillators	16	2	1 month	384
Oscilloscopes and multi-channel recorders	8	2	6 months	32
pH meters and blood-gas analyzers	8	3	6 months	48
External pacemakers	34	0.75	6 months	51
Cardiac monitors	60	0.5	2 months	180
Marquette System	1	6	1 week	312
EEG	4	1	1 year	4
Other instruments	70	2	6 months	280
Max cart	1	2	1 month	24
Intercommunication equipment	all	20	6 months	40
Entertainment equipment	all	15	6 months	30
Electrosurgical units	17	3	3 months	204
Operating room setup	all	4	daily	1000
Repair and overhaul—estimated workload				2000
Totals	279			6149

* These figures do not include supervision, record keeping, clerical tasks nor support of research programs.

lated conductors all have stray or "phantom" capacitance. Also, a wire's insulation resistance is never infinite. Both finite leakage and phantom capacitance permit some of the alternating current to seek ground. The instrument case is at ground potential when it is not hot. Either a broken ground connection or a resistive ground connection will allow a voltage on the case which is above ground. A resistance between case and ground above 0.1 ohm (Ω) will produce a hot case. A person touching the case and ground will provide a leakage-current path for between 2 and 200 μA. Battery-operated equipment has no leakage current. Excessive electric interference or artifacts in the instrument is often one clue that a ground fault has occurred.

The green wire is the ground lead. A short will cause fault current to take the path of least resistance through the ground wire. Although the circuit breaker may sometimes trip, the hazard occurs before the breaker can trip. Checking green-wire (ground) continuity to below 0.1 Ω gives the instrument a clean bill of health. However, the instrument's ground may not be at exactly the same electric potential as other grounds nearby. Leakage-current measurements are discussed in Sec. 2-6.

If every conductor or conductive surface in the hospital is at the same electric potential, no current flows through an object or person in contact with two conductors. However, a check of a facility often reveals that there are several volts between different grounds, such as between the power ground of an electrical three-prong outlet and an electronic monitoring ground. A short between these grounds would carry a current flow of several hundred milliamperes. Different voltage levels at different ground points are inevitable; they are caused by leakage currents, electric noise, inductive pickup, and other side effects. Using one ground point nearly eliminates the problem.

THE THIRD WIRE

The third wire is a ground circuit intended to safely carry away fault currents. In older buildings the function of the third wire was often performed by the wiring conduit (metal casing); since this metal casing can rust, corrode, and possibly not provide a safe return for fault currents, a third wire of appropriate size should always be used. If at all possible, it should be added where it does not now exist.

Even the best ground wire offers finite resistance. If a fault current of 20 A occurs and the resistance of the ground wire and the myocardium are 0.05 and 500 Ω, respectively, then $\frac{1}{10000}$ (0.0001) of the fault current, or 2 mA, could flow through the myocardium until the circuit breaker opened. Special construction practices are called for in the case of electrically sensitive patients. The diameter and length of the ground wire, the resistance of its connections, and the magnitude of possible fault currents must be carefully controlled. These problems may be dealt with by employing a *power center* for each bed. This consists of a set of nearby electrical outlets intended for devices serving a particular patient in a particular bed. All must have identical phasing. Because of the proximity of the outlets, the ground connection between them is very short, and very heavy-gage wire can be employed at little cost. Other metal surfaces within reach of the patient or anyone attending the patient must be connected to the same ground point, as must receptacles elsewhere in the room that could be used in connection with the patient, i.e., those for taking an electrocardiogram (EGG) or an x-ray. If more than one bed is in the room, the ground point for the room must be connected to each power-center ground by a separate heavy-gage conductor. Separate isolation transformer units have been proposed as a further means of making the electrical environment safer. Such transformers are intended to serve individual beds or even individual rooms. Despite considerable discussion by engineering authorities there remains significant disagreement as to their value. Isolation transformers having the capacity required for these applications are costly, require maintenance, and do not eliminate certain types of hazards. Additional hazards are introduced by the ground-fault detectors which these systems incorporate. Medical electronic devices should incorporate them anyway. Therefore, while there are potential benefits of isolation transformers, they are not at this time required by the National Electrical Code and are not considered mandatory in view of their expense and imperfections.

THE SNOWFLAKE

Figure 2-1 shows a ground system in the form of a snowflake. The room or area subground point is connected to a system main ground through a heavy-gage insulated wire (No. 6 or 8 gage), as illustrated. The subground point must be as close as possible to the patient. All equipment and accessories are connected to this ground point with short, heavy-gage wire forming the snowflake ground system. Frequently, it is necessary to disconnect existing grounds to power outlets and to insert plastic insulator tubing into air or vacuum lines to eliminate ground loops, which may result in excessive noise or interference during ECG or EEG (electroencephalogram) monitoring.

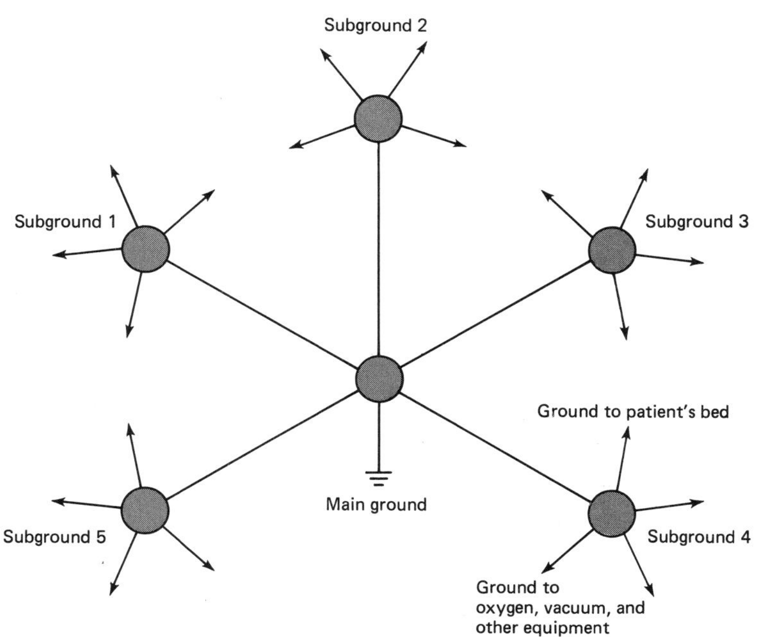

Fig. 2-1 The snowflake grounding system. Each subground should be as close as possible to the patient.

Proper installation of the ground wires and interconnection and the connection between ground and equipment are very important factors. Dependence on the built-in ground wires of the power line and the power plug is not sufficient, since the ground connection in the three-prong connector can break or be of high resistance. For this reason, it is important that an external grounding cable be connected firmly to all electric equipment. This grounding cable should be of No. 6 or 8 gage with firmly attached connections such as solder lugs. These solder lugs must be screwed with a $\frac{1}{4}$-in diameter bolt, for example, to the equipment to be grounded.

Figure 2-2 shows a ground system for a typical intensive-care ward, with the snowflake ground system. The central monitor, normally located midway between rooms, forms the midpoint of the grounding system. Heavy-gage wires come from this location to form subgroups at the bedside wall plate, which can also be used as a junction box for different transducer connectors and ECG-EEG electrodes. Permanent ground connections should be soldered or securely made with heavy copper lugs and noncorrosive hardware. The patient's bed, the electronic monitoring cabinet, ground pins of three-way electrical outlets, permanently installed electric accessories, vacuum lines, oxygen lines, and any other metallic accessories which may come in contact with the

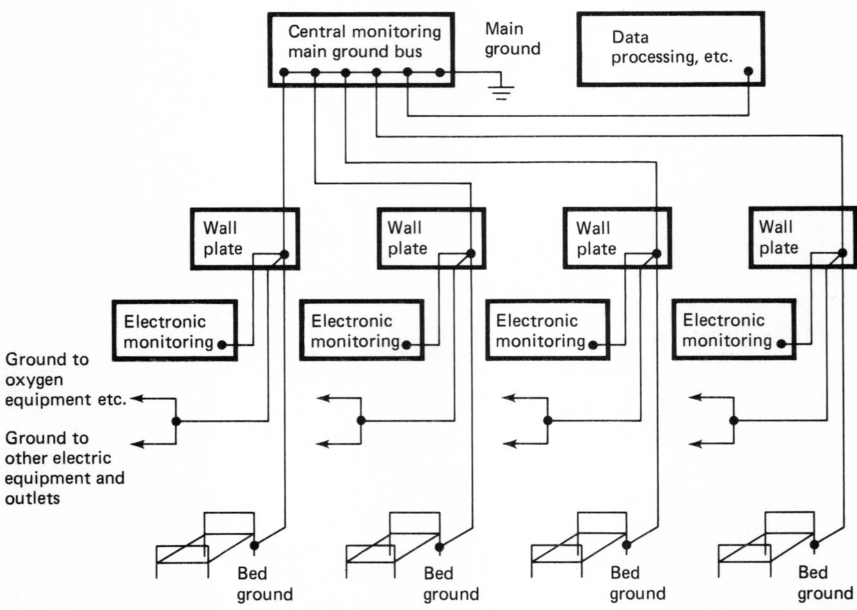

Fig. 2-2 Ground system in a typical intensive-care ward. Heavy-gage wires are used from the central monitor to all subgroups. The wall plate also becomes part of the grounding system.

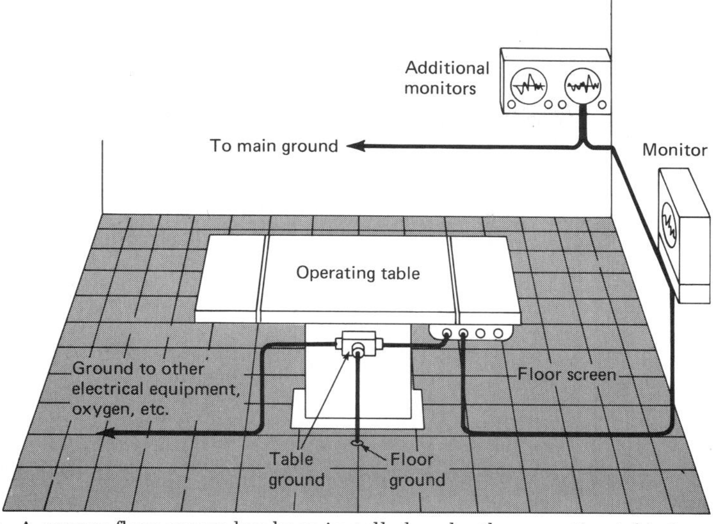

Fig. 2-3 A copper floor screen has been installed under the operating table to minimize interference and to ground currents. Its ground connection to the operating table, various monitors, and to the main ground is shown.

power line, water line, or floor must be connected to this patient-safety ground.

Figure 2-3 shows a ground system for a simple operating room installation. Again, the snowflake ground system is applied. A main ground is provided somewhere in the building and is fed through a heavy-gage wire to the monitoring system, operating table, remote monitor oscilloscope, junction box, electric equipment, oxygen equipment, and a floor screen.

Frequent problems with ECGs arise in operating rooms because of line interference. A simple floor screen (approximately 12 by 12 ft) under the operating table will reduce the interference considerably. The screen can be provided during the construction of the floor or can be added later under or above the floor covering. The material for the screen is not critical, although a good conductor such as copper is preferred. Where the screen is exposed to traffic, stainless steel plates are acceptable.

AVOIDANCE OF HAZARDOUS CURRENTS

Hazardous currents result from the patient or operator coming in contact with the power line. Because one side of the power line is grounded, the other wire is essentially 115 V (or 220 V) above ground. Even a brief contact with the "live" wire can be fatal. To minimize this danger from shocks, an ungrounded system should be employed, using an isolation transformer at each bedside station or operating room. These transformers should be of low leakage and low primary-to-secondary capacity [100 picofarads (pF) or less], and they should be installed close to the individual monitoring station. In operating rooms it is standard practice to monitor the ungrounded system to minimize the possibility of shocks or sparks. This ground detector provides an audio-visual alarm in case the leakage from either of the power lines to ground exceeds the value established by the codes.

THE OPEN GROUND

Isolation transformers and other protective devices cannot eliminate a serious problem if a ground wire breaks in a power cord. The patient can be placed in immediate danger. Power cords are constantly subject to abuse. Casters are rolled over them, and they are flexed and often yanked out of the wall socket. Thus the power cord is often responsible for a variety of problems.

Should one of the power conductors open, the equipment will not function. If the two power conductors short, a circuit breaker or fuse will blow. However, when a ground wire breaks, the staff is not alerted because the instrument continues to function.

In a typical situation, a patient could be connected to two instruments, with electrodes from one going to the leg as shown in Fig. 2-4*a*. The second instrument is connected to the chest as shown. Both instruments usually have radio-interference filters connected between the case and the power line. These suppression filters are seen in Fig. 2-4*a* as RF_1 and RF_2. Bypass capacitors in those filters constitute a current path to the instrument case when the ground lead of instrument 2 has broken. The dashed line shows the new current path. Another important factor is the stray capacitance that exists between the power line and the case, shown as C_1 and C_2. With the ground lead in instrument 2 broken, the leakage current that would normally flow to ground flows through the patient. It continues on to the case of instrument 1. From there, the current will finally reach ground via the intact ground wire of instrument 1.

THE OPEN GROUND AND THE WHEATSTONE BRIDGE. In Sec. 3-4, Pressure Transducers, we will learn how the Wheatstone bridge operates. Any imbalance in one of the bridge arms will produce a voltage output, either in the connected amplifier or in the voltmeter connected across the bridge. The open ground in Fig. 2-4*b* is actually a Wheatstone bridge. Only this time, the patient replaces the amplifier or voltmeter in the bridge output circuit. Any imbalance between C_A, C_B, or C_D creates a voltage across the patient. The patient then becomes the

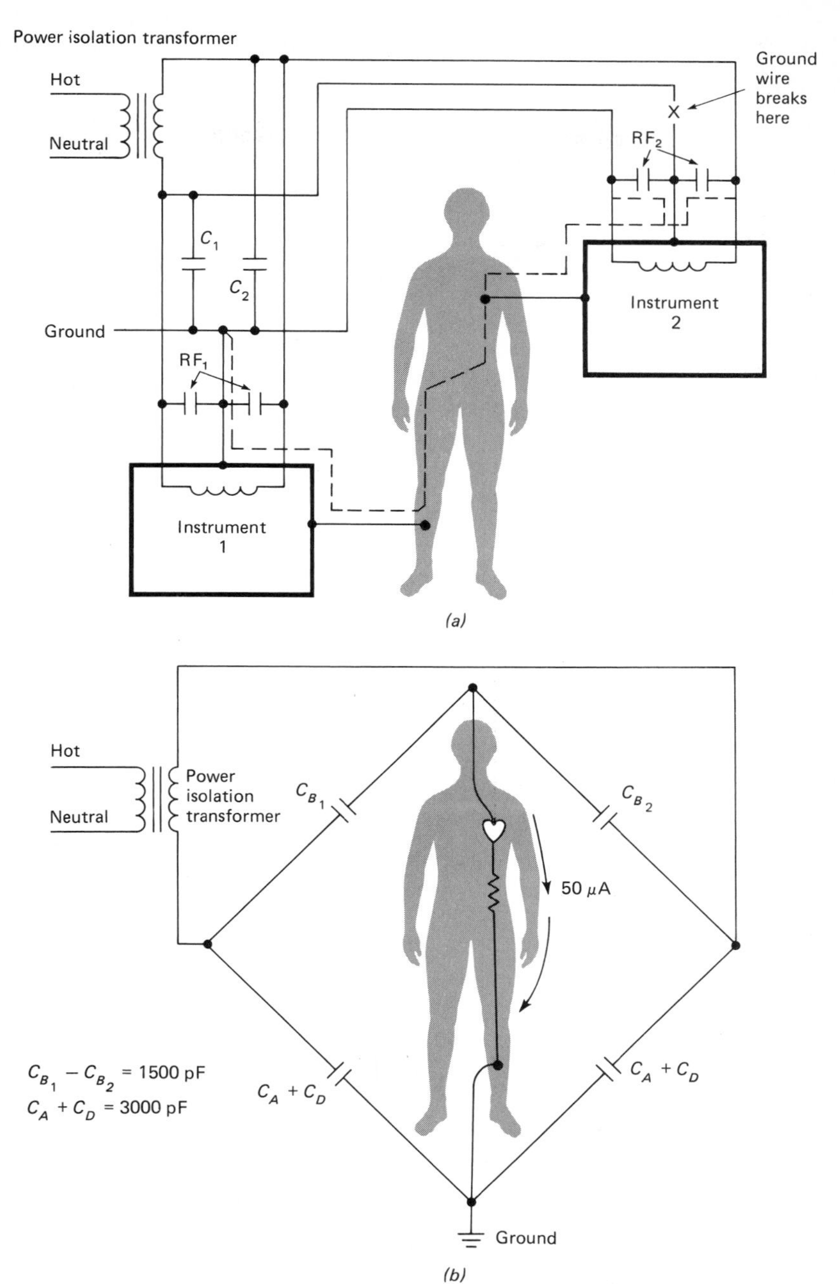

Fig. 2-4 When a ground fault (open ground wires) occurs, the patient becomes the "sensing element" of a capacitive Wheatstone bridge. Current flows through the patient according to the imbalance of the bridge capacitors. Capacitors C_d represent leakage currents to ground.

sensing element across this capacitive Wheatstone bridge. In the dc Wheatstone bridge we calculate resistance ratios to determine the voltage output of the bridge. To determine the voltage across the patient, use the capacitive reactance values at 60 Hz which can be found in any reactance table.

2-5 PATIENT ISOLATION

The patient in the typical intensive-care unit (ICU) or cardiac-care unit (CCU) is exposed to the danger of microshock when high patient-circuit impedance is not maintained. This requires care by the medical personnel in their handling of an internal conductor that is passed into, or close to, the heart; it also requires the choice of instrumentation whose patient circuits are adequately isolated from both the power line and ground. This can be accomplished by designing isolated input circuits into ECG instruments (as shown in Fig. 2-5) which are normally connected to the patient with in-dwelling electrodes.

The isolated circuits, which connect directly to the patient, are phys-

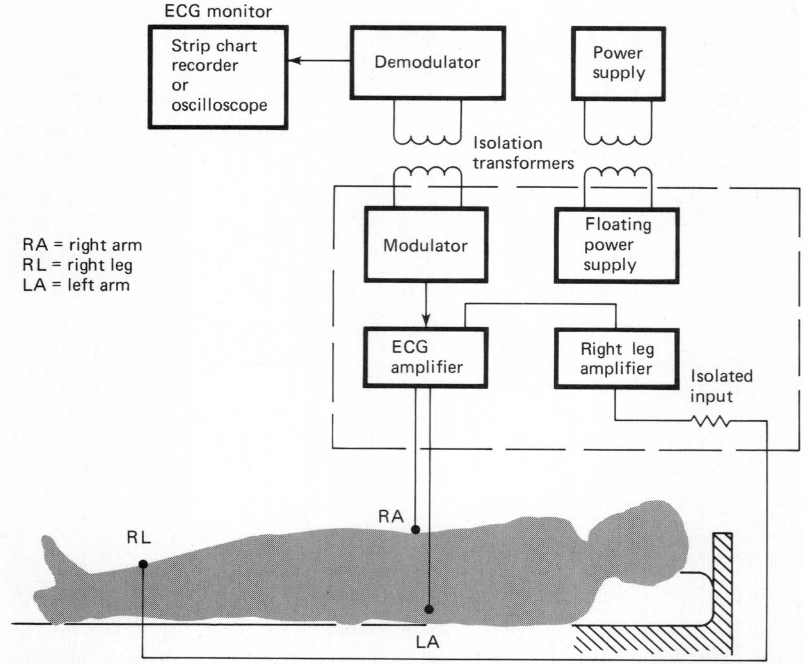

Fig. 2-5 Patient in cardiac-care unit. All circuits that connect to the patient's body must be fully isolated from both the power line and the ground. The isolated input circuits provide more than 10 MΩ of isolation impedance between the input and ground terminals.

ically insulated from ground and other portions of the ECG or patient monitor. One isolated circuit, for example, receives its power through a small isolation transformer (operating at high frequency) inside the instrument and transmits the ECG signal through another isolation transformer (operating at the same high frequency) to the display and recording sections of the device. No conductive path is present between isolated and other sections of the instrument.

If it were possible to make the circuit infinitely small or to separate it by an infinite distance from other portions of the device, perfect isolation could be achieved. Since this is not possible, a small amount of capacitance remains between the isolated and grounded sections of the circuits. Yet, with present techniques, at 50 or 60 Hz, more than 10 megohms (MΩ) of isolation impedance between input and terminals ground can be achieved.

Other monitoring devices that are connected to the patient can also be isolated. For instance, transducers for arterial- and venous-pressure measurement can be designed so that the saline column in the catheter is not connected to the chassis of the pressure monitor through the shield in the transducer cable. Also, sensors such as temperature probes, heart-sound microphones, and respiration transducers are available in isolated versions.

The advantages of isolating the ECG leads from a patient in an ICU can be seen when the patient is connected to an ECG monitor that grounded the patient's right leg, and this electrode becomes part of a hazardous current path when the attendant touches an electric bed (with a broken ground connection) and the pacemaker catheter terminals simultaneously (Fig. 2-6). If we substitute a monitor, with isolated input circuits and with 25-MΩ isolated impedance, the quantity of current flowing through the monitor will be less than 5 μA—a considerable reduction when compared with 100 μA when using the ECG monitor directly.

POWER ISOLATION TRANSFORMERS

The power-isolation-transformer approach to a safe environment for the patient is based on eliminating low-voltage hazards (in contrast to the patient isolation concept just discussed, which eliminates possible current paths through the patient). Although the concepts are different, they are complementary, and the combination of both can produce a safe patient environment. The objective of both concepts, however, is the same: preventing currents greater than 10 μA from passing through the heart muscle from in-dwelling electrodes.

The power-isolation-transformer concept assumes that the externally exposed end of the electrode or catheter will be grounded either inten-

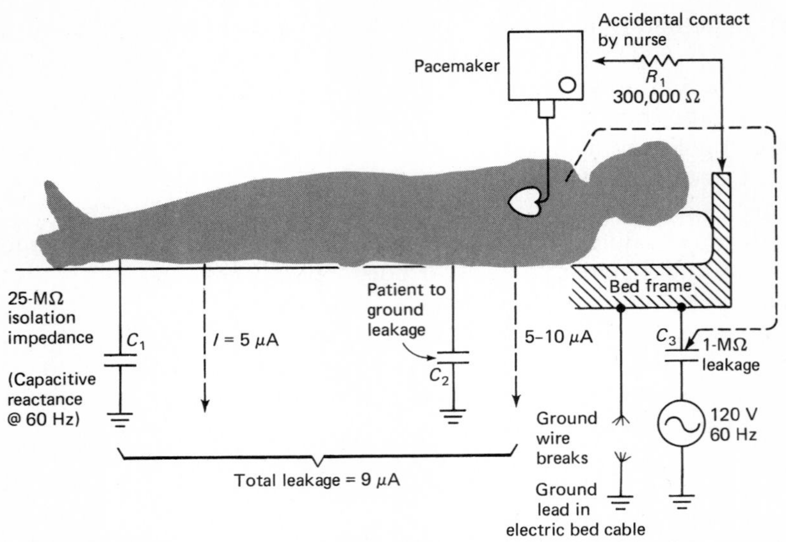

Fig. 2-6 Equivalent circuit when ground wire from bed frame breaks and nurse accidentally touches bed frame and patient at the same time. Although the patient is protected by 25-MΩ isolated input impedance, slightly under 5 μA flows through the patient. Use $I = E/R$ to calculate the exact current. Thus $I = 120\ \text{V}/[25\ \text{M}\Omega\ (C_1) + 300{,}000\ \Omega\ (R_1) + 1\ \text{M}\Omega\ (C_3)]$.

tionally or by accident. Further, if we assume that the resistance to current flow, measured from the catheter terminals to a point on the surface of the patient's skin, can be as low as 500 Ω, it then becomes necessary to limit the potential difference between the catheter terminals and any other surface or instrument in the vicinity of the patient to less than 5 mV if the current is to be below 10 μA.

But successfully achieving and maintaining such low levels of potential difference in a patient is not easy. If the leakage current from a device near the patient exceeds 5 mA and the grounding connection to it exceeds 1 Ω (not improbable conditions), then the potential on the outer case of the appliance will exceed the 5 mV defined as hazardous. Further, if an internal insulation failure occurs in the appliance, permitting a live power wire to touch a grounded part, the resulting fault-current flow can reach many amperes before the circuit breaker in the branch circuit supplying power to the appliance trips out. Larger fault currents will cause potential differences of several volts. This would be intolerable in the vicinity of a patient with a grounded internal catheter.

To understand the operation of isolation transformers, we must consider the modern three-wire branch circuits in hospitals where:

1. The current-carrying wire is at 110/120 V above ground (in the United States and Canada).
2. The neutral wire, carrying the return load current, is near ground potential.
3. The grounding wire is at ground, or zero, potential.

The grounding wire provides a safe return path for any leakage currents from the appliances (or other devices supplied by the branch circuit). The assumption is that ground is connected to the outer case of these devices. The ground wire also serves to carry large fault currents if a current-carrying part in the appliance comes in contact with the case, thereby preventing the case from becoming hot with respect to ground. In this type of power circuit, the amount of current that would flow if the hot wire were to contact a grounded part of a device is limited only by the branch circuit fuse or circuit breaker.

In the power isolation transformer, shown schematically in Fig. 2-7, note that both sides of the circuit are isolated from ground and that either line *A* or line *B* can be short-circuited to ground without a large

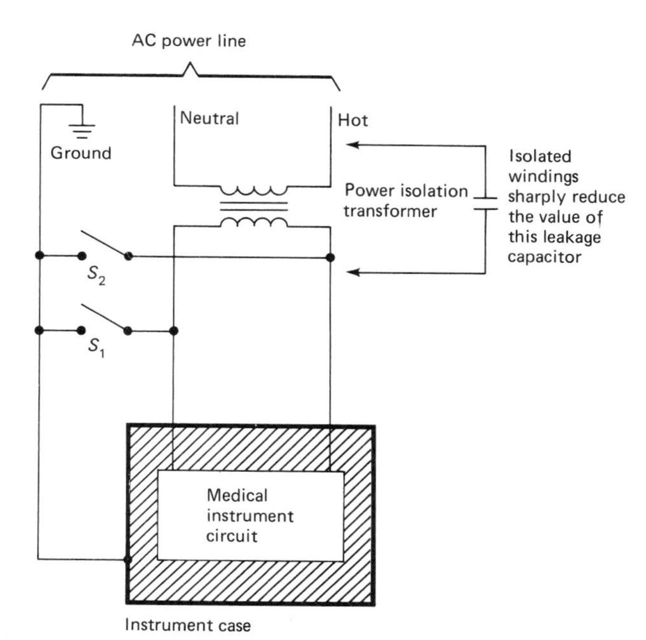

Fig. 2-7 A power isolation transformer has been installed. Switches S_1 and S_2 represent a short circuit between either side of the ac line and the grounded instrument case. Only a few milliamperes of current flows through either short circuit because of the low capacitance between the primary and secondary of the isolation transformer.

current flowing through the connection. Actually, the current that will flow in a short circuit to ground is limited by the leakage capacitance in the transformer and associated wiring. It is generally no more than a few milliamperes.

The transformer also affords a high degree of protection against electric shock to medical personnel. Since an operating room staff and all conductive equipment are grounded to prevent static discharges (and possible fires or explosions in the presence of anesthetic fumes), it is possible that such personnel could receive a serious shock if a live power wire were accidentally contacted.

MONITORING LINE ISOLATION

An additional protective feature, used in conjunction with the power isolation transformer, is the line isolation monitor (Fig. 2-8). It is con-

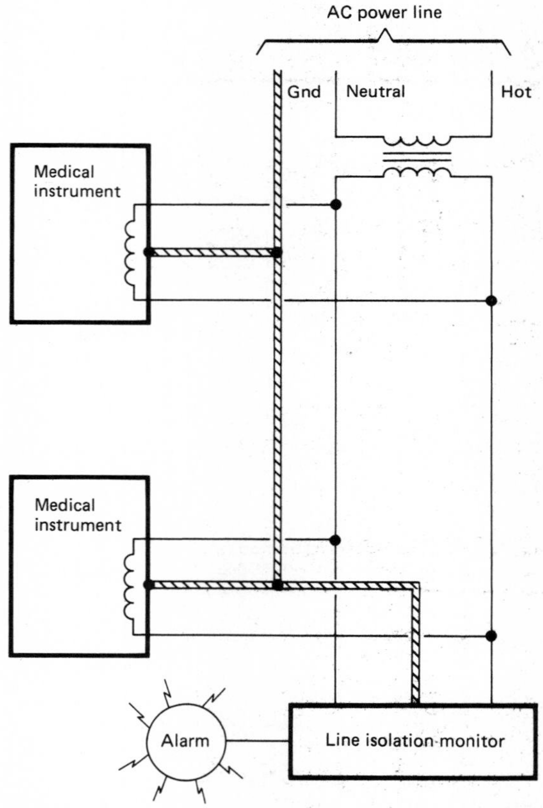

Fig. 2-8 When the impedance of either leg of the ac line drops below 60,000 Ω above ground, the line-isolation-monitor detector is activated. The detector then trips the alarm to its left.

nected to a detector that is set to trip an appropriate alarm if the impedance drops below a predetermined level (usually 60,000 Ω). Thus, as long as each power line is at least 60,000 Ω above ground, if either line is short-circuited to ground, not more than 2 mA will flow through the fault in a 120-V 60-Hz system.

Isolation techniques reduce the inherent hazards of electrically powered equipment to a degree. Isolation transformers can help to protect the patient if devices that ground the implanted electrode are used. As we have learned, the patient is not protected if a grounding connection fails. Therefore, routine inspection and testing of the quality of these connections is essential.

A CASE SITUATION

The reader may get a better understanding of isolation transformer performance in the actual operational situation. Figure 2-9 shows a patient connected between two devices. Here, we assume that:

- The catheter leading to the patient's heart is connected to the outer case of device *A*, while another part of the patient's body is connected to the case of device *B*.
- Devices *A* and *B* are connected to a common ground point, with wires each having 1 Ω of resistance, and the patient represents 500 to 1000 Ω of resistance. This is the range often assumed for patient-safety calculations.

The power for each device is supplied from an isolation transformer that, under single-fault conditions, will limit the current flowing in the fault to less than 1 mA. If a fault now occurs in device *B* (such as an insulation breakdown in the power transformer, which permits the live power line to touch the case), the isolation transformer limits the fault-current flow to 1 mA. Because of the 500 to 1 ratio between the patient and ground-wire impedances, 998 μA will flow in the ground wire and only 2 μA will flow through the patient. Meanwhile, the isolation monitor would have triggered an alarm to indicate an equipment failure. As a step toward avoiding these conditions, several companies now manufacture a grounded-line outlet cluster for a one-bed safe-patient environment. This cluster has several bedside outlets. There is a reference ground near the bed which connects the system to the metal building structure.

GROUND-FAULT INTERRUPTERS

Another device, the ground-fault interrupter, detects the current flowing through the neutral wire and the current flowing through the hot wire. The interrupter compares these two currents. If it detects

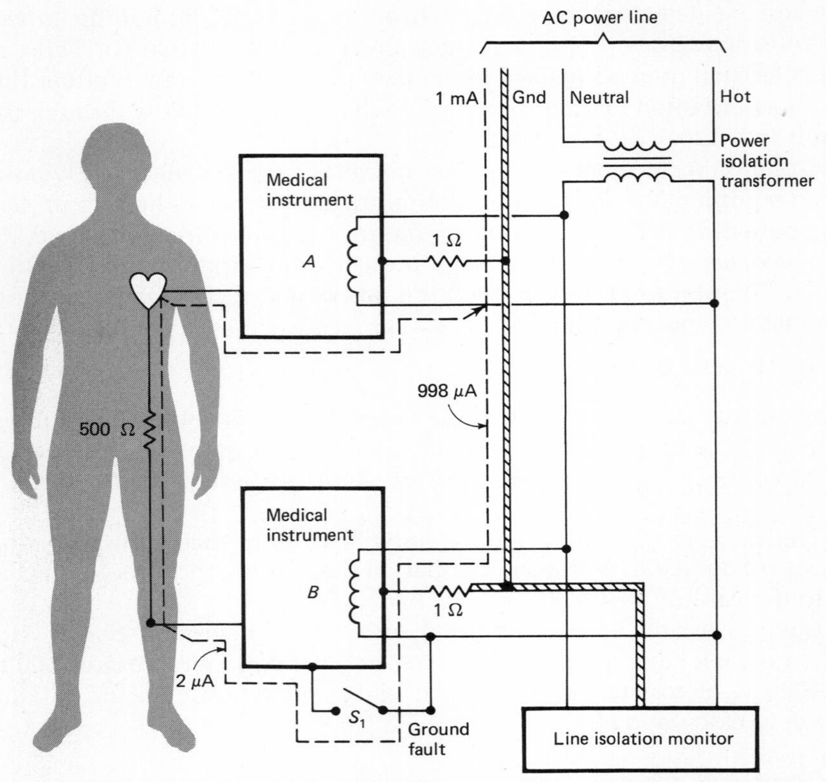

Fig. 2-9 Medical instrument *B* develops a short (S_1) from the line to its grounded case. Only 1 mA flows through the ground circuit because of the isolation transformer. The patient impedance (500 Ω) is 500 times the ground-wire impedance (1 Ω). Thus only $\frac{1}{500}$ (0.002) of the total fault current flows through the patient, or 2 μA.

more than a 3-mA current difference, it interrupts all power. The interrupter is based on the principle that all current flowing in the hot wire returns through the neutral wire. When a person touches an instrument with a ground fault, current will flow through the higher body. In that case, the neutral-wire current will be smaller and the circuit-breaking interrupter will be triggered.

OPTICAL ISOLATION

A power isolation transformer will reduce ac leakage between the patient and the power source to a considerable degree, as we have seen. In addition, monitoring and alarm devices can open circuits as soon as a high leakage condition is detected. Nevertheless, even the small amount of current entering the patient (when using an isolation transformer) might prove harmful. Furthermore, leakage monitoring and

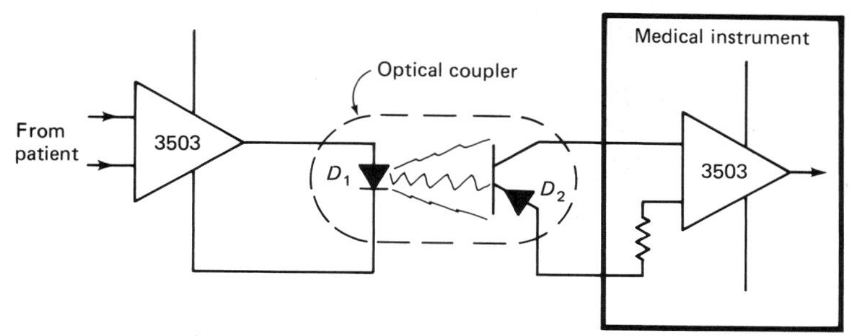

Fig. 2-10 A Burr-Brown integrated circuit amplifies the patient data which feeds the light-emitting diode D_1. Then the light-sensitive diode D_2 changes the optical impulses back into electrical data.

alarm systems require a finite time to trip circuits. The patient could suffer adverse effects even during this brief period. This dangerous condition can be seen in Fig. 2-4*a*.

Optical isolation prohibits the passage of even the smallest electric currents. Data from the patient is preamplified, then converted to light waves by an optical transmitter. In Fig. 2-10, the light-emitting diode (LED) converts the amplifier output into low-intensity light. In the same (lighttight) solid-state package is an optical receiver. In Fig. 2-10, the optical sensor receives the light impulses. Its output is then fed to another preamplifier in the medical instrument itself. The patient is thus completely protected against any leakage, insulation breakdown, or short in the medical instrument.

2-6 LEAKAGE-CURRENT MEASUREMENTS

We have discovered that leakage current flows from the live electric circuit of an instrument to the accessible case. As we have seen, an open ground wire can produce large amounts of leakage currents. However, even when the ground wire is intact, harmful leakage currents often exist.

Leakage currents have both a capacitive and a resistive nature. When capacitive, the air between two wires carrying power becomes a dielectric. Also, there is capacitance between power-cord conductors and ground, and the primary of the power transformer has a capacitance to the instrument case. In Fig. 2-4*a* we saw how the capacitors in RF suppression filters can pass leakage currents. The resistive component of leakage current is established by the finite resistance of insulation surrounding conductors carrying alternating current. However, this factor is relatively negligible due to the high quality of insulation material currently in use.

Leakage measurements may be divided into four general categories. These are illustrated in Fig. 2-11 and consist of:

1. Instrument case to ground
2. Instrument case to line
3. Instrument case to patient lead
4. Between patient leads

Leakage meters are available from several sources. One manufacturer is Neurodyne-Dempsey, Napa, Calif. Their meter has autoranging; that is, it will automatically switch scales according to the measured current so that the meter cannot burn out. The meter scales are 0–10, 0–100, and 0–1000 A. In addition, a 500-mA constant-current source allows four terminal resistance measurements of 1 Ω or less. We have seen how even small resistances in the ground path can create a voltage drop. A resistance between case and ground above 0.1 Ω will produce a hot case. A person touching this case may carry from 2 to 200 μA.

A good leakage meter will measure leakage from the hot ac lead to ground and also from the neutral ac lead to ground. It will automatically respond to reversed polarity where the hot and neutral ac power leads have been incorrectly wired.

Several medical and instrumentation groups have established standards concerning "worst case" leakage currents. These standards are continuously undergoing changes, and they are difficult to apply under all medical applications. For example, during cardiac catheterization,

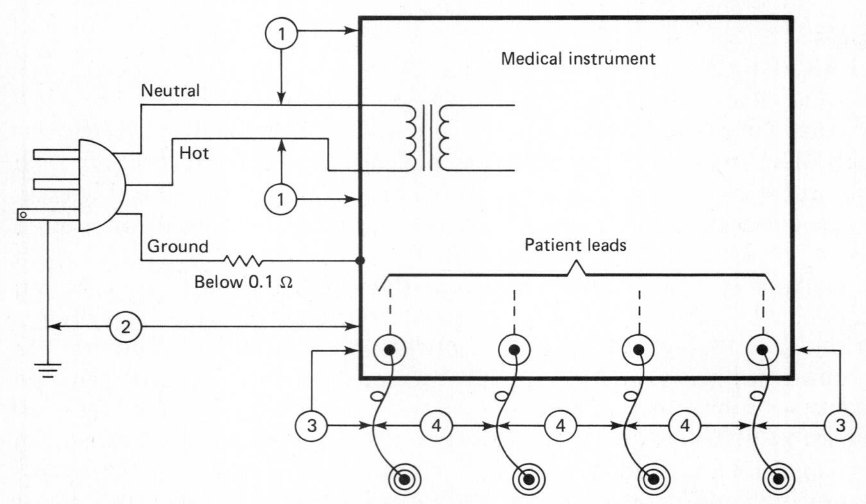

Fig. 2-11 The four categories of leakage measurements are shown. The meter is numbered according to the particular measurement. For example, 1 is case to line, 2 is case to ground, 3 is case to patient lead, and 4 is between leads.

leakage above 5 A from case to ground can be harmful to the patient. At the other extreme, in nerve-conduction tests of a limb, leakage currents of 40 A can sometimes be tolerated. How then can the BMET protect the patient and the hospital staff under such wide and varying conditions of permissible leakage currents? To confuse matters further, several medical instruments may be connected to the patient simultaneously.

One solution to this problem is simply to refer to the instrument operating manual. Most operating manuals will list worst-case leakage current for that particular instrument. In instances where the manufacturer fails to specify leakage current, the BMET can always find out from the manufacturer what the leakage current should be.

When new instruments arrive in the hospital, good practice dictates that the leakage current be checked. Referring to the preventive maintenance schedules (Table 2-2), item 3 shows that leakage current and power-cord condition should be checked on a routine basis every 3 months. In addition, whenever there is any danger of an electrosensitive patient, precautionary leakage measurements should be taken. This is especially true where a potentially hazardous environment exists. Table 2-1 supplies a complete listing of such hazardous environments, the most hazardous being a low-impedance conductor in contact with the heart. At the other extreme, a hazardous electrical environment may exist when patients are exposed to either wet or otherwise conductive bodies.

QUESTIONS

1. Which body mechanism limits the duration of an electric shock?
2. Another name for the return path of a current source is a(n) ________.
3. One milliampere of 60-Hz ac flowing in the body will produce ________.
4. What effect can result from current over 80 mA flowing through the body?
5. As little as 20 μA of alternating current leaking into a pacemaker catheter can cause ________.
6. Is the fibrillation threshold for direct current higher or lower than that for alternating current?
7. What biological effects can high-frequency alternating current create?
8. Which types of electric and magnetic fields can be hazardous to persons wearing an artificial pacemaker?
9. How short a period of power interruption to life-support equipment can cause a fatality?
10. When is an instrument case "hot"?
11. On an electric bed, describe the current flow that might result from a ground fault.
12. How would you connect a low-resistance ohmmeter to check for a faulty ground on a biomedical instrument?
13. In performing the check in Question 12 you measured 15 Ω. As this is quite

a low resistance, the medical instrument may be operated as is. True or false? Explain your answer.

14. Six instruments are all connected to the same patient. Each one tests below 0.1 Ω from the instrument case to the ground pin. Is it safe to assume that no ground current can exist between any of the six instruments? Explain your answer.

15. In cardiac catheterization, even circuit-breaker protection can present a problem. A momentary fault current of 15 A occurs with a ground-wire resistance of 0.1 Ω. Myocardium resistance to ground is 1000 Ω. What current would flow through the myocardium before the circuit breaker opened up?

16. Draw an illustration of the snowflake system.

17. Can the bedside wall plate be used as a junction-box ground for different ECG-EEG electrodes and for a variety of transducers?

18. When making a permanent ground connection, list three good practices to observe.

19. Explain the function of the copper floor screen in the operating room.

20. Briefly describe the hookup and operation of a line isolation monitor.

chapter 3
Converting Physiological Changes into Electric Signals

3-1 MEASURING PHYSICAL AND ELECTRICAL PARAMETERS

We saw in Chap. 1 how the tiny cell produces electrical activity. When these cells are combined in specialized tissue, large amounts of signals can be produced. The heart and the brain are excellent examples of this. In addition to these electrical changes, a number of mechanical changes are constantly occurring within the body. The body has been compared to a plumbing system full of a maze of pipes. As with the plumbing system analogy, there is a continuously changing pressure, changing flow, and changing fluid resistance. Indeed, if we were plumbers measuring large amounts of water pressure, simple mechanical indicators could be used. As biomedical engineers we are not so fortunate.

The pressure parameters to be measured can be as low as −100 mmHg, the electrical parameters as low as a microvolt, and the fluid-flow parameters as low as 5 milliliters (mL). Because of the instrumentation sensitivity required for these measurements, the galvanometer has been abandoned in favor of complex electronics. However, at the heart of the most sophisticated electronic system is the device that picks up the body's electrical activity or converts other physiological parameters into electric signals. Even when measuring impedance variations within the body, the pickup electrodes are a key factor in the entire system.

THE BIOELECTRIC RECORDING RANGE

In recording the various types of physiological activity, there are differing wavelengths or frequencies to be encountered. If we used instrumentation that was sensitive in the range of 5000 Hz to measure electroencephalogram (EEG) activity, we would certainly be wasting our time. Likewise, if we used instrumentation that was sensitive in the 1- to 10-Hz range to measure sensory nerve impulses, we would again be wasting our time. We must match the measurement to the spectrum characteristics of the physiological signals we desire to investigate. Equally important is a knowledge of the levels of activity we can expect.

Figure 3-1 illustrates both characteristic frequency ranges and amplitude levels of the various physiological specialties. We find that EEG recording requires the most sensitive instrumentation since EEG potentials can be as low as 1 μV. For these applications, the gain, stability, and noise level of the entire system must be critically evaluated. On the other hand, we find that electromyograph (EMG) signals can vary all the way from 20 μV up to 4000 μV, or 4 mV. This is a ratio of 200 from the smallest possible EMG signal to the largest possible EMG signal. Care must be taken to determine that our complete instrumentation system, including the input device, will reproduce the full dynamic range without introducing distortion or nonlinearity.

Figure 3-1 illustrates eight distinct types of medical data. In many applications, it is imperative that we compare one data channel with another. We might even wish to observe all eight data channels simul-

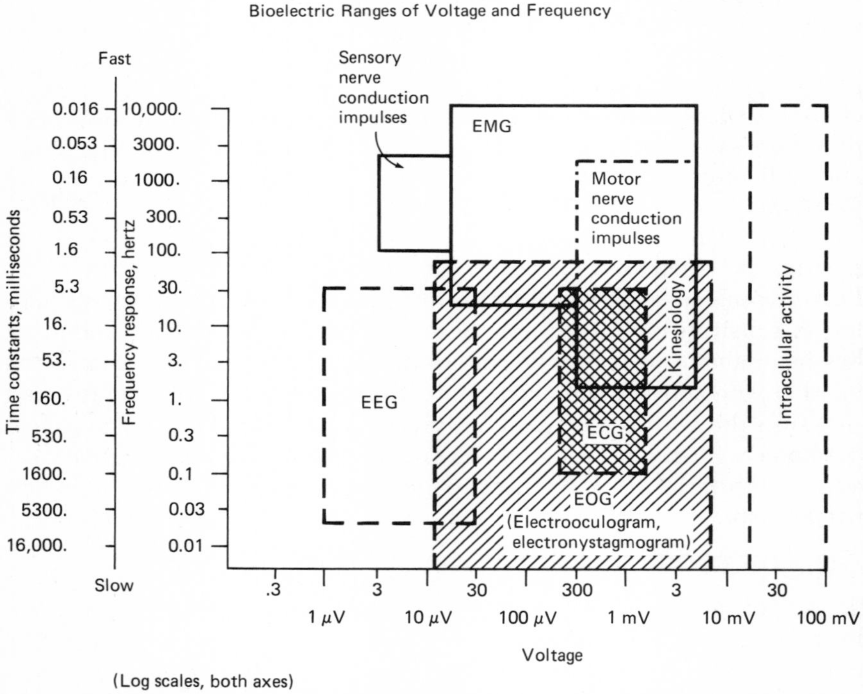

Bioelectric Ranges of Voltage and Frequency

(Log scales, both axes)

Fig. 3-1 Bioelectrical activity is seen increasing in amplitude as it moves horizontally to the right. Activity increases in rate or frequency as it moves up toward the top. EEG can have the lowest amplitude (1 μV), while EMG and intracellular activity can have the highest frequency (10,000 Hz). It is interesting that motor-nerve activity has a higher amplitude and a lower frequency than sensory-nerve impulses.

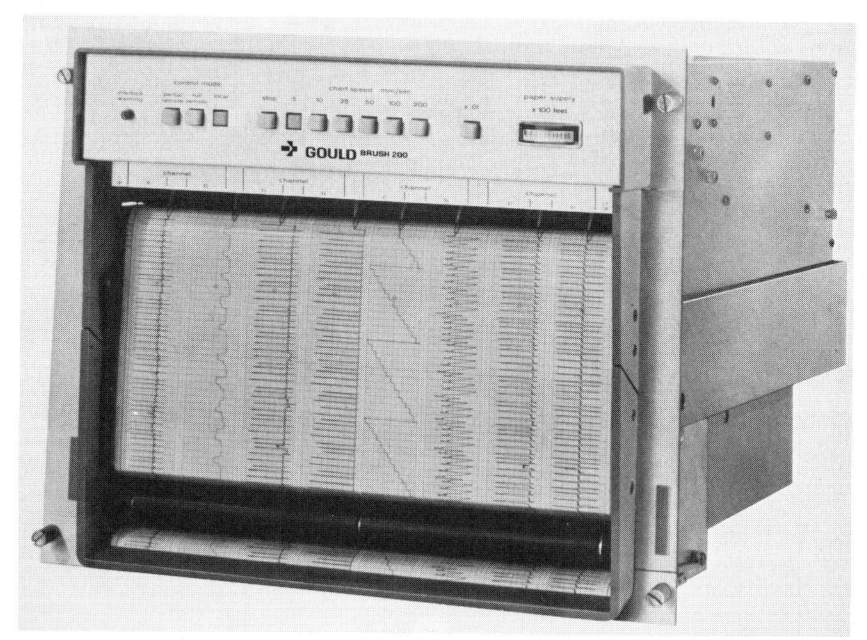

Fig. 3-2 The various types of bioelectrical activity that were described in Fig. 3-1 have different waveshapes. Here we see an eight-channel chart recorder displaying different types of biological data. In addition, one channel carries a calibration test pattern.

taneously. The Gould chart recorder shown in Fig. 3-2 makes this possible.

3-2 THE INPUT DEVICE

Regardless of which physiological parameter we are working with, some type of device is necessary to convert physiological changes into electric signals. Surface electrodes, needle electrodes, strain gages, flowmeters, thermistors, accelerometers, and microphones are all examples of such devices.

Since there are more than 30 biomedical applications, the BMET must understand the various conversion devices available for a particular application. Table 3-1 lists the more common biomedical applications, their primary signal characteristics, and the type of transducer, or conversion device, required. Just as it would be useless to attempt to use surface electrodes to measure temperature, it would be equally useless to use a thermistor to measure EMG activity. EMG activity is electrical and originates in the muscle tissue. If the muscle we are interested in is close to the body's surface, then we will have no trouble using surface electrodes to convert EMG changes into electric signals.

Table 3-1 **Primary Signal Characteristics and the Transducer* Required for Common Biomedical Applications**

Application	Primary Signal Characteristics	Transducer Required
	Cardiovascular Systems	
ECG or EKG (electrocardiogram)	Frequency range: 0.05 to 1000 Hz, 0.05 to 100 Hz usually adequate. Voltage: 10 μV to 5 mV covers fetal range.	Surface electrodes are used with jelly, paste, or cream. Needle electrodes are less noisy.
VCG (vectorcardiogram)	Same as for ECG	Same as for ECG
Heart rate	Rate: 25 to 600 beats per minute. Normal human rate (at rest): 60 to 90 beats per minute.	Obtained from ECG, VCG, arterial blood pressure, or blood-pressure pulse wave amplifiers
Blood pressure: Arterial direct	Frequency range: dc to 200 Hz, dc to 60 Hz usually adequate. Pressure range: 20 to 300 mmHg.	Strain-gage pressure transducer (Statham P23 series recommended
Derivative dP/dt	Frequency range: dc to 200 Hz, dc to 60 Hz usually adequate.	Output of left ventricular pressure channel
Arterial indirect	Pressure transducer: dc to 5 Hz; 0 to 300 mmHg. Microphone: 10 to 100 Hz; voltage depends upon type used.	Strain-gage pressure transducer (Statham P23 series recommended). Any good, low-frequency microphone.
Venous direct	Frequency range: dc to 40 Hz. Pressure range: −5 to +20 mmHg.	Strain-gage pressure transducer (Statham P23 series recommended)
Pulse waves, indirect, arterial, peripheral	Frequency range: 0.1 to 60 Hz usually adequate. Pulse trace similar to blood arterial pressure, but ac-coupled.	Finger or ear lobe pickup (light source and photocell). Piezoelectric.
Blood flow, aortic or venous	Rate: 0 to 300 mL/s. Frequency range: approximately 0 to 100 Hz.	Tracer methods, electromagnetic flowmeters, Doppler flowmeter, and thermistor-tipped catheter.

Table 3-1 (Continued)

Application	Primary Signal Characteristics	Transducer Required
Cardiac output (blood flow)	Frequency range: 0 to 60 Hz, 0 to 5 Hz usually adequate. Blood flow in liters per minute.	Dye-dilution methods. Integration of aortic blood-flow function.
Phonocardiogram (heart sounds)	Frequency range: 16 to 2000 Hz. Voltage. Depends upon microphone used.	Crystal or magnetic microphone
Ballistocardiogram (BCG)	Frequency range: dc to 40 Hz.	Infinite-period platform with strain-gage accelerometer
Impedance cardiogram (rheocardiography)	Frequency range: dc to 60 Hz. Impedance range: 15 to 500 Ω.	Surface or needle electrodes
EEG (electroencephalogram)	Frequency range: 0.1 to 100 Hz. Voltage: 2 to 200 μV.	Surface and needle electrodes
Cerebral potentials, intracranially recorded	Pulse duration: 0.6 ms to 0.1 s. Voltage: 10 μV to 100 mV.	Deep needle electrodes
EMG primary signal (electromyogram)	Frequency range: 5 to 2000 Hz. Voltage: 20 to 5000 μV.	Surface or needle electrodes
Electrogastrogram (smooth muscle)	Frequency range: dc to 1 Hz. Voltage: 0 to 80 mV.	Needle electrodes
Electroretinogram	Frequency range: 0.01 to 200 Hz. Voltage: 0.5 μV to 1 mV.	Corneal electrodes
EOG (electrooculogram, electronystagmogram)	Frequency range: dc to 100 Hz. Voltage: 10 to 3500 μV; high input impedance required.	Miniature surface electrodes
	Respiratory Systems	
Spirogram	Frequency range: dc to 50 Hz.	Spirometer with electronic outputs
Pneumotachogram (respiratory flow rate)	Frequency range: dc to 50 Hz.	Fleisch pneumotachograph head with strain-gage transducer (Statham PM)

Table 3-1 (Continued)

Application	Primary Signal Characteristics	Transducer Required
Impedance pneumograph	Frequency range: dc to 30 Hz from demodulated carrier.	Surface or needle electrodes
Respiration rate	0–50 breaths/ minute (human).	Output of respiratory function channel
Tidal volume (volume/ breath)	Frequency range: dc to 5 Hz. Adult human: 600 mL/breath.	Direct from spirometer. Integrated from pneumotach or flow channel.
Minute ventilation (volume/minute)	6 to 8 L/min.	Integrated from pneumotach or flow channel.
Mercury (Whitney) strain gage	Frequency range: dc to 30 Hz.	When in series with a fixed resistance it forms one leg of a bridge circuit.
Pulmonary gases	Frequency range: dc to 5 Hz.	Appropriate P_{O_2}/P_{CO_2} analyzer
Dissolved blood gases and pH	Frequency range: dc to 5 Hz.	Appropriate analyzer
	Physical Quantities	
Temperature	Frequency range: dc to 1 Hz.	Thermistor (Yellow Springs Instrument 400 Series)
Isotonic muscle contraction	Frequency range: dc to 10 Hz.	Gould Isotonic Muscle Transducer
Tocogram	Frequency range: dc to 5 Hz.	P23Db + Saline Catheter
Plethysmogram (volume measurement)	Frequency range: dc to 30 Hz from demodulated carrier.	Surface or needle electrodes

* For many applications a number of transducers may be used. The transducers listed here are the most readily available commercial units.
Source: Gould Instruments.

3-3 ELECTRODES

SURFACE ELECTRODES

If a pad of gauze is soaked in saline solution and attached to a piece of wire, it can be used as a surface electrode. As the solution evaporates, the conductivity of the gauze will change, affecting our measurement. Early researchers in electromyography sought to eliminate this difficulty by preparing a large container filled with saline. Wires were attached to the container at several points. A finger or even a hand or foot could be immersed in the container to pick up EMG activity. Evaporation of the saline solution was no longer a problem. As EMG research developed, however, signals were sought from a particular muscle. The saline-solution containers soon became obsolete.

Metal electrodes were developed to be placed on an individual muscle. The hair on the skin surface was shaved, the skin was rubbed with emery cloth until red, and the electrode was held tightly against the skin. The tissue-electrode interface impedance was somewhat reduced by these methods, but it was still too high to measure small biopotentials. An electrode paste made of a saline compound further reduced the interface impedance. Again the problem of evaporation arose as the compound evaporated. Since those early experiments, electrode jelly with far greater stability has been developed. Another problem was that the pressure of the surface electrode against the skin would squeeze the conductive paste out.

To overcome those early problems, electrodes have been developed which have a spacing between the electrode and the skin to hold the jelly. Figure 3-3 shows a type of disposable disk electrode. The Gel Applicator injects jelly into the electrode until the space is filled. The Applicator can measure the amount of jelly injected. Changing skin-electrode interface impedance due to the jelly drying up does not be-

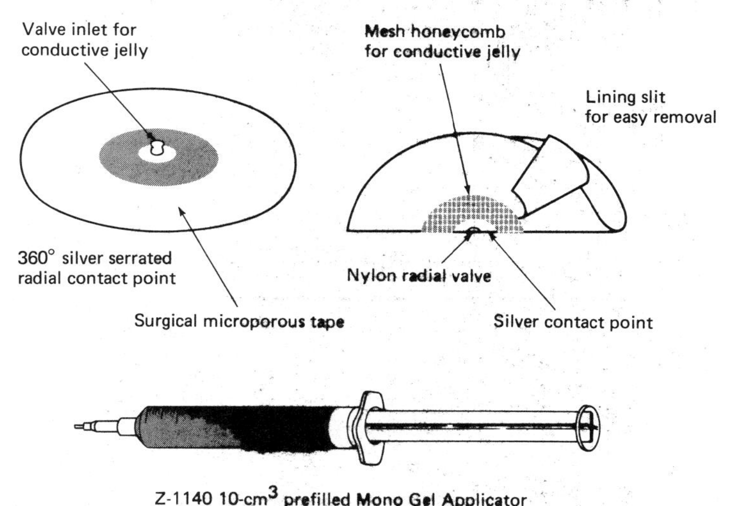

Fig. 3-3 Disposable Mono-Disc surface electrodes manufactured by Zenco Engineering Corp. The Mono Gel Applicator inserts conductive jelly into the electrode valve inlet. Instrument accuracy is increased because the precise amount of applied jelly is known.

come a problem as the complete electrode is disposable. In Chap. 4, Interference and Instability, we will learn how important it is to keep the tissue-electrode interface impedance as low as possible. The weaker the biological signal is, the more critical the tissue-electrode impedance becomes.

When the application is long-term monitoring or exercise testing, the surface electrode becomes an especially important part of the system. An effective gel for silver chloride electrodes will last over a 4- to 6-day period. It should be transparent to permit detection and elimination of trapped air bubbles. To ensure stability the pH of the gel should be 7.0 and should be buffered. Some silver–silver chloride electrodes use a shielded cable to reduce interference. The only drawback in using a shielded cable is that it may degrade the sharp risetime of a very fast muscle potential. However, to observe general EMG activity, the shielded cable does not present a problem. This is illustrated in Fig. 3-4. In each of the recordings silver–silver chloride electrodes (Mark II Biode electrode made by Biocom) with a shielded cable were used. When making use of surface electrodes it is important to bear in mind that signals are being observed from a relatively large section of tissue. The activity we see is the total product of millions of nerve or muscle cells working as a team. If it becomes necessary to evaluate the activity of a small section of tissue, or of cells themselves, then we can no longer use surface electrodes.

NEEDLE ELECTRODES

To observe signals from discrete portions of tissue it is necessary to use needle electrodes. These electrodes may be made of zinc, stainless steel, tungsten, or a platinum alloy fine wire. Metals like copper and silver kill living cells, so they cannot be used for electrodes. Glass tubes filled with a paste or fluid containing ions will also make good electrodes. The fluid may be a salt solution. Wicks of cotton soaked in this solution and wrapped around a wire can conduct electricity away from nerve or muscle tissue. The size of the electrode becomes critical when data from only a small section of tissue are desired. A single human red blood corpuscle measures 7 μm across (0.0007 cm). Human nerve fibers measure between 1 and 20 μm, and the largest spinal cord nerve cells about 150 μm in diameter.

To measure the electrical activity of such cells, microelectrodes of stainless steel or tungsten wire must be sharpened to a fine tip. Fluid-filled glass pipettes with an opening of 1 μm at the sharp end can also be used. These microelectrodes are pushed into the nerve cell and come to rest inside the cell.

In the early days of biological research, the string galvanometer perfected by Einthoven was used to record the signals picked up by needle electrodes. A few years later a fine quartz fiber was stretched between two poles of a strong magnet. This fiber was gold-plated. The biopotential compelled the fiber to move as it was placed within a magnetic field. A beam of light interrupted by the fiber registered these movements. The frequency range these mechanical devices would respond to was extremely limited, as was their sensitivity.

Today's recording instrumentation has input impedances up to $10^{11}\ \Omega$. This allows extremely high frequencies to be faithfully reproduced. But to take advantage of well-designed instrumentation, the needle electrode must have an extremely minute active pickup area with the remainder being a high-quality insulator. Such an electrode is called a *Teflon-coated needle electrode.* The electrode is dipped several times in liquid Teflon. After each dip, it is baked at a very high temperature. This results in a smooth coating of high electric resistance. The extreme tip is then bared and etched. This type of electrode has a very low noise level. Needle electrodes are divided into four general categories: monopolar, bipolar, multilead, and concentric.

THE MONOPOLAR NEEDLE ELECTRODE. This needle electrode is a solid wire, usually stainless steel, coated except at its tip with an insulating varnish or plastic. Variations in voltage between the tip of the needle (exploring electrode), the muscle, and a metal plate on the skin surface or a bare needle in subcutaneous tissue (reference electrode) are measured.

BIPOLAR, BIFILAR NEEDLE ELECTRODES. Variations in voltage are measured between the bared tips of two insulated wires cemented side by side in a steel cannula. The bare tips of the electrodes are flush with the bevel of the cannula, which may be grounded.

MULTILEAD ELECTRODE. Three or more insulated wires are inserted through a common steel cannula. Their bared tips are arranged linearly at an aperture in the cannula which is parallel with its axis, the bare tips being flush with the outer circumference of the cannula.

CONCENTRIC NEEDLE ELECTRODE. Variations in voltage are measured between the bare tip of an insulated wire, usually stainless steel, silver, or platinum, and the bare shaft of a steel cannula through which it is inserted. The bare tip of the central wire (exploring electrode) is flush with the bevel of the cannula, which becomes the reference electrode. The concentric needle electrode is shown in Fig. 3-5.

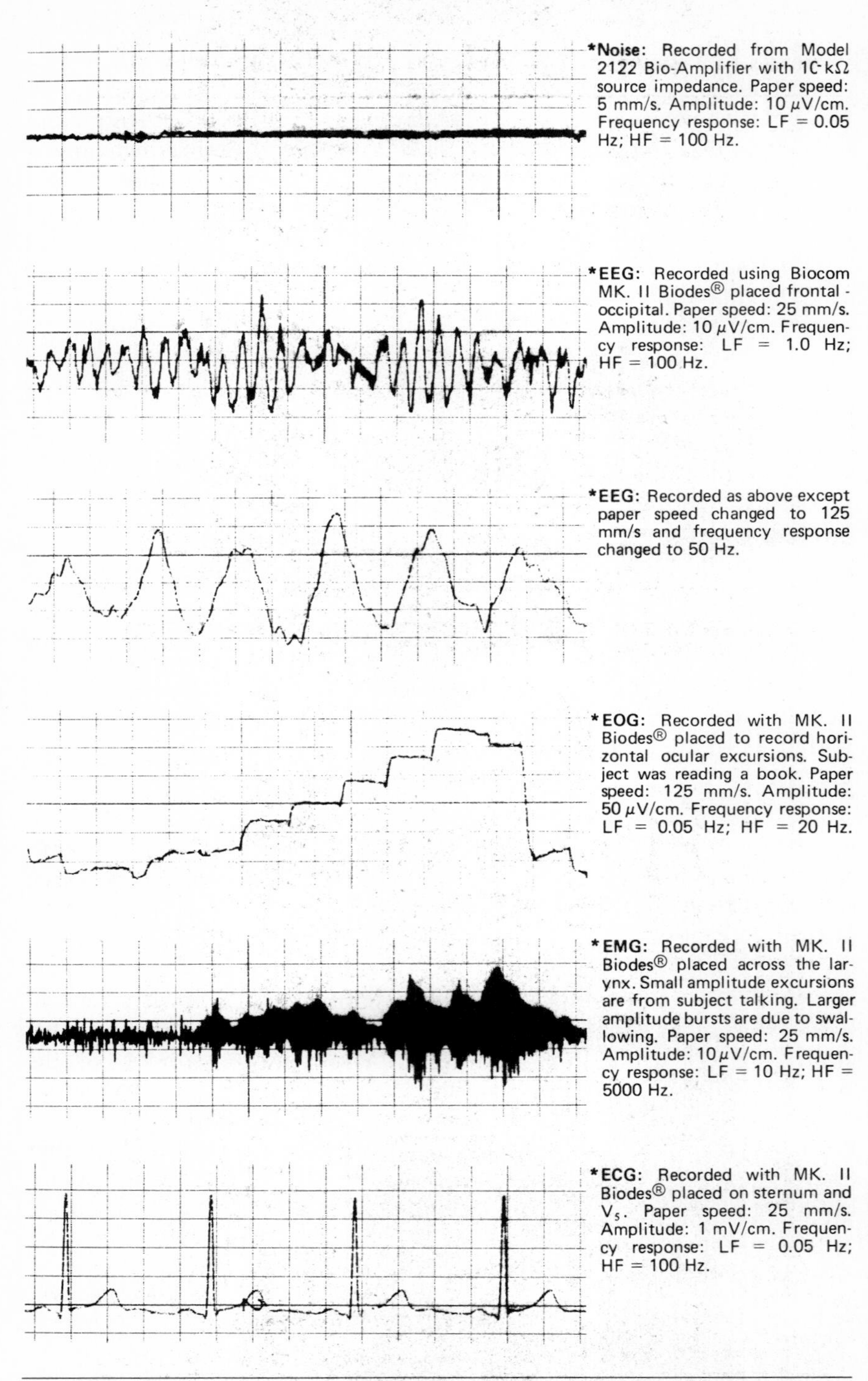

***Noise:** Recorded from Model 2122 Bio-Amplifier with 10-kΩ source impedance. Paper speed: 5 mm/s. Amplitude: 10 μV/cm. Frequency response: LF = 0.05 Hz; HF = 100 Hz.

***EEG:** Recorded using Biocom MK. II Biodes® placed frontal - occipital. Paper speed: 25 mm/s. Amplitude: 10 μV/cm. Frequency response: LF = 1.0 Hz; HF = 100 Hz.

***EEG:** Recorded as above except paper speed changed to 125 mm/s and frequency response changed to 50 Hz.

***EOG:** Recorded with MK. II Biodes® placed to record horizontal ocular excursions. Subject was reading a book. Paper speed: 125 mm/s. Amplitude: 50 μV/cm. Frequency response: LF = 0.05 Hz; HF = 20 Hz.

***EMG:** Recorded with MK. II Biodes® placed across the larynx. Small amplitude excursions are from subject talking. Larger amplitude bursts are due to swallowing. Paper speed: 25 mm/s. Amplitude: 10 μV/cm. Frequency response: LF = 10 Hz; HF = 5000 Hz.

***ECG:** Recorded with MK. II Biodes® placed on sternum and V_5. Paper speed: 25 mm/s. Amplitude: 1 mV/cm. Frequency response: LF = 0.05 Hz; HF = 100 Hz.

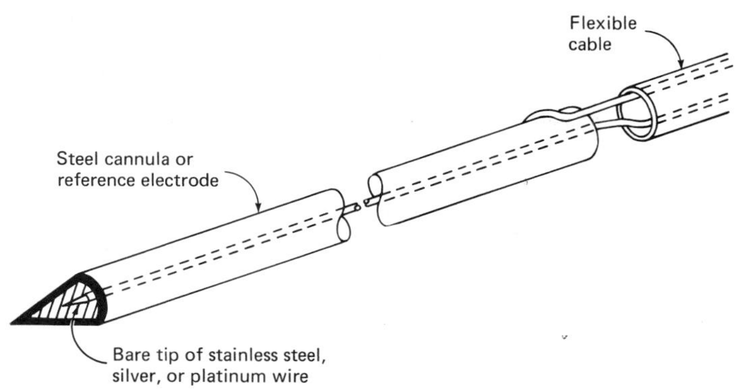

Fig. 3-5 Typical concentric needle electrode. This type of electrode is made from stainless steel hypodermic stock. The center insert can be platinum alloy wire (0.076 mm) embedded in epoxy. The tip is sharpened with a standard taper. A Silastic-covered flexible cable is attached which terminates in standard phone tips.

CAUSES OF DISTORTION

In any microelectrode there is always some current flowing at the metal and electrolyte interface. Some electrode configurations may minimize this problem, but it nevertheless exists. Even though an electrometer preamplifier were used, there would still be a finite input current. Other types of preamplifiers have an even larger amount of input current or a lower input resistance. The higher the current that flows in either the metal-electrode interface or the preamplifier input, the greater is the distortion of the signal being observed.

The use of silver–silver chloride pickup electrodes in glass-microelectrode systems does not eliminate the ac polarization impedance which causes distortion. Another cause of distortion is the series capacitance of the needle electrode. This is most harmful where fast, pulsed signals are involved. If a glass microelectrode is used, it can be thought of as a low-pass filter. Slowly varying potentials will pass easily, but fast signals may be distorted. To record fast potentials such as the activity of an axon, it is best to use metal microelectrodes. Metal microelectrodes may be thought of as high-pass filters. While glass microelectrodes pass slow signals, metal electrodes pass fast signals more easily. The explanation for this is based on the *RC* components involved and the ac polarization. Glass systems have a much higher shunt capacitance and series resistance. If needle electrodes are picking up the output of a stimulus, true reproduction of the stimulus

---

Fig. 3-4 (page 74) Unretouched recordings using a Biocom Model 2122 bioamplifier. The pickup electrode was a silver–silver chloride electrode (Mark II Biode electrode), and electrostatic interference has been minimized with a bioshield cable.

waveshape may be important. This is especially true in conduction-velocity measurements. To minimize distortion, the impedance of the stimulator must be matched to the stimulator output. The impedance the needle electrode sees must also be properly matched. The coupling coefficient, within the tissue, between stimulator and needle must also be considered. A lack of coupling will create difficulties in picking up the stimulator pulse. Overcoupling will distort the shape of the stimulus pulse. Stimulators should have a constant-current output.

3-4 PRESSURE TRANSDUCERS

PIEZOELECTRIC TRANSDUCERS

Measuring the pulse is a prime application of the piezoelectric transducer. Many methods have become available to convert the force of the human pulse into an electric signal. One method makes use of a piezoelectric element. A piezoelectric phonograph pickup will produce signals whenever it is vibrated by a phonograph record. Likewise, a piezoelectric pulse transducer will produce signals whenever it is vibrated by the force of peripheral pulse pressure. In order to measure force, a piezoelectric transducer must have an opposing force against which to react. This opposing force is supplied by taping the transducer to the subject, as illustrated in Fig. 3-6. The tape must be taut enough to hold the transducer without cutting off circulation. The tip of the finger must rest on the transducer button. The position of the transducer on the finger pad is important. Viewing both transducer and finger from the side, the correct position will be found when the edge of the transducer corresponds to the edge of the fingertip.

Like the phonograph pickup, the piezoelectric transducer has an extremely high electric impedance. Its output must be fed into equipment with a very high input impedance, at least 1 MΩ or higher. With a vacuum-tube amplifier this is usually the case. However, with solid-state equipment, high-impedance FET or MOSFET input must be

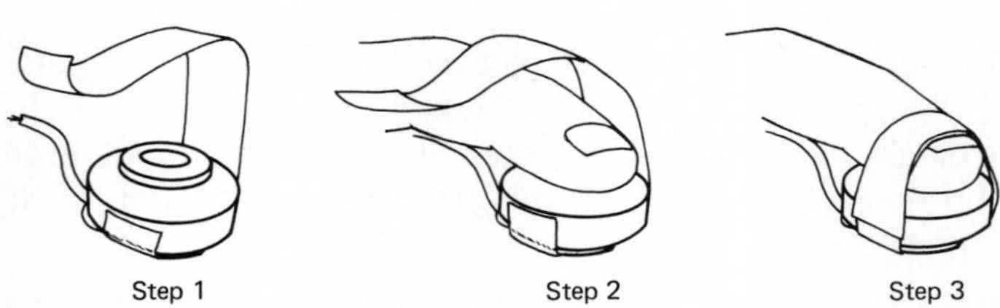

Fig. 3-6 The three steps required in taping a piezoelectric transducer to the finger. The preferable tape is Johnson & Johnson Dermicel. However, Scotch brand masking tape may also be used.

available. Low-impedance transistor input will not function with these devices.

Another important system requirement is that the amplifier does not easily saturate, in other words, that it has a wide dynamic range and will respond faithfully to extremely strong signals. Cardioscopes, for example, will saturate on signals over 4 or 5 mV. The output of a typical piezoelectric transducer can be 100 mV. Where a strong force may produce a high output, a resistive attenuator must be inserted between the transducer and the amplifier. Biocom, the manufacturer of the transducer shown in Fig. 3-5, makes an adapter for this purpose. With a phonograph pickup, the low-frequency response of your amplifier need only be from 25 to 60 Hz. However, with a pulse transducer, the low-frequency output will be down to 1 Hz.

PRECAUTIONS. Piezoelectric transducers are extremely sensitive. It is important for the BMET to observe strict precautions when using them. The transducer must never be exposed to temperatures above 120°F. If you attempt to measure the resistance of these transducers with an ohmmeter, the voltage from the ohmmeter will damage the crystal. Never expose the diaphragm to volatile solvents such as ether or carbon tetrachloride. Do not press the button on the diaphragm between the fingers. Too much direct stress will fracture the transducing element.

THE VARIABLE-RELUCTANCE PRESSURE TRANSDUCER

The piezoelectric pressure transducer, as we have discovered, will not withstand a strong shock or vibration. It has a poor overload tolerance. Its extremely high impedance limits the length of connecting cable that can be used if noise and interference are to be kept low. To measure interthoracic, pulmonary, vascular, and other respiratory pressures, large variations are encountered. The transducer must have a wide dynamic response, have a high overload tolerance, and be operator-proof. The variable-reluctance transducer has been found to be valuable for such applications.

Reluctance is the ratio of magnetomotive force to the total magnetic flux. It is measured in ampere-turns per weber, or At/Wb. By using a diaphragm which will deflect under pressure, a coil's magnetic reluctance can be made to change. Figure 3-7 shows such an arrangement. The diaphragm is magnetically permeable stainless steel. It is clamped between two blocks and deflects when pressure difference is applied through the pressure ports. The core and coil assembly is embedded in each block with a small gap between the diaphragm and the *E* core. The arrangement is symmetrical, resulting in a condition of equal inductance with the diaphragm in an undeflected position. Diaphragm de-

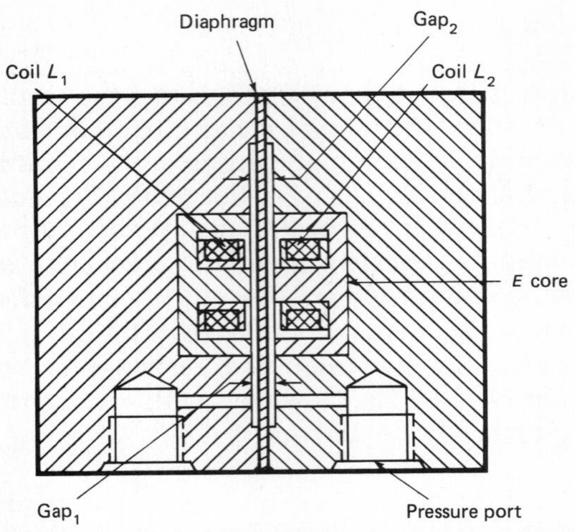

Fig. 3-7 A simplified cross-sectional diagram of the differential pressure transducer. A dc voltage is produced proportional to the difference between pressure at the pressure port and at the reference port. The movement of the diaphragm creates a difference in inductance (reluctance) between coil L_1 and coil L_2.

flection results in an increase in the gap in the magnetic flux path of one core and an equal decrease in the other. The reluctance varies with the gap, determining the inductance value. Thus the effect of the diaphragm motion is a change in the inductance of the two coils, one decreasing and the other increasing.

The low volumetric displacement and the low internal volume results in the extremely wide dynamic response. The high mechanical natural frequency is a key factor in this wide dynamic response, as shown in Fig. 3-8. Coil L_1 is excited by 115 V ac or 28 V dc, and the output is taken from coil L_2. The output is amplified and demodulated. It is then a dc voltage which is proportional to the flow or volume being measured.

The transducer in Fig. 3-7 is of the differential type. That is, its output indicates the difference in pressure between the two pressure ports. One such differential variable-reluctance pressure transducer, manufactured by Validyne Engineering, is shown in Fig. 3-9. Chapter 8, Common Biomedical Circuits, will discuss the electronics associated with this type of transducer. Its prime applications are to measure mouth pressure, airway resistance, airway closure, and all respiratory parameters. A complete system using this device, with recorded data indicating pneumotachography measurements, is shown in Fig. 3-10. Flow and volume are determined for FVC (forced vital capacity), FEV (forced expiratory volume), FEF (forced expiratory flow), MVV (maximal voluntary ventilation), and TV (tidal volume). Refer back to Sec. 1-20 for the significance of each of these respiratory parameters.

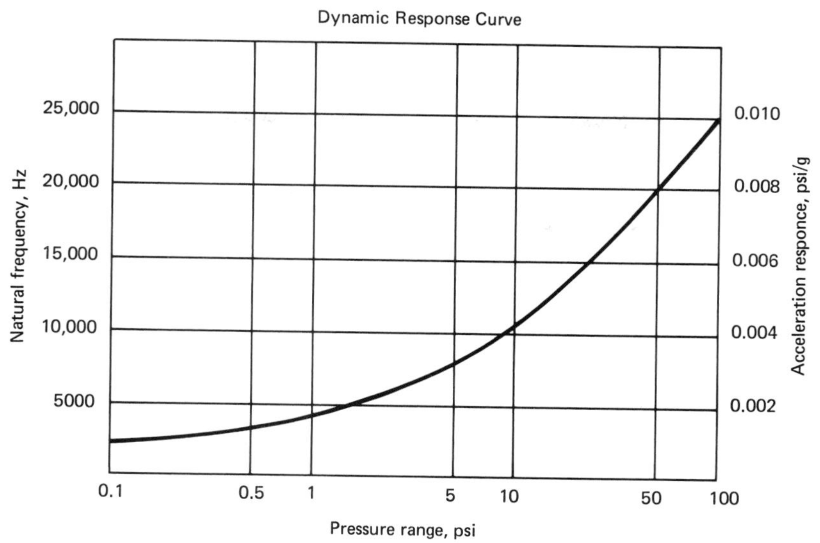

Fig. 3-8 The dynamic range of the differential transducer accelerates rapidly at the higher frequencies. At 25,000 Hz, its pressure range is up to 100 lb/in².

THE STRAIN-GAGE TRANSDUCER

When measuring arterial pressures, and when increased waveform detail is important, the transducer must have very low volume displacement. This is especially essential when fine-bore catheters are used. When measuring venous pressure, sensitivities as low as −50 mmHg,

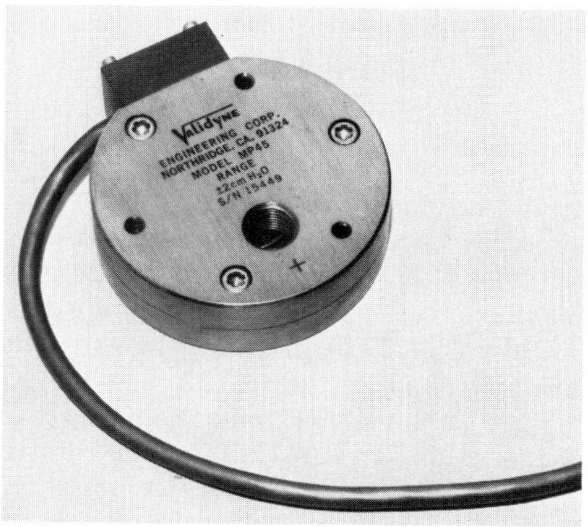

Fig. 3-9 The Validyne Engineering differential pressure transducer. The flexible cable carries the excitation voltage to the transducer and also carries the transducer input data signal. The positive differential input is seen in the lower center.

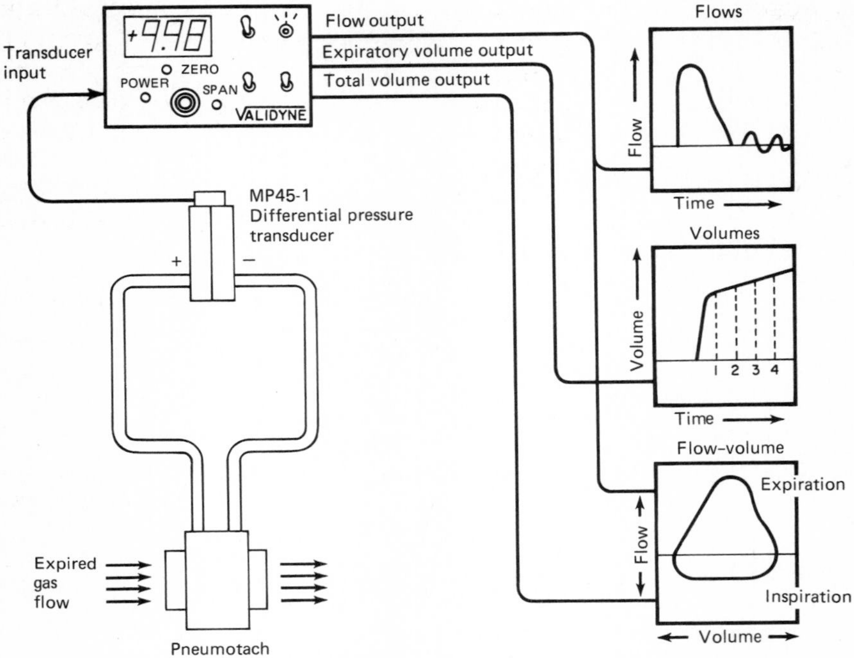

Fig. 3-10 A carrier excites the differential pressure transducer. Its differential output is then amplified and demodulated. A dc voltage is produced which is proportional to the flow function. Expiratory and total volume are obtained by integrating the flow signal in an integrating amplifier. Flow function, expiratory volume, and total volume are displayed on individual chart recorders.

and extreme stability, are required. For the long-term monitoring of arterial, venous, and cerebrospinal fluid, the transducer must be extremely small and lightweight. This is necessary for patient comfort. The strain-gage transducer is capable of meeting all these stringent demands.

Some strain-gage transducers are designed to withstand voltages up to 10,000 V which may be found during electrocautery and defibrillation. In addition, they provide isolation between the internal mechanism and the transducer case and between the transducer case and the patient's body fluids. The Statham strain-gage transducer shown in Fig. 3-11 is an example of a transducer with these special features. The unbonded strain gage can be seen in the bottom center part of the illustration. It consists of a fine wire (stainless steel) tightly held between two supporting posts. When the pressure across this wire changes, there is a proportionate change in its electric resistance. How is this change in electric resistance translated into a voltage?

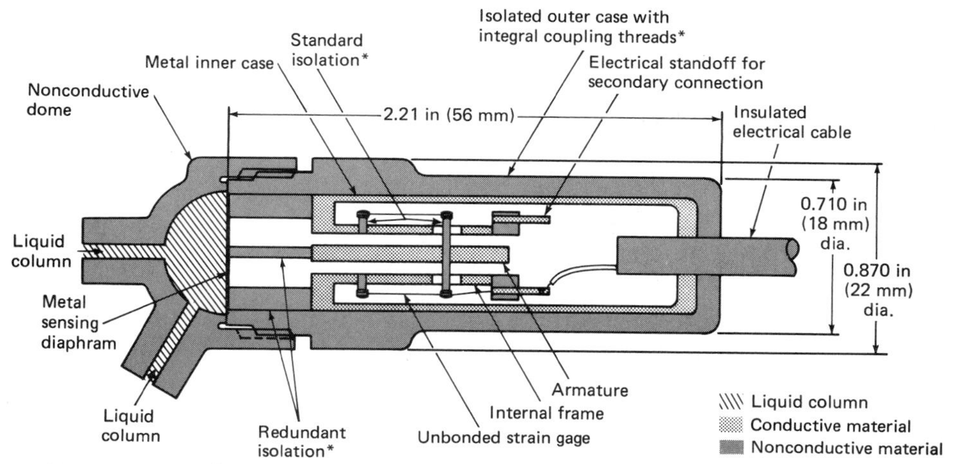

Fig. 3-11 A Statham strain-gage pressure transducer. The bridge elements are isolated from the inside of the case and from the frame. This provides protection from extraneous voltages, such as defibrillation voltages. The unbounded strain gage can be observed along the bottom center of the illustration.

THE WHEATSTONE BRIDGE. The Wheatstone bridge is essentially a balanced circuit. The voltages at two different points in the circuit are balanced against each other so that zero potential exists between them. However, when the bridge is not balanced, a definite voltage will be created between these two points in the bridge. In Fig. 3-12*a*, a voltmeter is placed across these two points. R_1 through R_4 are called the bridge arms. When the voltage across R_3 and R_4 adds algebraically to zero, then $E_1 = E_2$ and the voltmeter reads zero. R_1, R_3 and R_2, R_4 form voltage dividers across the excitation voltage. When

$$\frac{R_3}{R_1 \text{ and } R_3} = \frac{R_4}{R_2 \text{ and } R_4}$$

then $E_1 = E_2$ and there will be zero voltage output. In Fig. 3-12*b*, R_4 becomes R_X, the strain gage, and R_3 becomes R_s. The equation can now be restated as

$$R_X = R_s \frac{R_2}{R_1}$$

The arms of the bridge, R_1 and R_2, are made equal. The calibrated, adjustable resistor R_s will have the same value as R_X when the voltage output is zero. R_s can be adjusted to compensate for barometric pressure changes or positional artifacts.

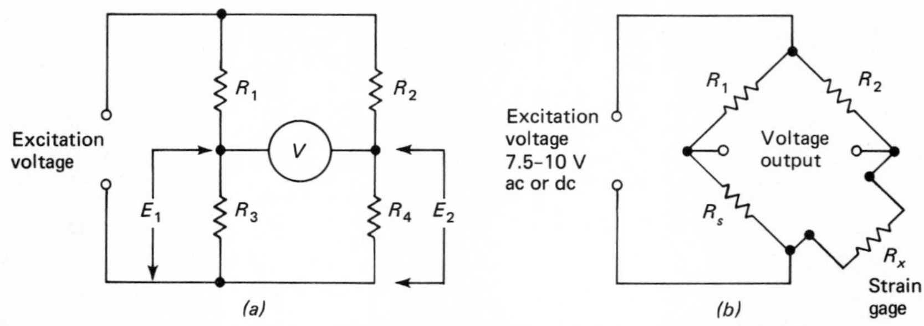

Fig. 3-12 The strain gage becomes one leg of the Wheatstone bridge. Changes in the strain-gage resistance are converted into an output voltage.

When ordering a strain-gage transducer, it is important to specify the make and model of the recording system. This will ensure that the appropriate connector, wired with the required voltage-adjusting resistor, will be furnished.

STERILIZATION OF STRAIN-GAGE TRANSDUCERS. Transducer sterilization is accomplished by immersing the transducer (except for the connector) in chemical disinfectants and sterilizing solutions. Ethylene oxide or Cidex may be used, followed by proper aeration.

SOLID-STATE STRAIN-GAGE TRANSDUCERS. In cardiac catheterization and precise chronic blood-pressure measurement, difficult-to-reach areas can be explored with the complete transducer mounted on the distal tip of a catheter. With the entire bridge in the catheter tip, there is no time delay (catheter leg) through the length of the catheter. In addition, the internal capacitance of the catheter lead does not degrade the high-frequency response of the system. The subminiature size (1.0-mm diameter) is facilitated by the use of a silicon semiconductor element. Four strain gages are atomically diffused to this element. The semiconductor is reacted upon by a diaphragm force-pressure collector. The diaphragm is bonded to the case and sealed at 1 atmosphere reference pressure. The transducer case is made from pure titanium, which is inert and nontoxic to body tissue. This implantable transducer is shown four times actual size in Fig. 3-13.

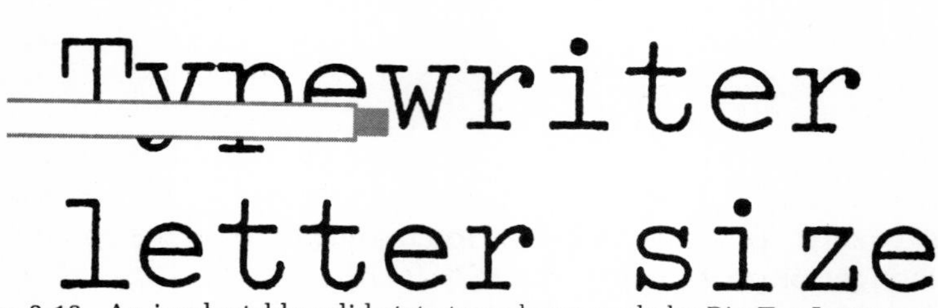

Fig. 3-13 An implantable solid-state transducer made by Bio-Tec Instruments.

3-5 ULTRASONIC TRANSDUCERS

We have seen how various types of transducers are needed to measure blood pressure, depending on the medical technique which is used. A method of blood-pressure measurement which has been gaining in popularity is based on the shift of ultrasonic waves. This frequency shift or Doppler effect occurs whenever the moving blood flows between the transmitting and receiving transducers. The Doppler effect is a frequency change caused by a time rate of change in the effective length of the wave's path of travel. The Doppler effect is proportional to the blood's velocity. Thus pressure can be measured.

Ultrasonic techniques are becoming popular because they are noninvasive, and data can be collected from specific blood vessels. To do this effectively, extremely high frequencies must be utilized. A typical system would focus a 10-megahertz (MHz) ultrasonic wave into the blood stream. This energy sent by the transmitting transducer is reflected from the individual blood cells, then received by the receiving transducer. Both transducers use piezoelectric crystals.

PIEZOELECTRIC CRYSTALS

In nature we find certain crystalline materials that can change mechanical strain into an electric charge. The piezoelectric transducer used to pick the blood-pressure pulse off the finger (see Fig. 3-6) worked on this principle. That transducer could transduce a broad range of frequencies from 1 Hz up to several thousand hertz.

If special care is taken in choosing the kind of crystal, how it is cut, and the dimensions of the crystal plate, we can make it work at only one frequency. The transducer sensitivity at that particular frequency (its natural resonant frequency) will increase many times over that of the untuned, broadband transducer. The crystal is now said to have an extremely high Q or quality factor. We could no longer use it as a microphone or as a phonograph pickup. Those applications (just as fingertip blood-pressure readings) require that a broad frequency range be received. What we now have is the equivalent of a finely tuned resonant circuit. In Fig. 3-14, the equivalent L and C tune the crystal. R, or the mechanical resistance, detracts from the sharply tuned characteristic of the LC circuit. C_h is the capacitance between the plates (or contacts) holding the crystal in place, and the capacitance of the connecting wires. This circuit has a series resonant frequency determined by L and C. Its impedance is largely determined by R, provided the reactance of C_h is large compared with R. However, the same circuit also has a parallel resonant frequency determined by L and the equivalent capacitance of C and C_h in series. Since the equivalent capacitance

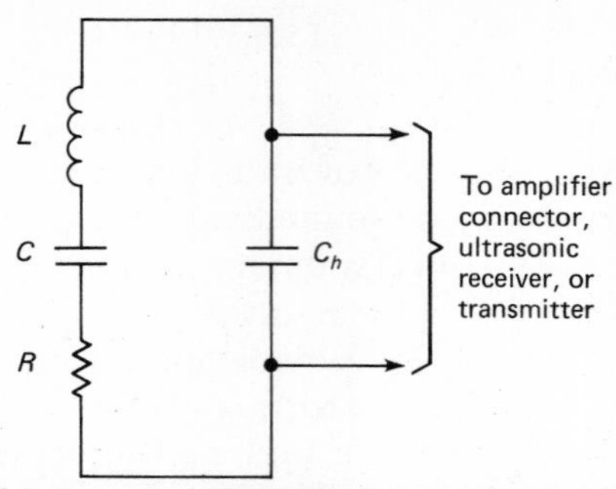

Fig. 3-14 Equivalent circuit of a transducer crystal resonator. *L*, *C*, and *R* are the electrical equivalents of mechanical properties of the crystal. C_h represents the capacitance that is always present in the cable from the transducer to the instrument.

is smaller than C alone, the parallel resonant frequency is higher than the series resonant frequency. The separation between the two resonant frequencies depends on the ratio of C_h to C. When this ratio is large (as is the case of the crystal resonator), the two frequencies will be quite close together. This can be seen in Fig. 3-15, which shows the reactance and resistance of the transducer vs. frequency. Using the series reso-

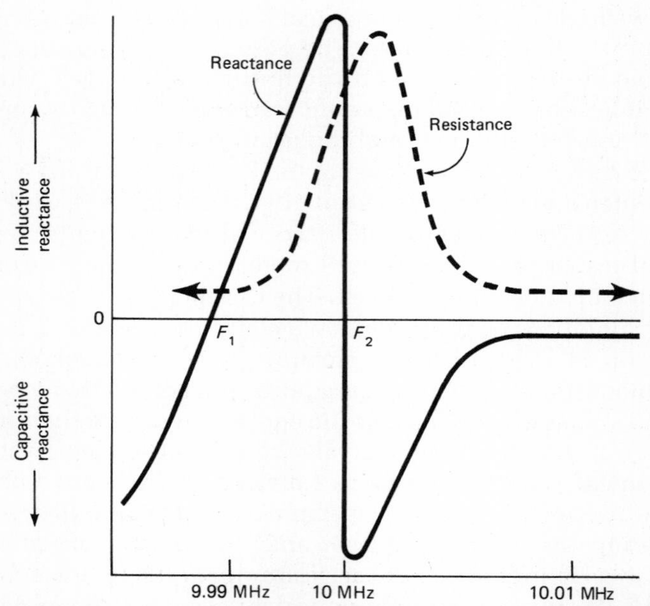

Fig. 3-15 A resonant piezoelectric transducer will function on either its series resonant frequency (F_1) or its parallel resonant frequency (F_2). The *L*, *C*, and *R* of Fig. 3-14 determine the actual separation between the series and parallel resonant frequencies. The transducer's impedance is expressed in either inductive or capacitive reactance. Both reactances are equal at F_1 and F_2; thus there are two resonant frequencies.

nant mode of operation, the crystal receives reflected ultrasonic signals from the transmitting transducer.

The transmitting transducer often uses the parallel resonant frequency. In the 10-MHz ultrasonic system used for blood-pressure measurements, a 10-MHz signal is generated by an oscillator. This signal is amplified and fed to the transmitting transducer. The transmitting transducer (unlike the receiving transducer) must be capable of handling a considerable amount of power. The greater the distance between the transmitting and receiving transducer, the greater the transmitting power required.

In Chap. 8, Common Biomedical Circuits, an isolated power supply is described. It makes use of a transmitting and receiving ultrasonic transducer. In Chap. 10, Troubleshooting the System, a test procedure is described to determine the functional status of piezoelectric transducers.

3-6 FLOW PROBES

The measurement of fluids in the body can be divided into several distinct applications:

- Monitoring blood flow during cardiopulmonary bypass
- Flow measurement of conductive liquids such as urine or saline
- Intracorporal measurements during surgery to give immediate indication of effectiveness of a reconstructive procedure or an organ transplant
- Comparing the flow before and after peripheral vascular reconstruction and myocardial revascularization
- Extracorporeal flow measurements with perfusion systems

BLOOD-FLOW MEASUREMENTS IN STUDIES OF SHOCK AND INTRAVASCULAR DRUGS

The entire flowmeter system begins with the probe. The probe (transducer) picks up the flow signal and must fit over the vessel being measured. Thus the proper size probe must be used. Figure 3-16 shows only a small portion of flow probes manufactured by Carolina Medical Electronics. Probe size is specified in millimeters of lumen circumference because the vessel circumference can be easily determined. A suture is tied around the vessel. The suture is cut and its length is measured with millimeter scale. Electrodes inside the probe must make contact with the vessel wall. Thus an oversize probe is not reliable. If large blood-pressure changes are anticipated, the probe must be small enough to maintain good contact at the lowest pressure. Too small a

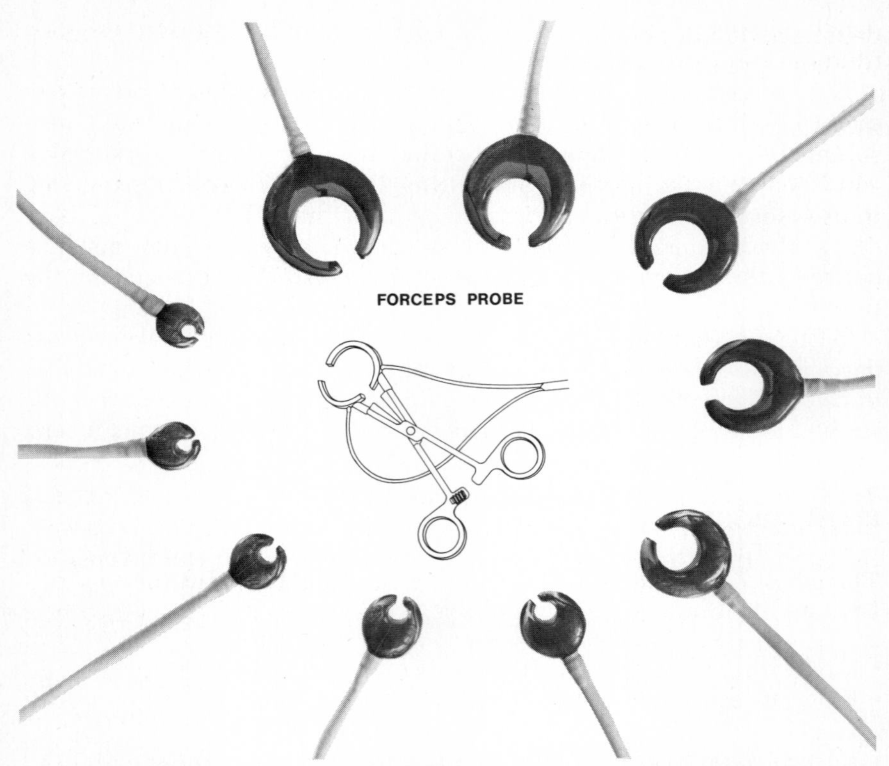

Fig. 3-16 Some of the many blood-flow probes manufactured by Carolina Medical Electronics. In the center is a flow probe attached to a forceps.

probe will alter the arterial pulsatile flow pattern. Constriction beyond 50 percent may cause a reduction of mean flow; however, constriction up to 20 percent does not alter the flow pattern. Atherosclerotic vessels require special caution. When selecting a probe, consideration should be given to the vessel length which is exposed, space around the vessel, proximity of adjacent organs, and depth of vessel location.

The probe cable is connected to the flowmeter electronics. This system must supply an energizing signal to produce the magnetic field in the probe. The flowmeter receives the flow-induced signal. This signal is amplified and converted into a dc voltage proportional to the volumetric flow rate. This signal is made available for visual presentation, computation, or storage. The electronics may amplify several channels of flow data simultaneously. The output is indicated in milliliters or liters per minute. Full-scale range may vary from 10 to 30,000 mL/min. The actual pulsatile flow-rate signal is provided for recording and display. The mean signal time constant is 5 s, and the frequency response or roll-off of the pulsatile display is typically 50 Hz. Zero flow determination can be made without vessel occlusion. Mean and pulsatile flow can be seen simultaneously.

PRINCIPLE OF PROBE OPERATION

Modern flow instrumentation is based on Faraday's law of electromagnetic induction:

$$E = (MLV) \times 10^{-8}$$

where E = electromotive force, V
M = magnetic field, gauss (G)
L = lumen diameter, cm
V = velocity of the liquid, cm/s

The law states that when a conductor (body fluid) moves through a magnetic field, a voltage is induced at right angles to the direction of motion and to the magnetic field. Polarity of the induced voltage depends on the direction of the fluid's motion. The magnitude of the induced voltage is determined by the velocity of the fluid's motion. The theory is illustrated in Fig. 3-17.

The probe is basically an electromagnet to produce the field, and two electrodes (180° apart) are held rigidly in the inner circumference of the lumen. These electrodes pick up the flow-induced signal. Electrodes in the extracorporeal (cannulating) and intravascular (catheter) probes

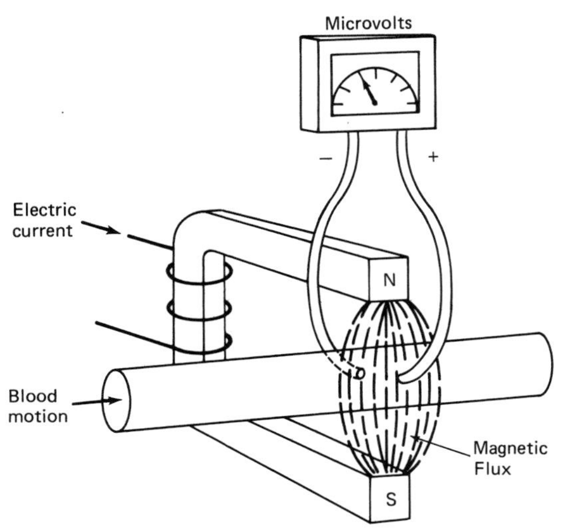

Fig. 3-17 Output, proportional to blood flow, is taken from electrodes at right angles to both blood flow and applied magnetic field.

make direct contact with the blood. The electrodes in the extravascular (noncannulating) probes make contact with the outer surface of the vessel wall. An arrow on conventional-type probes indicates the direction of flow which will produce a positive flowmeter output when the flowmeter polarity switch is in the + position.

Different types of flowmeters are identified according to the type of waveshape that produces the magnetic field in the probe. A square-wave excitation current is desirable to permit separation of the flow signal from unwanted artifacts. Typical current used for magnetic-field excitation would be 1 A with a pulse width of 0.4 ms. The probe amplifier should have a sensitivity down to $\frac{1}{2}$ μV p-p at 1 Hz, and 1 μV p-p at 50 Hz.

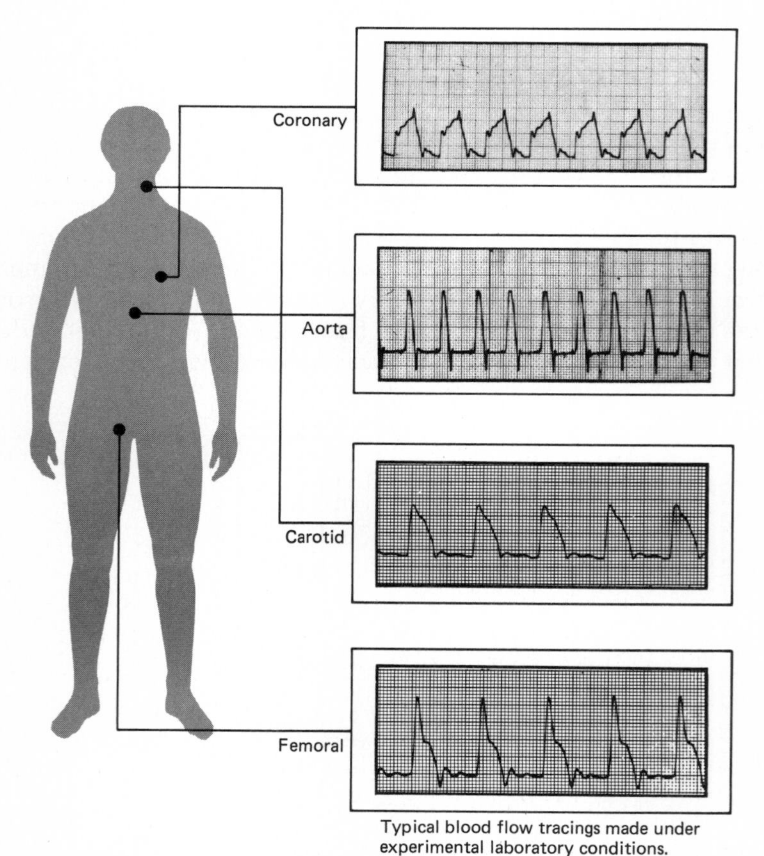
Coronary
Aorta
Carotid
Femoral
Typical blood flow tracings made under experimental laboratory conditions.

Fig. 3-18 The pattern of blood-flow pulsation will vary according to the part of the body. Here, blood-flow tracings from four different arteries can be seen. These recordings were made with Statham Blood Flowmeters.

INTRACORPOREAL FLOW PROBES

Intracorporeal flow transducers must be small and thin. When the lumen is very narrow, they are suitable for aorta and coronary applications where space is a factor.The cannulating type of probe is designed for cannulation of small and large vessels. They have a thin wall. These types of probes are best for acute applications.

RECORDING FLOW-PROBE DATA

Many portable, lightweight strip-chart recorders are available for use with flowmeter systems. A typical example is the Statham Series SP2006, SP2007, and SP2008. Recordings from different vessels will produce various types of tracings. Coronary flow will appear broad with a sharp peak, whereas femoral and aorta flow will tend to be narrower. These variations in flow tracings are illustrated in Fig. 3-18.

3-7 THERMISTORS

The electric resistance of a thermistor will go up when the temperature goes down and go down when the temperature goes up. The temperature coefficient of resistance is said to be high and nonlinear. Characteristics of a typical commercial thermistor are shown in Fig. 3-19. Between 0 and 20°C, the resistance drops very rapidly. However, above 50°C, the resistance drop is much more gradual.

Thermistors are made from metallic oxides, including those of nickel, copper, and zinc. Thermistor sensitivity is of the order of 1 to 6 percent/°C. A higher sensitivity would increase the problem of reproducibility and drift. Although there are many physical configurations in which thermistors are found, four are the most common. These are the bead, washer, disk, and rod, as illustrated in Fig. 3-20.

Thermistors are usually small and flat so that they will not be influenced by connective heat transfer but only by conductive transfer from the measured device. The sensing element is a metal wire wound around a thin insulating card or a coiled wire cemented to the base. All thermistor designs seek to expose the maximum area of sensing surface within a minimum size.

For fluid-temperature measurements, immersion probes with a platinum wire element (can be nickel or nickel alloy) are utilized. The probe-type transducer has a ceramic encapsulated element within a perforated, protective sheath to be usable for a variety of fluids over a wide temperature range. In stagnant fluids, an exposed thermistor element is used to provide a shorter time constant.

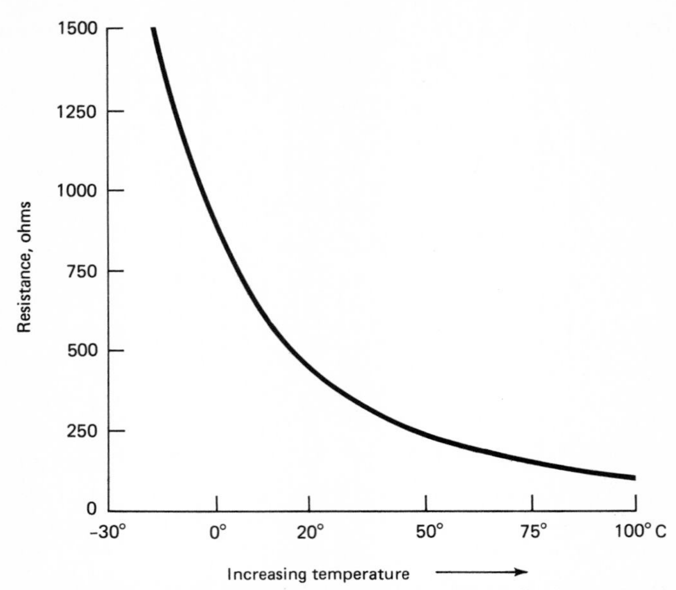

Fig. 3-19 As the body temperature increases, the resistance of a thermistor decreases. If the thermistor were used over the temperature range shown in this illustration, the data would not be reliable because of the nonlinearity. Close to 0°C, resistance change is far greater than it is at higher temperatures.

Thermistors are used for both surface- and fluid-temperature measurements. A large resistance change occurs within a small temperature change. When a short time constant is required, a glass-coated thermistor bead (as small as 0.2 mm in diameter) can be suspended on metal-alloy leads. A general rule for all thermistors is that excitation current is maintained at the lowest possible level to avoid heating the sensing element and causing an erroneous reading.

Thermometers made of germanium crystals mixed with highly controlled impurities are used for cryogenic measurements below −190°C. Carbon resistors and gallium arsenide junction diodes are also used for these applications. Silicon-wafer transducers are used for temperature

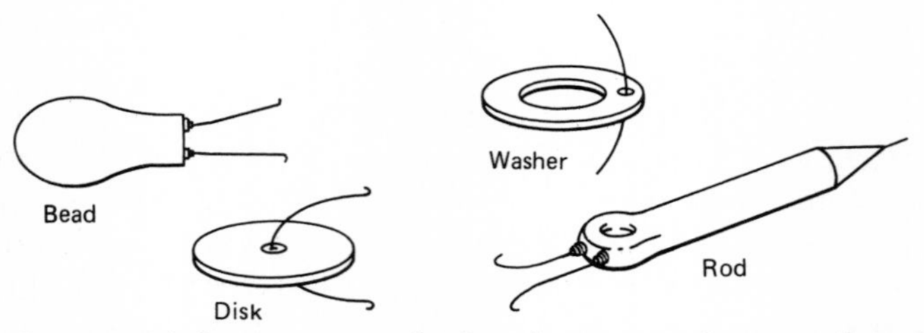

Fig. 3-20 Commercial thermistors can be found in over a dozen configurations. The bead, washer, disk, and rod are the most common physical shapes.

measurements from −50 to +275°C. Their resistance vs. temperature characteristics are similar to those of some metallic wire elements.

SELECTING THE RIGHT THERMISTOR

The selection of a thermistor requires more consideration than the selection of most other types of transducers. The prime objective is that of finding a sensing element that will attain the temperature of the surface or fluid within the time available to make the measurement. In other words, it is important that the temperature-range limits and the required response time (time constant) be taken into account. The sensitivity of the available instrumentation should be considered, as well as the available excitation voltage.

THERMISTOR PLETHYSMOGRAPHY

This is a technique whereby temperature change is converted into electrical data. These data are then used as a factor in determining arterial-blood pulsations. A simple cuff is used as a finger-arterial systolic-pressure recorder. A constriction of diameter 0.030 in is introduced into the air line to the cuff. A 0.010-in-diameter thermistor bead is mounted in the constriction and heated by direct current. Finger pulsations cause a rapid expulsion of air at the commencement of the pulse and a slower return at cessation. The flow of air past the thermistor gives rise to temperature changes, which are reflected as a change in resistance. This is converted into a pulsatile voltage which modulates the dc voltage. Since ac coupling is used, the dc voltage is abandoned. The resultant alternating current is then analogous to the arterial pulsations of the subject.

3-8 BIOCHEMICAL TRANSDUCERS

There is a delicate balance in the body between enzymes, proteins, metabolites, ions, dissolved gases, and waste products. An abnormal proportion of any of the body's chemicals signals possible trouble on a cellular level. It is possible to trace this chemical balance through exhaled breath or perspiration. However, the best method is directly through the blood supply.

The pressure of oxygen (P_{O_2}), or oxygen tension, as well as carbon dioxide pressure (P_{CO_2}), varies in different parts of the body. P_{O_2} is lowest in the heart and liver, where oxygen is quickly consumed, and highest in the kidneys and resting muscles. We know the proper amount of P_{O_2} that we should find in any particular part of the healthy body. Normal determinations can be made using a technique called *photometry*.

PHOTOMETRY

Oxygen in the blood supply combines with hemoglobin (H_b). The product formed is oxyhemoglobin, or H_bO_2. Photometry detects the amount of light reflection at various parts of the light spectrum. H_bO_2 absorbs much less orange light than H_b, giving oxyhemoglobin a bright red appearance. The photometer operator calibrates the instrument and installs two light filters, one for hemoglobin and one for oxyhemoglobin. Then the optical density or light reflection is measured at these two wavelengths (corresponding to the two light filters). Light reflection at the H_b and the H_bO_2 wavelengths then indicates how much oxygen is in the blood. Blood oxygen is directly proportional to oxygen tension. P_{O_2}. Thus the photometry technique, using an optical transducer, has given us a P_{O_2} determination.

SPECTROPHOTOMETRY

While reflection photometry uses only two wavelengths of reflected light, spectrophotometry uses infrared, ultraviolet, and the entire visible spectrum. The angstrom (Å), equal to 10^{-10} m), is the unit of measurement in this part of the spectrum. For example, visible light consists of wavelengths from 3600 to 7700 Å. In spectrophotometry, the blood sample is heated to incandescence, causing ions and elements to emit light. The concentration of a particular substance in the blood is determined by the intensity of its characteristic emission line. The emission line is that part of the spectrum at which the unknown substance emits light. A broad emission line at a particular color corresponds to a particular chemical element. Calcium, potassium, sodium, and other substances are thus measured.

MEASURING pH

The acidity or alkalinity of blood or urine depends on the hydrogen-ion concentration. For example, a strong alkali has only 10^{-14} g H+/L, a strong acid has 1 g H+/L. Converting to the logarithm of that ratio, then converting the algebraic sign, we get 0 to +14. That range is called the *pH scale*. Its neutral point is 7, which is the pH of pure water. Acids, H+, measure from 0 to 7. The alkalies (low in H+) range from 7 to 14 on the pH scale. The pH range in a healthy person will vary from 7.35 to 7.45. This is above the neutral 7 because most body fluids are normally slightly alkaline. pH measurements taken from venous blood will be close to the lower limit (7.35) because of the additional CO_2 in venous blood. Metabolism's end product is acidic. The process starts with the lactate chain as glycogen or starch is changed into lactic acid. Then 80 percent of the lactic acid is reconverted to glycogen. The remainder ends up as carbonic acid (CO_2 + H_2). The body will furnish buffers that will clean up the acidity or the H+ ions. The bicarbonate ion is such a buffer. The kidneys maintain the H+ ion gradient between blood and urine. Here also, the blood's acidity is weakened.

THE pH ELECTRODE. The biochemical transducer that converts ion information into an electric signal is the pH electrode. In Fig. 3-21 we see a glass tube with a thin glass membrane which passes only hydrogen ions in the form of H_3O+. This is a membrane interface for hydrogen. A highly acidic buffer solution is found inside the glass bulb. The potential across the glass interface is developed by placing a silver–silver chloride electrode in the solution inside the glass bulb. A reference electrode is in the solution being measured.

Special pH electrodes used for stomach pH have a glass electrode at the end of a tube for entry into the stomach via the mouth and esophagus. Typical impedances for the glass pH electrode range from 50 to 500 MΩ. To match this extremely high impedance, the amplifier input impedance must be at least equal or greater. The ion currents we are interested in measure 10^{-16} mA. A solid-state device that allows the pH electrode with its low currents and high impedance to be matched to conventional instruments is the metal-oxide semiconductor field-effect transistor (MOSFET). Figure 3-21 shows the electrode and a cutaway of

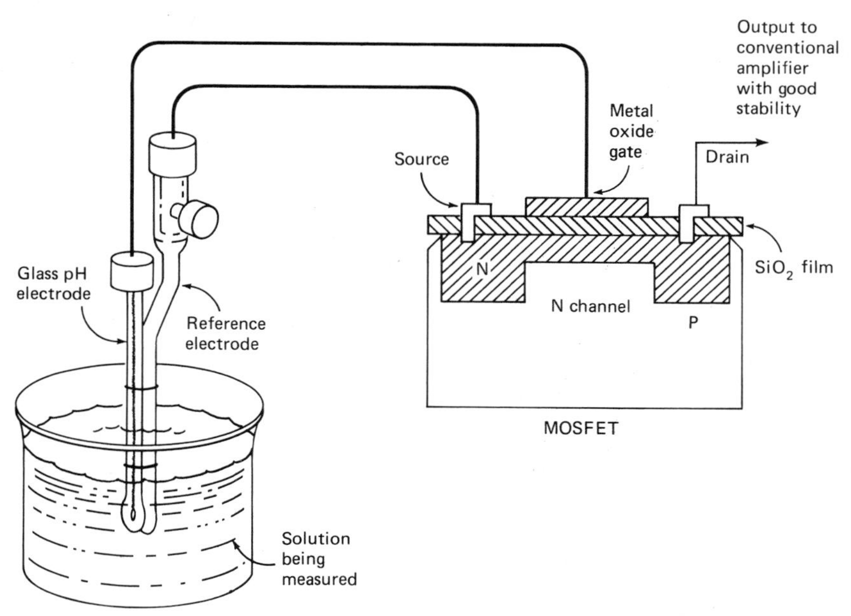

Fig. 3-21 Before the discovery of high-impedance solid-state devices, complex current-balancing circuits were used with pH electrodes. Here, a simple metal-oxide semiconductor field-effect transistor (MOSFET) provides a stable high-impedance input for a pH electrode. The MOSFET output is fed to conventional amplifying equipment.

the MOSFET matching device. These are the most critical components of the complete pH system.

AUTOMATED BLOOD ANALYZERS

These analyzers can perform up to 100 analyses per hour. Each serum or urine sample is drawn through a long tube and separated by distilled water and air bubbles from the other samples. A pump and manifold mix the air bubbles with the sample and allow precise quantities of each sample to be measured. A dialyzer (similar to an artificial kidney) removes protein molecules that might interfere with the measurement. A colorimeter (optical transducer) senses the color change created by the sample. This change reveals the substances which make up the sample. Automated sampling systems are costly. The BMET will most likely encounter simple pH-measuring instrumentation using glass pH electrodes.

BLOOD-GAS TRANSDUCERS

P_{O_2} and (P_{CO_2}) in the blood are important parameters. Gas pressure in the blood is in direct proportion to the quantity of that gas in the blood supply.

To measure P_{O_2} a fine piece of wire (encased in glass) with only its tip exposed is placed in an electrolyte into which oxygen has diffused. A reference voltage is supplied to the platinum electrode and also to a reference electrode (see Fig. 3-22). Any available oxygen in the electrolyte solution collects around the platinum wire, which is now a negative cathode. The extent of the current that flows via this process (oxidation-reduction current) indicates the proportion of P_{O_2} in the solution being measured. The separate cathode and reference electrode can be made into one electrode. Subminiature versions of this electrode can be placed at the tip of a catheter and inserted into the vascular system or even directly into the heart itself.

3-9 TRANSDUCERS FOR RADIOACTIVITY TRACING

After radioactive material has been injected into the body, the technician must determine how much of this injected material exists at various locations throughout the body. If radioactive iodine is injected, for example, we will want to determine how fast it is being assimilated by the thyroid. A Geiger counter placed over the thyroid will monitor approximately how much material the thyroid has absorbed. However, to determine how much material is taken up by other parts of the body, it is necessary to scan the body so that regions of accumulation can be discovered. A carriage-mounted radiation transducer is moved across

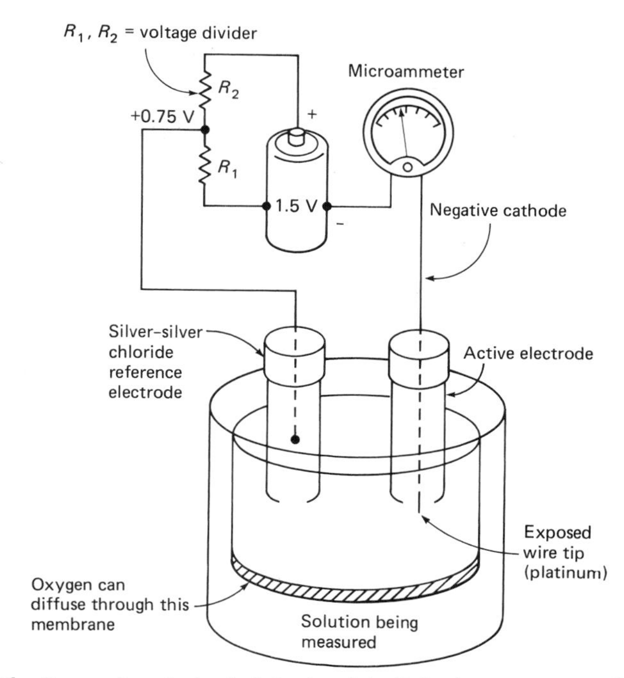

Fig. 3-22 The P_{O_2}-sensing electrode is broken into its basic components. Oxygen in the solution being measured diffuses through the membrane, determining how many electrons are collected at the exposed wire-tip cathode. An indication of this is then read on the microammeter scale.

the patient. The detector is shielded against any radiation except that which is parallel to its own axis. Any radiation which arrives at an angle is absorbed by this shield. A count of radioactivity is taken from each small area. These data are arranged to make up a radioactive map of the body. From 3 to 10 min is required to make a complete scan.

To update the older scanning technique, a more recent technique uses a gamma camera. The gamma camera is actually a scintillation detector. A radioactive particle passing through a transparent crystal generates a minute flash of light. This instantaneous flash is then detected by a sensitive photocell called a *photomultiplier*. The light flash generated by the crystal is close to the radioactive particle that originally caused the light flash. The gamma camera actually has a large, circular, flat crystal surface with an array of photomultipliers mounted behind it. The photomultipliers closest to the light flash receive the strongest signal. By correlating the photomultiplier output with their positions over the body, the exact position of maximum radiation is discovered. A picture of overall radiation intensity is built up on photographic film.

Radioactive tracings can reveal the patient's total blood volume. Dye is injected into the bloodstream. A blood sample is taken to determine how much dye is present. The particle-generated crystal flashes, or the scintillation effect, are converted into an electric signal through photoelectric transducers.

3-10 PHOTOELECTRIC TRANSDUCERS

In the language of electronics, frequency is no longer cycles per second; it is now hertz. This was the same Hertz who in 1887 discovered that electrons are liberated from certain materials under the influence of light. Hertz' discovery has come to be known as the *photoelectric effect.* This effect includes the liberation of electrons from a metallic surface, called *photoemission,* and the generation of hole-electron pairs in semiconductors exposed to radiation, called *photoconductivity,* the *junction photoeffect,* or the *photovoltiac effect.*

PHOTOVOLTIAC SENSORS

These solid-state transducers make use of a junction between two dissimilar materials when a voltage relative to the illumination on the junction is generated. Light particles or photons pass through a thin conductive layer and on to the junction itself. This creates an electron flow across the junction area. The flow influences polarity so that the conductive layer becomes the negative terminal of the sensor. Such sensors use single-crystal materials which resemble a light-sensitive resistor. Its resistance decreases as incident illumination increases. Commonly used materials are cadmium sulfide (CdS) and cadmium selenide (CdSe). These materials yield a high output. Their spectral response peaks in the visible-light region (0.6 μm).

PHOTOCONDUCTIVE JUNCTION SENSORS

These devices actually generate a photocurrent which increases with the intensity of light. Examples of photoconductive junction sensors are phototransistors and photodiodes. The silicon junction in these types of devices has a spectral peak near 1 μm.

PHOTOEMISSION

The gamma detector, used to locate radioactive material (see Sec. 3-9), uses a crystal surface backed up by an array of photomultipliers. These devices function on the principle of photoemission. Photoelectrons emitted from the photosensitive surface are emitted at all velocities. Their maximum velocity is calculated by

$$\tfrac{1}{2}MV_{\max}^2 = eV_r$$

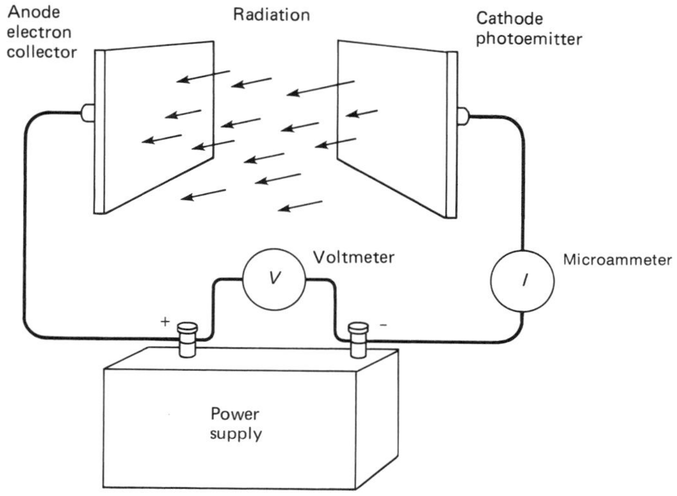

Fig. 3-23 The microammeter measures current L. If the spacing between the photoemitter and the anode collector is fixed, then the current I becomes a function of the voltage measured between the photoemitter and collector.

where V_r = retarding potential, V, needed to reduce the photocurrent to zero

When the accelerating potential is increased, electrons flow to the collector. They increase until saturation is reached. A simplified circuit is shown in Fig. 3-23. The variation in photocurrent vs. the anode potential V and the light intensity can be plotted. These curves appear in Fig. 3-24. They show that V_r and V_{max} are independent of the light

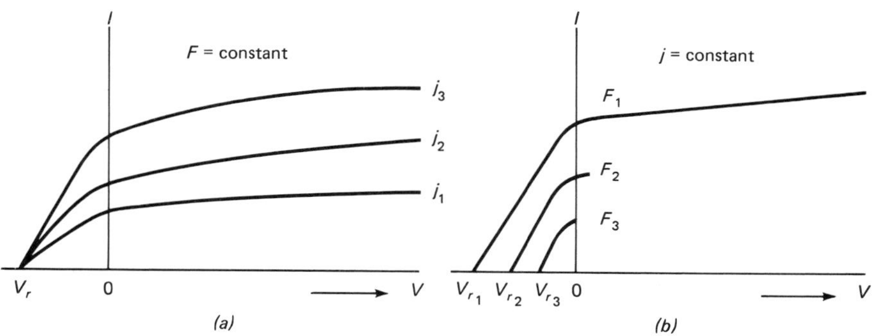

Fig. 3-24 Both illustrations show what happens to photocurrent as anode voltage is increased. (*a*) The light intensity *j* is varied in three increments. The frequency of the incident light is always constant. (*b*) The light intensity *j* is constant but the frequency of the incident light is varied in three increments. F_1, the highest frequency, is closest to the spectral response peak of the photoemitter and collector. Thus an increase in voltage results in an increase in current. However, F_3, the lowest frequency, is farthest from the spectral response peak of the photoemitter and collector. In this case, even though voltage is increased, there is no corresponding increase in current.

intensity. Figure 3-24*b* shows the photoelectric current measured as a function of the anode potential for different light frequencies *F* and equal intensities of incident light.

The greater the incident light, the more retarding potential is needed to reduce the photocurrent to zero. Maximum velocity of emission of photoelectrons increases with the frequency of the incident light. A linear relationship exists between V_r and F. Maximum energy of liberated electrons is independent of light intensity but varies linearly with the frequency of the incident light.

PHOTOTUBES

A phototube has a sensitive cathode surface and a collecting electrode. This cathode may be a semicylinder of metal upon which the photosensitive substance has been evaporated. Figure 3-25 shows typical phototube curves. The current at zero accelerating potential is a result of the initial velocity of the electrons. A retarding potential is applied to reduce this current to zero. The current increases very rapidly but soon reaches saturation. Saturation occurs when the field becomes sufficient to attract all electrons liberated from the cathode under the influence of the incident light.

The phototube glass envelope is filled with neon or argon. This increases the current yield for a given illumination because of ionization of the gas for voltages above the ionization potential V_i. The potential across the tube should never be raised to the point where a glow discharge occurs. That will cause cathode sputtering and damage the cathode surface.

Phototubes are available which peak in various portions of the spectrum. A silver–cesium oxide–cesium surface is sensitive throughout the entire visible range and also has a high sensitivity in the infrared region. The silver–rubidium oxide–rubidium surface is sensitive in the

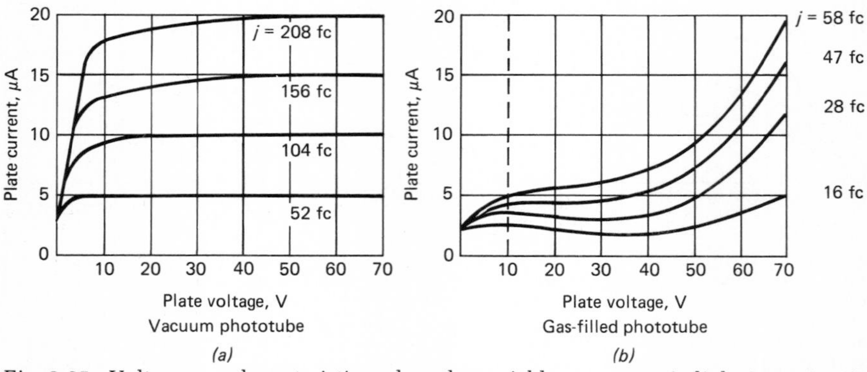

Fig. 3-25 Voltampere characteristics when the variable parameter is light intensity. A vacuum phototube and gas-filled phototube are compared in this illustration.

visible region only, with the peak at the blue end of the spectrum. While the antimony-cesium surface is very sensitive to the green, blue, and near-ultraviolet end of the spectrum, it is insensitive to red and infrared. When choosing a photocell, make sure the source emits strongly in the frequency range where the photocell is most sensitive. Thus the largest possible photocurrent is obtained. The gas photocell has the greatest sensitivity. However, the current in the gas-filled device increases more rapidly than the illumination for anode voltages that are higher than the ionization potential of the gas. Thus, once the gas becomes ionized, the gas phototube does not serve as an effective transducer.

PHOTOMETRY AND COLORIMETRY

In blood-oxygen determinations, the technique of photometry is used. In determining calcium, potassium, and sodium, the technique of spectrophotometry is used. Both techniques depend on the response of a photodevice to light in various parts of the spectrum. In other words, a given amount of illumination is being measured. As incident light changes, photocell output current changes. This results in a different voltage across the voltmeters (or instrument system input) in Fig. 3-26.

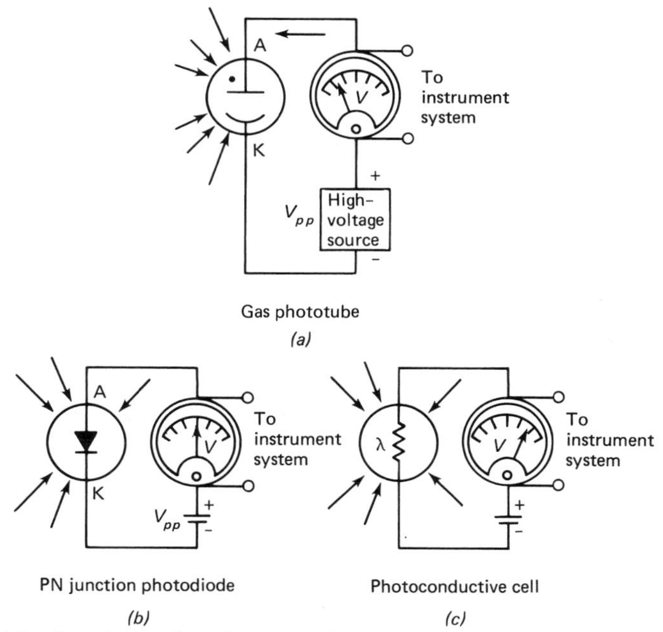

Fig. 3-26 The three basic photodevices and their circuits. The gas phototube requires a high-voltage source. The photodiode is used with a low-voltage source. The photoconductive cell may be used with a low-voltage source if it is solid state. Unless a high light intensity is available, amplifiers must be added to these circuits.

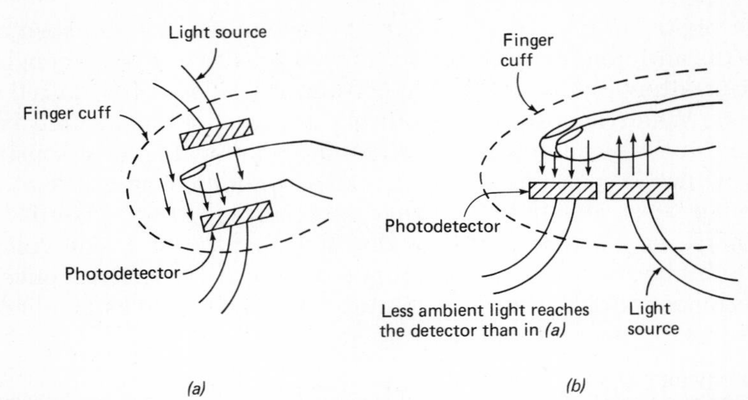

Fig. 3-27 Photodetection of blood pulse. (*a*) The light source transmits light through the finger. The optical density of this light is then modulated by the blood pulse. (*b*) Another method of pulse detection. The light source transmits light through the finger. Its reflection is then altered by the blood pulse.

These circuits are a basic starting point for numerous types of biomedical systems, aside from photometry and spectrophotometry. A popular application is detecting the blood's pulse with an optical transducer. In Fig. 3-27*a* light emitted from the source must penetrate through the finger. This light encounters pulsatile blood-volume changes. These changes modulate the optical density of the finger. Consequently, the emitted light reaching the photodetector varies in proportion to the blood pulse. One problem with this method is that some ambient illumination may reach the photodetector from outside the finger cuff. A modification of this system, which partially solves the ambient light problem, is the reflected light–finger pulse detector. In Fig. 3-27*b* both light source and detector are tightly held on the same side of the finger. Emitted light is reflected within the finger according to optical density. As the blood pulse modulates optical density, reflected light varies according to blood pulse.

THE PHOTOMULTIPLIER

So far we have seen three simplified photodevice circuits (Fig. 3-26). In colorimetry, nuclear-radiation detection, and other medical systems, the light intensities are very weak. In these applications, secondary emission is used to amplify the current from the photoelectric surface. The principle of operation of the photomultiplier is shown in Fig. 3-28. Light first reaches the cathode, causing the cathode to throw off photoelectrons. These photoelectrons are directed to dynode A, causing secondary electrons to be emitted by A. These electrons travel to dynode B, releasing additional secondary electrons. This process may be repeated with more dynodes. Secondary electrons from the last dynode are finally collected by the anode. R is the ratio of the number of sec-

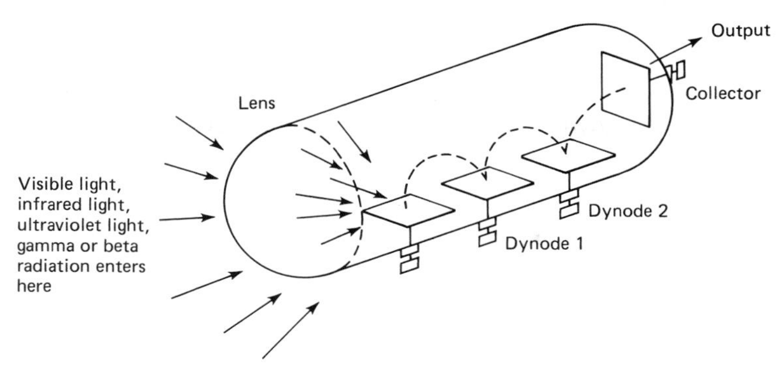

Fig. 3-28 In this photomultiplier, secondary emission takes place. Each dynode generates a magnetic field to cause deflection of the beam. The magnetic field and the beam's path is perpendicular to the plane of this paper.

ondary electrons to primary electrons. N tells us how many dynodes exist. The collector current can be determined by the equation

$$\text{Total collector current} = \text{initial collector current } R^n$$

The initial current is the original photocurrent at the cathode. The current gain may be said to be R^n. An electrostatic (or electromagnetic) field directs the secondary electrons in Fig. 3-28 from dynode to dynode and then, finally, on to the collector. A photomultiplier with nine dynodes (RCA931) has a current amplification of 200,000. This highly sensitive, circular photomultiplier is shown in Fig. 3-29.

THE PHOTOCONDUCTIVE CELL

When radiation falls on a semiconductor, its conductivity increases. Light energy causes covalent bonds to be broken, increasing charge carriers and lowering the material's resistance. The presence of 100 footcandles (fc) of light can change a photoconductor's resistance by several kilohms. Silicon and germanium photoconductors do not have the same spectral response. Cadmium sulfide (CdS) is most commonly used for photoconductive cells. CdS may contain some silver, antimony, or indium impurities.

In absolute darkness, the resistance may be as high as 2 MΩ. When stimulated with a strong light, the resistance drops to about 10 Ω. Cadmium sulfide has a spectral response which is very similar to that of the human eye. Its response tapers off in the infrared and ultraviolet regions. CdS is outstanding in its high dissipation capability. These devices will dissipate 300 milliwatts (mW) and can even handle several watts. Thus a CdS photoconductor can operate a relay directly without the use of an amplifier. A lead sulfide (PbS) cell has a sensitivity peak at 2.9 μm and is used for infrared detection and absorption, whereas

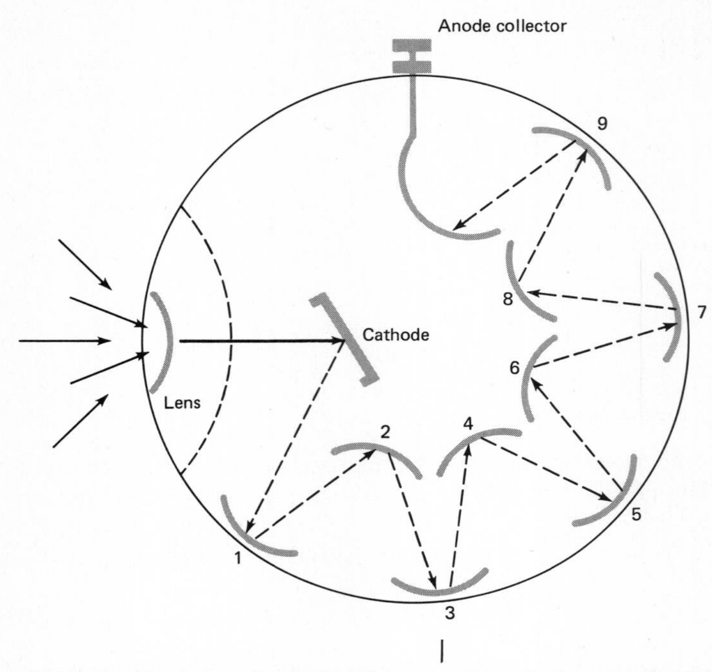

Fig. 3-29 RCA circular photomultiplier. Light energy from the lens causes electrons to be set free at the cathode. These electrons move to dynode 1, creating secondary emission. This emission is focused to dynode 2. The process repeats itself until secondary emission from dynode 9 is collected by the anode. The original optical radiation has now been converted into its electrical analog and is taken off the anode collector.

the selenium cell is sensitive to the visible wavelength and particularly the blue end of the spectrum.

THE PHOTODIODE

Light reaching a reverse-biased PN junction diode will cause its current to vary linearly with the illumination. The primary advantage of the photodiode is its size. These devices can be manufactured as small as 0.02 in. The light-sensitive junction is embedded in clear plastic with a small opening for light on one side of the device. The spectral response of the photodiode is the same as that of other semiconductors made of germanium or silicon. These light-sensitivity curves are shown in Fig. 3-30.

PHOTO-DUO-DIODE

If an N junction is joined to a P junction, and that P junction is then joined to another N junction, current flows from one N region over the forward-biased barrier into the P region, then to the second reverse-biased N region. The illuminated area should be close to this

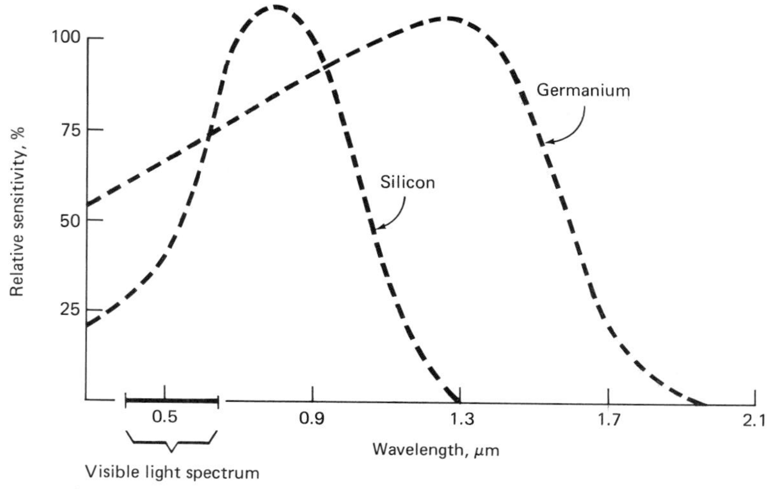

Fig. 3-30 The relative sensitivity of silicon and germanium photoconductors at various wavelengths is compared. The spectral response of germanium is greatest (most sensitive) in the longer, infrared wavelengths, at approximately 1.3 μm. While silicon has its greatest sensitivity in the visible-light spectrum, it is most sensitive to yellow and orange light. Cadmium sulfide and cadmium selenide have a spectral response similar to silicon, peaking at 0.6 μA.

reverse-biased junction. The advantage of this device over the simple photodiode is that a large current gain takes place. The result of this current gain is that the photo-duo-diode can be 100 times more sensitive to light than the PN photodiode.

QUESTIONS

1. What problem would develop with surface electrodes made of gauze?
2. What should be the ideal pH for an electrode preparation gel? Explain your answer.
3. We wish to observe very fast EMG spike potentials with a 3-μs risetime. Interference is extremely high, so we will use shielded patient leads. Is this solution satisfactory? Explain.
4. Our investigation calls for the study of a small group of nerve cells. We decide to use surface electrodes. Is our choice of electrodes good? Explain your answer.
5. Name four materials that may be used for needle electrodes.
6. Which two metals should always be avoided for needle electrodes?
7. In a concentric needle electrode, a high capacitance between the insulated center conductor and the cannula is beneficial to reduce interference, especially when observing fast pulses. True or false?
8. An amplifier appears to be operational, but its piezoelectric transducer is suspect. Would we check the transducer with an ohmmeter? Explain your answer.
9. How does the dynamic range of the reluctance transducer compare to other transducers?

10. A small, lightweight transducer with low volume displacement and high sensitivity and stability is required to measure pressure. Which transducer would be used?
11. We stretch a stainless steel wire between two supporting posts. Which type of transducer have we made?
12. In Fig. 3-12*a*, $R_1 = 80\ \Omega$, $R_2 = 80\ \Omega$, $R_3 = 125\ \Omega$. What must R_4 be in order for the voltmeter to read zero?
13. Explain the purpose of the excitation voltage in the Wheatstone-bridge strain-gage transducer.
14. How is the piezoelectric effect used?
15. What are three factors that directly affect a crystal's resonant frequency?
16. True or false: An untuned (broadband) crystal transducer is more efficient than a resonant transducer.
17. Describe the consequences of using a blood-flow probe that is too tight around a blood vessel it surrounds.
18. To choose the right blood-flow probe, which factors aside from vessel size should be considered?
19. Use Faraday's law of electromagnetic induction to calculate the voltage induced in a blood-flow probe. Velocity of blood flow is 100 cm/s through a probe with a lumen diameter of 22 cm and a magnetic field of 0.5 G.
20. A cadmium sulfide photocell is suspected to be defective. In total darkness its resistance should be __________ Ω; in a strong light approximately __________ Ω.

chapter 4

Interference and Instability

INTRODUCTION

In the previous chapters we saw how there are numerous methods of translating raw physiological data into electric signals. If only these data were changed into electric signals and they were the only component of the electric signal, then there would not be an interference problem. Unfortunately, the high sensitivity of biomedical instrumentation also provides a path for unwanted signals of various types. You will learn how the patient's body, and the environment in general, contains both fundamentals and harmonics related to the power-source frequency. These signals are picked up by the medical instrument. When this activity becomes objectionable, filters and other techniques must be used to eliminate it. The power line itself is an excellent carrier for all types of electric signals generated by devices connected to it, even at remote locations. Once the specific type of line noise has been determined, it can be traced back to its source and either reduced or completely eliminated.

Another problem is that patient pickup leads are sensitive to very-high-frequency activity. This phenomena is covered under radio-frequency interference (RFI). Elaborate measures will be discussed to determine the frequency of such interference. With the frequency known, this high-frequency interference can be eradicated. As biomedical instrumentation ages, specific forms of interference may be generated within the equipment itself. Knowledge of the source of unwanted radiation can lead to circuit modifications to compensate for this mode of spurious activity and to quench it at its source.

If all these varied types of interference were not enough, there still remains the problem of instability. The most serious form of this troublesome problem is base-line shift. Several self-balancing systems are described that will automatically compensate for this kind of instability. In addition, a novel impedance-sensitive technique is discussed that depends on the changing load of a 50-kHz oscillator.

4-1
SIXTY HERTZ

By far the most common source of interference in biomedical recording and monitoring can be traced to the 60-Hz power-line frequency and its harmonic components. These ac potentials are always present. Although we cannot remove their presence, we can minimize their effects. Expensive shielded rooms have been built to overcome this source of interference in hospitals. Shielded rooms, however, are not always effective, and in most cases recording and monitoring must take place in unshielded areas. It has been common practice to search for instrument locations where the minimum amount of power-line interference exists. Unfortunately the elimination of power-line interference by this method is almost impossible, as the troublesome power line is used to provide lighting and to power the equipment itself. In spite of these difficulties, the BMET, working closely with medical personnel, can do a great deal to defeat this nuisance.

RECOGNITION

The ac power originating in the power line is, of course, a sine wave. However, should we attempt to recognize this form of interference by looking for a sine wave, our effort will seldom be rewarded. In Fig. 4-1, 60-Hz interference in electrocardiography is seen on a chart recording. There the thickening base line and heavy QRS complex are being modulated by power-line interference in spite of the fact that this ECG (electrocardiogram) recording system responds very poorly to frequencies as high as 60 Hz. The appearance of power-line interference

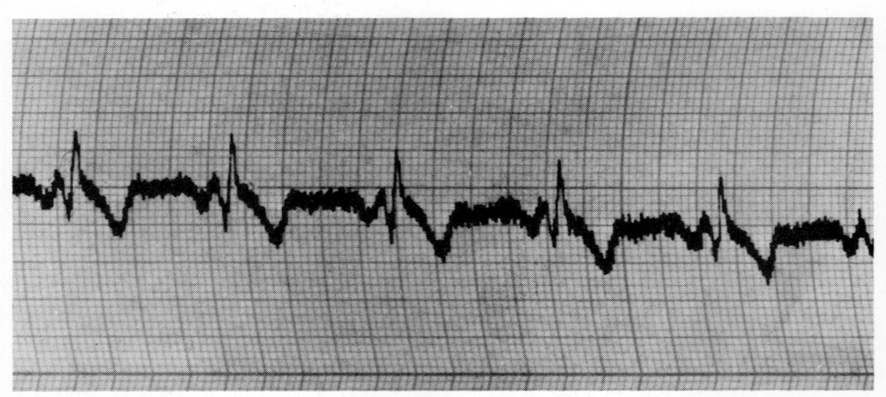

Fig. 4-1 ECG tracing with 60-Hz interference riding on the data. The high-frequency response of the ECG amplifier is only 30 Hz, and the chart-paper movement is very slow compared to the interfering signal. Thus the interference appears the same as high-frequency noise, causing the base line to thicken.

in EEG (electroencephalogram) recordings appears very similar to the ECG interference in Fig. 4-1. However in EEG recordings, the effects may be much more severe, causing the base line to wander as well as widen and creating other unstable factors. This is so because it is often necessary for EEG equipment to have 50 to 100 times more sensitivity than ECG instrumentation. Some EEG data may be of the order of only a few microvolts, whereas ECG data are many times stronger. The effects of interference from fluorescent lights as displayed on an EMG (electromyogram) oscilloscope are seen in Fig. 4-2. Unlike the case of ECG interference, here we can collect detailed data concerning the nature of the interference. It is possible to measure the time interval between successive peaks to determine the exact frequency of the interfering signal. The measured time interval here is slightly less than 8.5 ms. It can be calculated that 8.33 ms times 120 approximately equals 1000 ms, or 1 s. Thus the interfering signal is 120 Hz. This is the second harmonic of the 60-Hz power-line frequency. If the EMG oscilloscope sweep frequency has been calibrated, and the 50-ms time base is used, six peaks of the interfering pattern will be observed. This interference is less prevalent but sometimes seen. Nine peaks on the 50-ms time base would give a 5.6-ms interval between peaks. To find frequency, $\frac{1000}{5.6} \approx 180$ Hz. In this instance, the interference is the third harmonic of the 60-Hz power-line frequency. Of course, the most common source of interference is 60 Hz itself. On the 50-ms time base, only three peaks would be observed this time: $\frac{1000}{16.66} \approx 60$ Hz. This is the fundamental power-line frequency.

ALLOWABLE INTERFERENCE

When considering the effects of any form of interference, it is wise to look at the interference as a ratio of the total amplitude of the data we

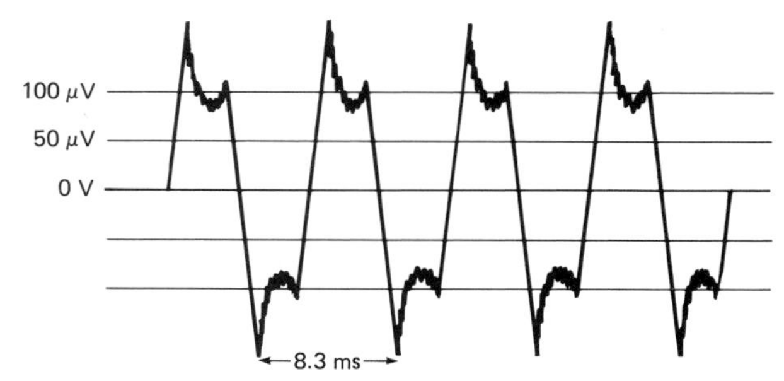

Fig. 4-2 Interference from a fluorescent light source is seen on an electromyograph tracing. The spacing between each peak is always 8.3 ms. The interfering frequency is determined by this repetitive spacing. If it were not for the phase-shift distortion, we would be able to see a well-defined sine wave. Unlike in the ECG tracing of Fig. 4-1, the high-frequency components of the interference pass through the EMG equipment. This is seen in the sharp, straight line at the beginning of each half-cycle, or the *leading edge*. However, in this case, the oscilloscope does not pass the low-frequency components too well. Thus the *trailing edge* of each half-cycle is clipped and jagged.

wish to observe. In this manner, a goal can be established regarding how much interference must be eliminated and how much can be tolerated. Starting with the ECG, for example, if the data being studied are of the order of 500 μV, then approximately 5 μV of interference can be tolerated. Thus the ratio of 5 to 500 μV is 1 percent, and 1 percent interference will create a negligible effect on our monitor or recorder. In other areas of work, the absolute value of interference will be sharply different. If EEG signals of 50 μV are being observed, then only 0.5 μV (1 percent) can be tolerated. In EMG and nerve-conduction studies, the data may vary over a large amplitude range. When watching large EMG signals of 1 mV, 10 μV of interference could be tolerated, but for a nerve-conduction response of 20 μV, only 0.2 μV of interference could be tolerated.

4-2 THE MAGNETIC COMPONENT

Whenever an electric current flows through a wire, a magnetic field is generated. This field surrounds the wire, as shown in Fig. 4-3. Should this wire be wound into a coil or a transformer, then the magnetic field would appear as in Fig. 4-4. Here a five-turn inductor has 4 A flowing through it. The magnetic flux or magnetomotive force is F.

$$F = NI$$

where N = number of turns
I = current, A

or

$$F = 5 \text{ turns} \times 4 \text{ A}$$
$$= 20 \text{ ampere-turns (At)}$$

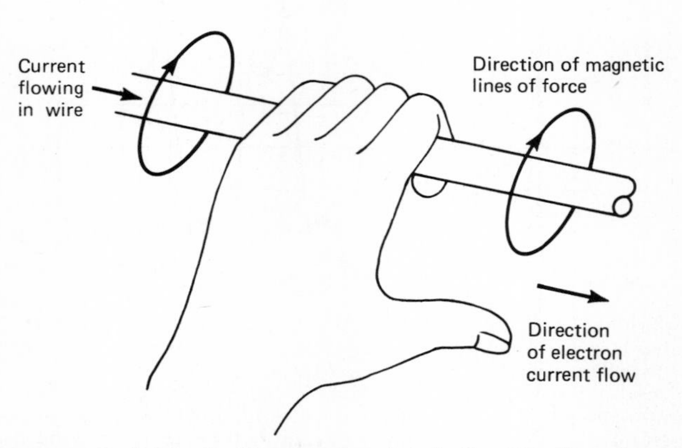

Fig. 4-3 The magnetic field rule. The thumb points in the direction of current flow. The fingers point in the direction of the magnetic field.

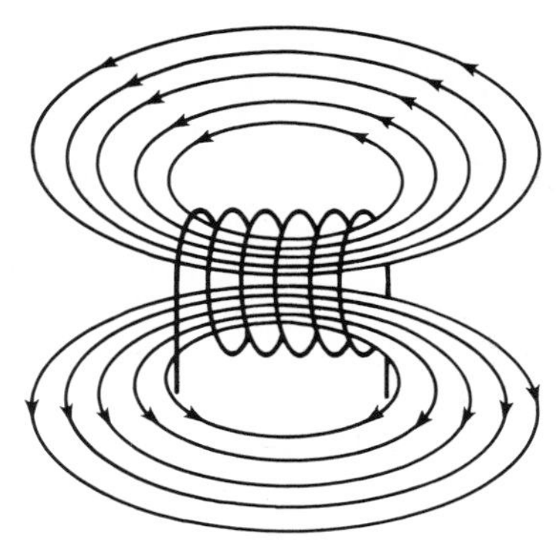

Fig. 4-4 The inductor seen here has five turns. The current flowing through the coil is 2 A. The magnetic flux is then 10 ampere-turns or maxwells.

From these figures it can be seen that equipment in which large currents flow can become excellent transmitters of magnetic energy. Only ferromagnetic materials will shield magnetic fields; copper or aluminum will not. Thus air conditioners, for example, enclosed in aluminum cabinets, will radiate a strong magnetic field. Any conductive or wire loop within a magnetic field will pick up magnetic energy by induction. For example, two or more leads from the patient to the instrumentation may form a magnetic receiving loop. To determine if this is in fact happening, vary the size of the loop by spreading the leads further apart from the patient's body. If the interference increases as a linear function of the increase in the loop size, then the loop is the culprit. Now rotate the loop. If changing the plane of the loop also changes the amplitude of interference, then we have a second verification of the loop's behavior as a magnetic receiver.

SOLUTION

Fortunately the magnetic component of interference can be eliminated by relatively simple precautions. Where the loop has been formed, twist the lead wires together so that the leads from the patient run along the surface of the patient's body where they are twisted together.

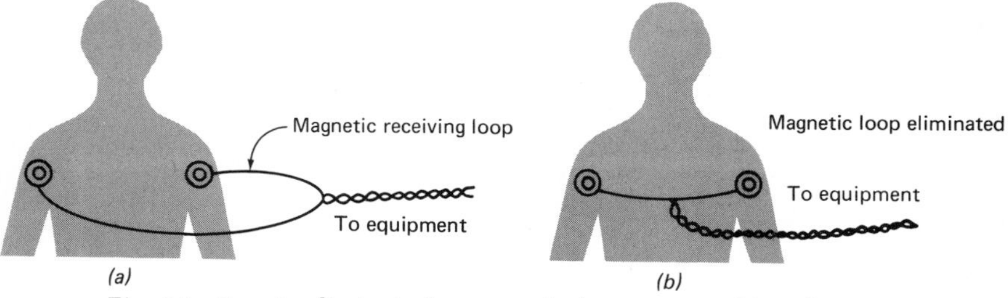

Fig. 4-5 How to eliminate the magnetic-loop source of interference.

Figure 4-5*a* shows the loop creating the problem, and Fig. 4-5*b* shows the solution. In cases where multiple leads have created several receiving-loop situations, merely perform the same procedure with each available pair of leads.

4-3 THE ELECTRIC COMPONENT

We have just learned that, in the case of the magnetic component of interference, the more current that flows, the greater the potential problem. Current must always flow or there is no magnetic radiation. The power line is a source of electric interference which is more complex than its magnetic counterpart. Even though no current is flowing in a circuit, the electric component of interference can create damaging effects. To illustrate this, place a lamp close to sensitive biomedical instrumentation. Although the lamp is switched off, it radiates a large amount of interference. Our test lamp may be unplugged to solve this problem, but the overhead lighting fixture is permanently wired to its source of power. Even the instrument itself may introduce power-source electric interference. Despite power-cord shielding, chassis shielding, and grounded shields, some interference from this source may result because grounding systems are usually far from ideal. Resistance paths exist all along the conduit which shields the power line and carries ground currents. Many terminations exist along the conduit's path, and each one may introduce resistance. As a generalization, the greater the distance between the instrumentation and earth ground, the greater the potential problem. With the trend toward high-rise hospital structures, this fact becomes more meaningful. However, a knowledge of the basics of this type of interference, along with good medical technique, can go a long way toward minimizing its effects. Refer to Chap. 2, Patient Safety, for several discussions concerning ground problems.

4-4 LEADS AS A PATH OF LEAST RESISTANCE

Going back to electronic fundamentals, it may be remembered that an electric current always follows the path of least resistance. The path of least resistance might be the leads connecting the instrument to the patient. Another path of least resistance might be the patient's body itself. If either situation develops, it aggravates the interference problem.

Patient leads are usually unshielded for several reasons. One is that any shielding or capacitance across the extremely high input impedance of most biomedical instruments might distort the very fast physiological events, as, for example, the fast risetime of an EMG biopotential.

Another reason for unshielded leads is that shielding may produce what is called *flexing artifacts*. This form of interference can reach an amplitude of up to 100 μV. It is caused by rapid motion or vibration (flexing) of the lead and can be compared to microphonics. Without shielding, even the smallest lead length from equipment to patient can pick up ac interference.

Earlier, in Sec. 4-1, we measured an oscilloscope pattern of the third harmonic of the power-line frequency, 180 Hz. Let us suppose that only 200 μV of 60-Hz energy existed in the vicinity of the patient leads. At the ninth harmonic, the potential could be one-ninth, or 22 μV at 540 Hz if nonlinear constants exist. Then the patient leads would act as capacitor plates, forming the capacitors C_1 and C_2 in Fig. 4-6. If only 20 picofarads (pF) of capacitance existed in C_1 and C_2, the capacitive reactance (X_c) would be only about 10 MΩ at 540 Hz. In this equivalent circuit, the input resistance (Z_p) is the resistance offered to the two surface electrodes by the patient's body.

It is true that there would be a ground electrode on the patient's body, but even if it were possible to locate this lead at precisely the right place to produce a perfect balance between Z_1, Z_2, and Z_p, the unequal resistance from electrode to tissue would offset this balance. This explains why Z_g (ground-lead impedance) comes from one side of Z_p. The term Z_o in Fig. 4-6 is the output impedance of the patient and lead combination. Z_o is fed into the biomedical instrument, which may have an input resistance of up to 100 MΩ, which is many times more than the impedance of Z_o.

Any current coupled into C_1 or C_2 flows along the path of least resistance, that is, away from the equipment through Z_1, Z_2, Z_p, and Z_g and on to ground. The voltage then developed across Z_o becomes the problem, for this voltage exists directly across the input of our recording or monitoring instrument. As R_1 and R_2 are balanced to ground,

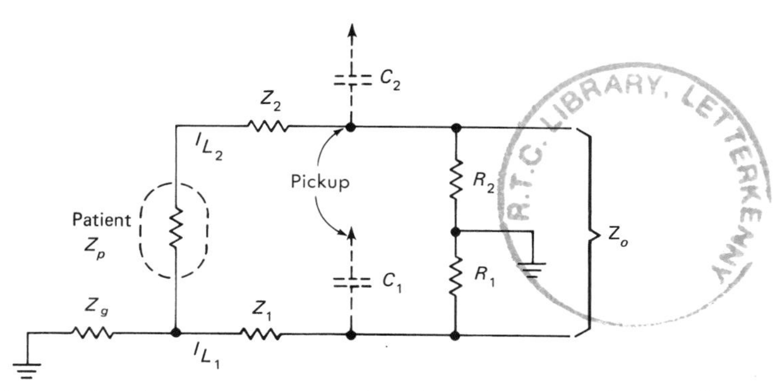

Fig. 4-6 Equivalent circuit of the patient, as well as the leads going to the recording instrument.

this input voltage becomes the algebraic difference between the voltage across the two resistors. $E = IR$, so that the voltage across either of these resistances will be the product of the resistance and current in that lead. Although Z_g and Z_p influence the interference voltage across Z_o, lead imbalance is our prime concern. Thus voltage across $Z_o = Z_1I_{L1} - Z_2I_{L2}$. Of course, if the impedance in both leads were equal, then no interference voltage would exist across Z_o. The problem is that even the smallest variation in least-resistance current or lead impedance will allow an interference voltage to develop. In a typical recording situation with electric lighting circuits and other electric equipment nearby, a patient lead 5 m long (No. 20 unshielded wire) will pick up almost 10 nanoamperes (nA) of least-resistance current. If both patient leads are equal in length (twisted together), the current in each lead will be fairly equal. Only the different lead impedances would then develop the interference voltage. With the patient leads picking up 10 nA, we would still have an electrode impedance of from 1000 up to 100,000 Ω. The imbalance between electrodes could easily be 4000 Ω. Thus we would have

$$\text{Voltage across } Z_o = (10 \times 10^{-9}\ \text{A})(4000\ \Omega)$$
$$= 40\ \mu\text{V}$$

Obviously, if we wanted to observe or record an EEG potential of 50 μV or an EMG fibrillation potential of 40 μV, the interfering voltage would obscure the data, making the task impossible.

4-5 MINIMIZING THE INTERFERENCE

A grounded surface between the plates of the hypothetical capacitors C_1 and C_2 in Fig. 4-6 will distort the electric field, drastically reducing the least resistance in either lead. The remedy suggested here is a grounded person or object between the lead and its source. This device would eliminate most of the least-resistance current in that lead. Increasing the size of the electrode area is another solution. A larger tissue-electrode area will reduce the tissue-electrode impedance. The interface-impedance imbalance will decrease. It would be possible to cut the 40-μV interference potential to approximately 20 μV merely by decreasing the tissue-electrode interface impedance from the previous 4000 Ω to 2000 Ω.

Another way of accomplishing the same thing is to better prepare the patient's skin to reduce interface impedance. In instances where there was no other way, skin has been rubbed with fine sandpaper and hair shaved off. Although this may produce reddening of the skin, it sharply reduces the resistance of the outer layer of skin. In Sec. 3-3, Electrodes, we found that dry electrode paste will contribute to sharply higher tissue-electrode resistance. Just as important, there may be a relatively large difference in electrode impedance with even fresh electrode paste made by different manufacturers. Remember, when comparing electrode paste specifications, take into account the procedure used by the paste manufacturer in writing this most critical specification.

THE PATIENT AS A LEAST-RESISTANCE PATH

It has been shown that leads can couple least-resistance currents, producing an interference potential. Whenever there is resistance, least-resistance currents will flow. Not only is there tissue-electrode resistance, but the patient is composed of various resistances. Although the patient may be grounded at several points along the body, there is still resistance to other points of the body. At one time or another we have all had the experience of touching the vertical input terminal of an oscilloscope with the vertical sensitivity turned up. The sudden flood of high-potential alternating current appearing all over the CRT display is proof that the human body makes an excellent pickup for power-line frequencies. The actual current flowing through your body could be measured if the oscilloscope input impedance at 60 Hz were determined. This can be found by the equation

$$Z_{in} = \frac{E_2}{E_1 - E_2}$$

where Z_{in} = oscilloscope input impedance
E_1 = voltage measured when your finger is touched to the input terminal
E_2 = voltage measured when your finger is touching the terminal through a 1-MΩ resistor

Current going through the body (I_b) is then

$$I = \frac{E}{R} \quad \text{or} \quad I_b = \frac{E_1}{Z}$$

In our biomedical situation, the body current I_b creates a common-mode voltage E_{cm} across the instrument differential-amplifier input terminal.

$$E_{cm} = I_b Z_g$$

E_{cm}, or common-mode potential, appears across our differential amplifier input and, ideally, should be canceled out by the differential amplifier. This is not always so, as we shall find out. If a body current I_b of 2 μA exists in Fig. 4-7 with a high ground-electrode impedance Z_g of 100 kilohms (kΩ), the maximum value of E_{cm} appearing on the body would be $E = IR$, or $(2 \times 10^{-6})(1 \times 10^5) = 0.2$ V. This is twice the value allowed by the American Heart Association. In a typical situation, however, between 1 and 10 mV would be found. The potential drop caused by the body's impedance is the largest factor in the induction of body current. This impedance, sometimes called *subcutaneous,* will cause different potentials to exist at different parts of the body. The E_{cm} that will exist across the input of our instrumentation will be ($E = IR$), or the product of body current I_b and body resistance Z_b. And $R = E/I$, or $Z_b = E_{cm}/I_b$. Placing the electrodes closer together will reduce Z_b, thus decreasing E_{cm}. When the leads are farther apart, the position of the ground electrode determines by what path current will flow to ground. If an unbalanced potential across the patient's body is suspected, the ground electrode may be moved to the position that yields the least interference. In an ECG, the ground electrode is often the right leg. It is possible that this ground location (Fig. 4-8) can create an imbalance. If

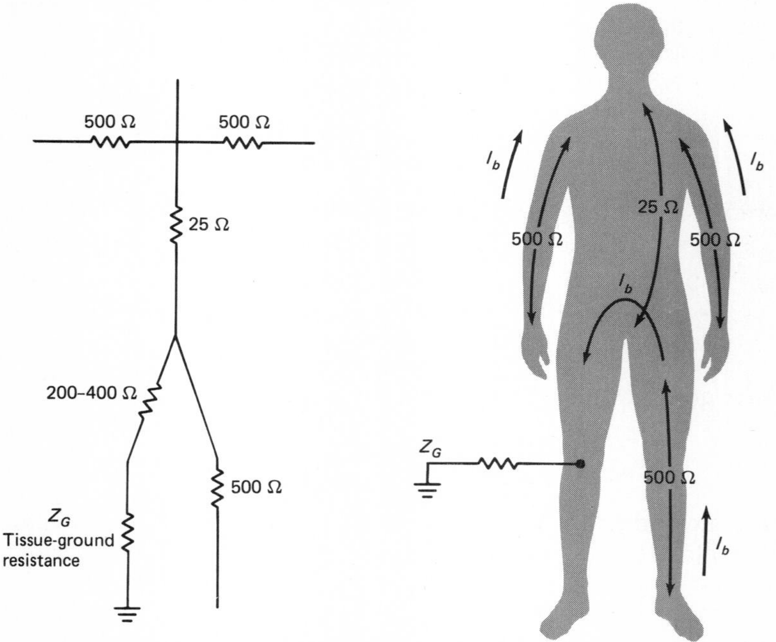

Fig. 4-7 How body currents (I_b) are created, with typical values of resistance. Electric currents see the patient this way.

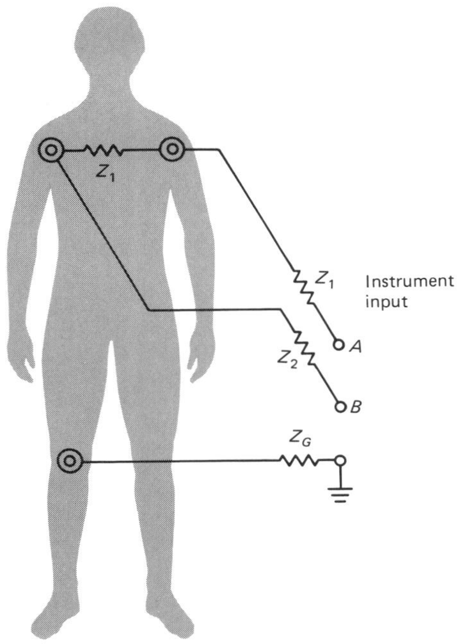

Fig. 4-8 Equivalent resistance within the patient and within each lead for an ECG with the right leg grounded.

body current pickup persists, try moving this ground electrode. If that fails, several manufacturers sell a grounded, conductive blanket which shields the body and prevents least-resistance currents from entering it.

COMBINING INSTRUMENTS

In surgical monitoring of the ECG, an internal catheter might be used. Here the body current is even more critical. As mentioned in Chap. 2, Patient Safety, values over 10 μA are considered unsafe, and ventricular fibrillation could result. An increase over normal 60-Hz interference could be the best indication that an unsafe condition exists. Should the equipment ground lead be open or broken, a high, unsafe leakage current would result. On many occasions it is necessary to connect the patient to several monitoring or recording instruments, for example, ECG, EEG, pulse, and respiration. If only one of the instruments in this group is not properly grounded, a high leakage current will exist between this instrument and other instruments in the system. This fault will be seen as higher than normal interference.

When one instrument is remotely located, a ground potential may exist between this instrument and the others. Instruments plugged into different receptacles might present high interference where a ground fault in the power line existed. Section 2-5, Patient Isolation, discusses the possibility of such occurrences taking place. The main point to be remembered is that if several instruments are included in a recording or monitoring system, make certain to ground each instrument to the same point on the patient's body.

4-6 FILTERS

When clinicians have been unable to remove 60-Hz interference by any other means, they have resorted to buffer amplifiers or cathode followers. These devices are placed at or near the electrodes. They convert high impedances into low impedances, making imbalances negligible. The problem with impedance converters or preamplifiers is that they must be perfectly matched, and remain that way. This handicap limits the use of such devices.

A more common solution to an otherwise insoluble problem is the use of 60-Hz filters. In considering a filter, a decision has to be made whether a passive or active filter is to be used. Passive filters use inductances, capacitances, and resistors as building blocks. Active filters use capacitances, resistances, and amplifiers, which are substituted for the omitted inductance. The active-filter approach will allow us to go to much lower frequencies, because the required inductances for passive filters would be too bulky and too costly. Many biomedical measurements are made in the 0.02- to 20-Hz range, and filters were unavailable in that low-frequency band before the development of the active filter. In addition, attenuation and impedance-matching problems have been eliminated by the use of active filters.

There is a drawback to active filters: They require their own power supply. Also the filter itself may introduce noise, limiting its dynamic range. The noise can be as high as 100 μV, which may be a serious obstacle in some low-level measurements. One way around this problem is to provide low noise amplification ahead of the filter. Thus, by raising the signal coming into the active filter to the volt range, a large increase in dynamic range can be obtained. Later, in Sec. 4-9, we will discuss radio, TV, and other high-frequency interference. In those situations, it is possible to construct our own passive filters without difficulty, as we shall find. However, in the case of very-low-frequency interference, it may be wise to consider the use of a commercially available active filter.

ACTIVE FILTERS

All filters can be classified into four general types: low-pass, high-pass, bandpass, and band-reject. Each of these categories is commercially available as fixed-frequency modules or as variable-frequency instruments. Active filters are particularly well suited to variable-frequency applications, and such variable-frequency filters are finding increasing application in the biomedical field. Where the frequency of interference is constant, an active notch filter may be used, as in the case of 60- or 120-Hz interference. Some biomedical engineers insist that low-frequency interference is by far the single most important problem in medical electronics. This is an indication of the future importance of the active filter in this field.

NOTCH FILTERS

The ideal notch filter is best described in terms of its response to a sinusoidal input-voltage signal of frequency f. Normally the filter is a three-terminal device, as shown in Fig. 4-9. We call the voltage transfer function of the device t_{21}.

$$t_{21} = \frac{E_2}{E_1}$$

The properties of the ideal notch filter are shown in Fig. 4-10.

The filter can be used as a 60-Hz eliminator in the biomedical field, as a frequency standard, and to eliminate spurious signals. See Fig. 4-11, where the presence of a 60-Hz component obscures the signal. The notch filter retrieves the signal. An unusual display is shown in Fig. 4-12, where the fundamental sine wave is removed from a square wave.

The ideal notch filter as shown in Fig. 4-10 does not exist. Instead the most common filter is a rather limited device. The circuit shown in Fig. 4-13 represents a notch filter which is less than the ideal. The limitation of this circuit is the large size of high-Q inductors in the low audio-frequency range. A more practical device is the symmetric twin T shown in Fig. 4-14. This circuit approaches a realistic filter extremely well. The attenuation curve for the notch filter is seen in Fig. 4-15.

Referring to Fig. 4-15, the intersection of the -3-decibel (dB) line with a particular curve is called the *breakpoint.* Note that for each curve of a fixed parameter $\mathscr{E}$ there are two breakpoints and the distance between

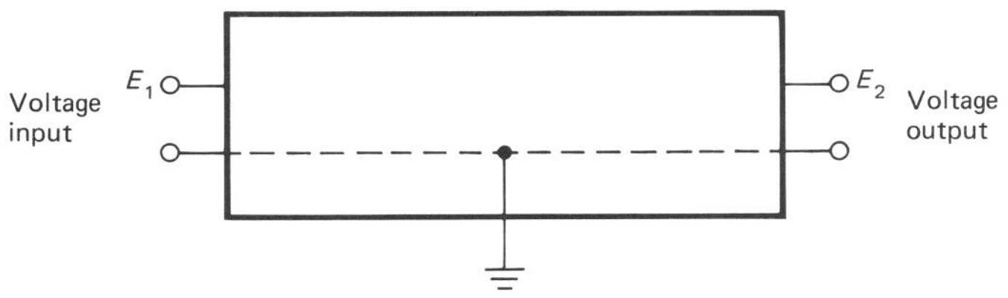

Fig. 4-9 A three-terminal network.

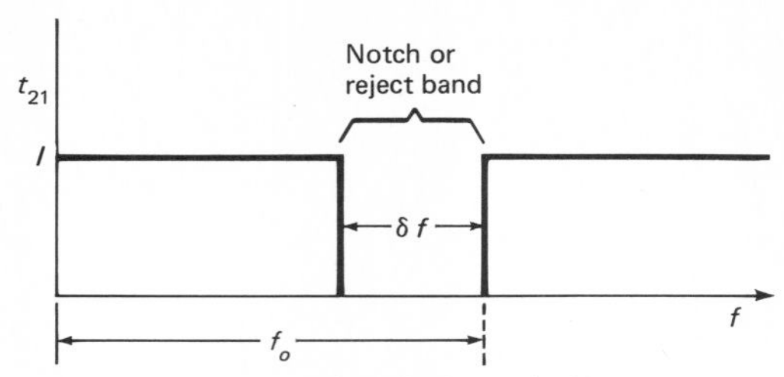

Fig. 4-10 The ideal notch filter.

them is denoted by $\delta f/f_0$. We call $\delta f/f_0$ the normalized *rejection bandwidth*. The inverse of the quantity, $f_0/\delta f$, is defined as the Q of the notch filter. Active filters which are capable of varying the characteristic number $\mathscr{E}$ are therefore also capable of varying the rejection bandwidth $\delta f/f_0$.

It is clear from Fig. 4-15 that the notch is symmetric on a logarithmic scale. This is different on a linear scale. For high-Q filters the normalized distance between the first breakpoint and the notch is half the rejection bandwidth.

PHASE DISTORTIONS. Unlike the magnitude characteristics, where most of the change occurs between the breakpoints, the phase changes are more spread out (see Fig. 4-16).

Further checking shows that the phase is $-45°$ at the first breakpoint

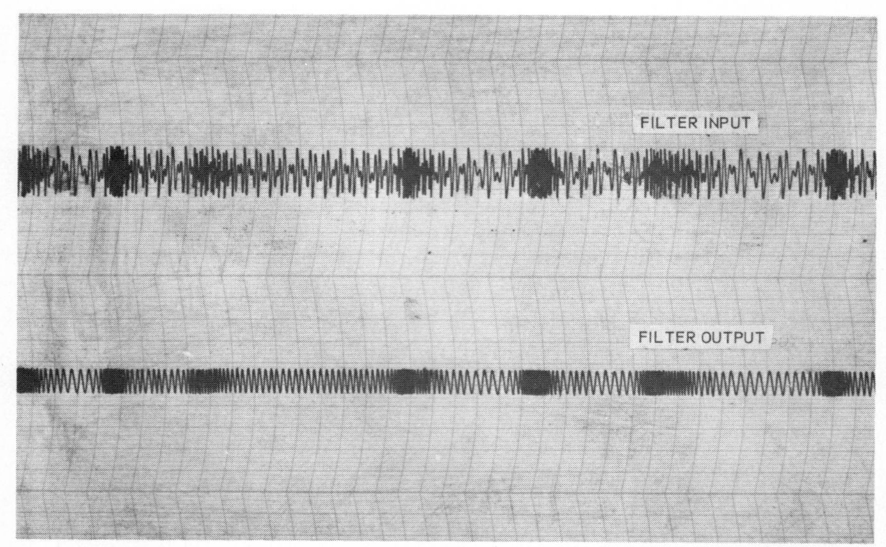

Fig. 4-11 In the top tracing, 60-Hz interference is modulating data which are entering the notch filter. In the bottom tracing, the data have already come through the notch filter. The desired data are now clean and free of the interference. (A. P. Circuit Corp.)

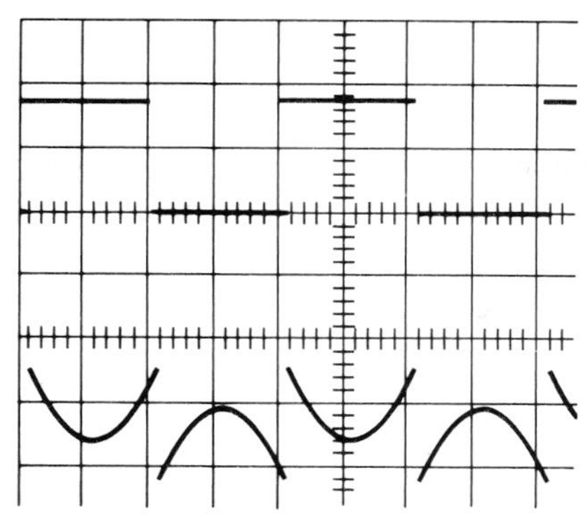

Fig. 4-12 In the top oscilloscope display is a square wave before it goes through a notch filter. The tracing below shows the same square wave after it has gone through the notch filter. Its fundamental frequency has now been removed by the filter. (A. P. Circuit Corp.)

and 45° at the second. This suggests strongly that to avoid excessive phase distortions the dominant frequency must be considerably away from the breakpoint. In Fig. 4-17 we show the effect of a notch filter on a triangular wave whose fundamental frequency is at the first breakpoint. For example, the notch frequency is 60 Hz, breakpoint is at 54 Hz, and triangular-wave frequency is 54 Hz. The output shows excessive magnitude and phase distortion. In Fig. 4-18 the same wave is passed through a filter whose breakpoint is $\delta f/f_0$ from the notch (for high Q's this is approximately twice the distance from the breakpoint). For example, the notch frequency is 60 Hz, breakpoint is 54 Hz, and triangular-wave frequency is 48 Hz. The Q of the filter is about 5. Note that the magnitude distortion is much reduced. Using Figs. 4-15 and 4-16, it can be observed that the respective magnitude loss and phase shift of the fundamental frequency of the triangular wave are -1 dB and 22°. The distorted effect of the triangular wave in Fig. 4-18 is now mainly due to the phase shift.

It follows from these considerations that the symmetric twin T shown in Fig. 4-14 would distort waveshapes that have components

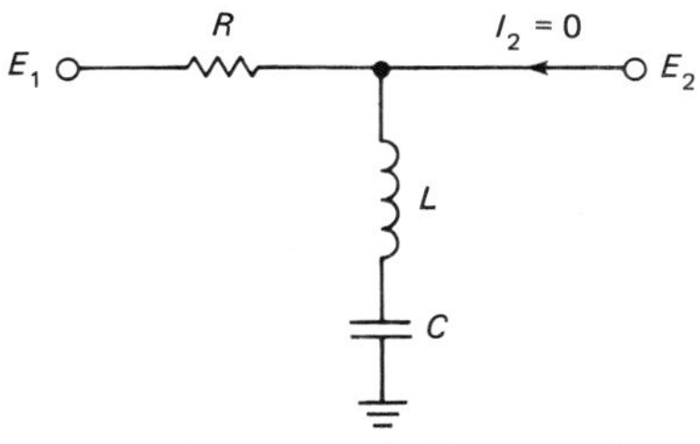

Fig. 4-13 The equivalent circuit of an *LC* notch filter. *R* is the insertion loss. *L* and *C* constitute a series resonant circuit which is tuned to the notch frequency. Minimum impedance (or a short circuit) then results at the notch frequency.

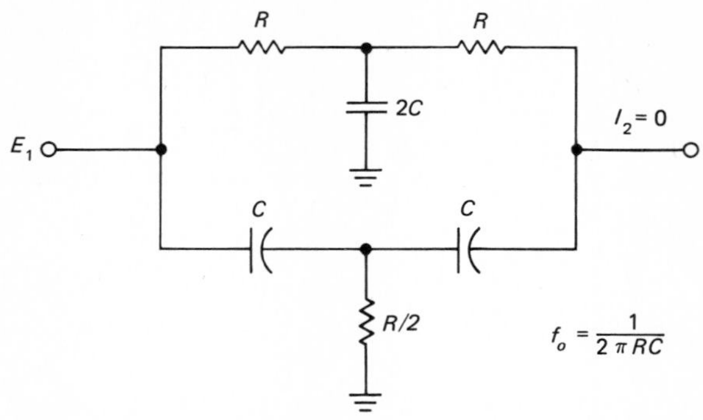

Fig. 4-14 Equivalent circuit of the twin T notch filter.

throughout the first decade from the notch. In summary, for distortionless transmission of waveshapes through notch filters, the rejection-bandwidth requirements should be determined from the notch phase-shift curves shown in Fig. 4-16.

PRACTICAL CONSIDERATION. This discussion regarding notch filters might seem to imply that high-Q filters are more desirable. This may be generally true, but there are some *side effects* that might require a compromise.

Referring to the display shown in Fig. 4-19, it is seen that the

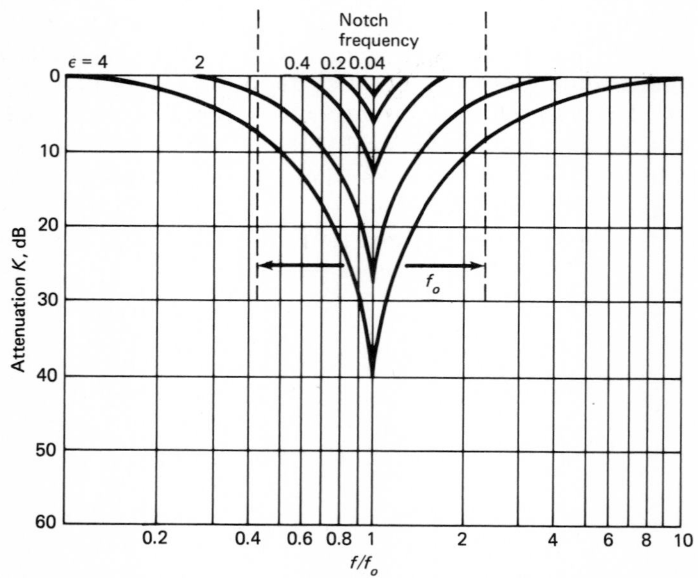

Fig. 4-15 Attenuation curves for a typical notch filter. The top line is 0-dB attenuation. At the notch frequency or point 1, the attenuation is 40 dB for E_4.

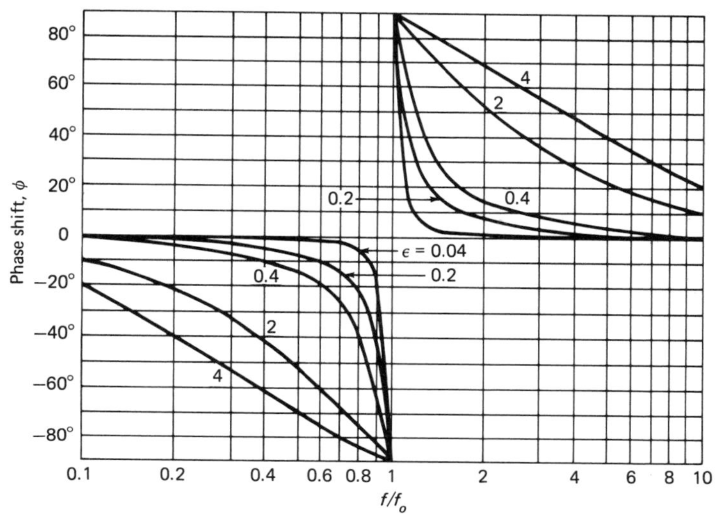

Fig. 4-16 Phase shift for the notch filter. These curves show how the phase-shift angle becomes more severe as the notch frequency is approached.

step function is producing some "ringing" in the response. The higher the Q, the smaller the amplitude of the ringing, but the rate of decay of the ringing is increasing. These two properties (overshoots and decay-time constant) are conflicting, and the best Q must be selected in each case for optimum performance.

High-Q notch filters are extremely sensitive to parameter variations. This may be both an asset and a liability. Suppose now that $Q = 100$ and that we are trying to reject a sine wave of frequency f_0. Of course the signal will be rejected completely. But if instead the signal's fre-

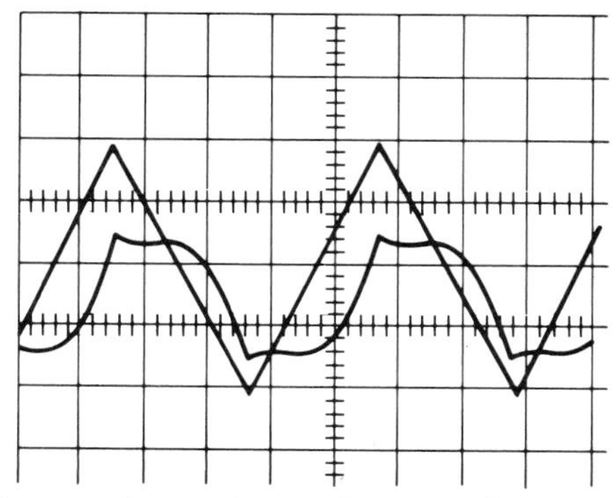

Fig. 4-17 A triangular wave is superimposed over another triangular wave which has passed through a notch filter. The wave's fundamental is seen at the first breakpoint below the undistorted wave's peak.

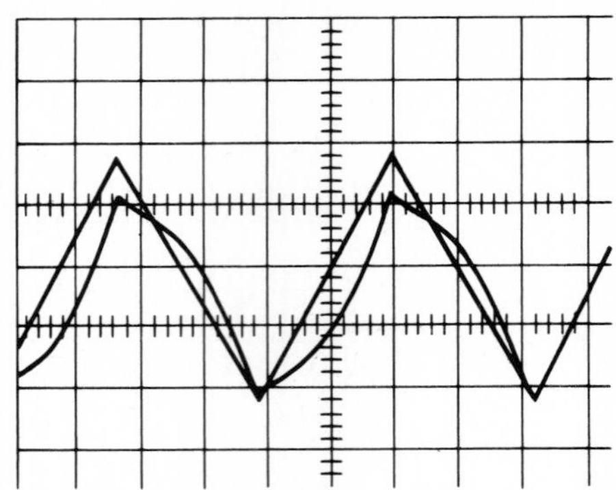

Fig. 4-18 A triangular wave passing through a notch filter. The wave's fundamental is one bandwidth, $\delta f/f_0$, from the notch.

quency drifts a little, say, $f_1 = f_0(1 + \gamma)$, we know that the breakpoint will occur at half the bandwidth:

$$\frac{f_0(1 + \gamma) - f_0}{f_0} = \frac{\delta f_1}{2f_0} = \frac{1}{20}$$

It follows that the attenuation—instead of being infinite—will vary correspondingly. In other words, a frequency drift produces an attenuation change away from infinite.

A similar situation occurs when some elements change in a filter network. Suppose that all the elements of Fig. 4-13 increase by

$$R = R(1 + \gamma)$$
$$L = L(1 + \gamma)$$
$$C = C(1 + \gamma)$$

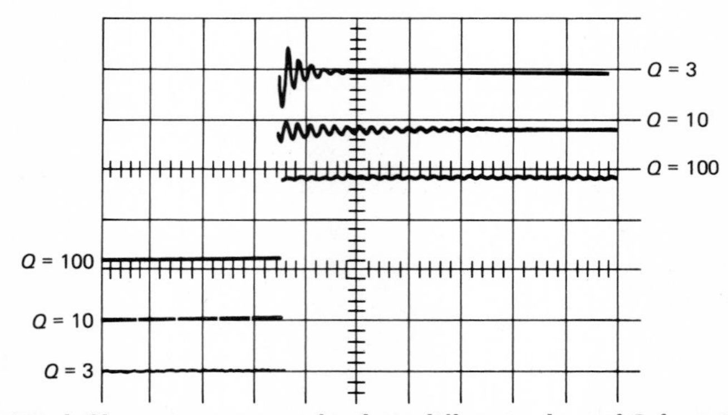

Fig. 4-19 Notch-filter step responses for three different values of Q from 3 to 100 are seen. The lines in the upper half show the rate of decay for the same three values of Q. The highest Q would give the sharpest notch frequency; the lowest Q would give the broadest notch.

It follows that $f_0 = f_0/1 + \gamma$. As would be the case with frequency drift, the attenuation here again will be less than infinite at the required frequency.

These considerations are generally valid and are applicable when elements change due to variation in temperature and age, or in tracking (when potentiometers are ganged).

Clearly a fixed-frequency, passive high-Q notch filter is excellent for frequency standards. The problem is that most audio-frequency signal generators (also the ac line) do not have frequency tolerances over extended periods due to temperature variations and other effects. However, an active notch filter can be adjusted to compensate for frequency drift, equivalent network, variation, etc.

AN ACTIVE NOTCH FILTER. A narrow-bandwidth band-reject or notch filter is analogous to an antiresonant inductance-capacitance circuit. The APN60 (Fig. 4-20) filter module, made by A.P. Circuit Corp., has been used in biomedical work. It is used to reject the 60-Hz line-voltage interference with minimum effect on the magnitude and phase of the signal being measured. In Fig. 4-21, we see the elimination of troublesome 60-Hz interference without degradation of the quality of the ECG tracing. A variable-frequency notch filter can be used to suppress carrier-frequency components of variable frequency. This type of instrument can be used to scan the frequency spectrum to detect and suppress unknown narrow-bandwidth interferences.

VARIABLE-FREQUENCY FILTERS

There are two types of variable-frequency filters: bandpass and band-reject. In one approach, the bandpass effect is achieved by connecting a high-pass filter in series with a low-pass filter. The band-reject effect is achieved by paralleling the output of a low-pass with the output of a

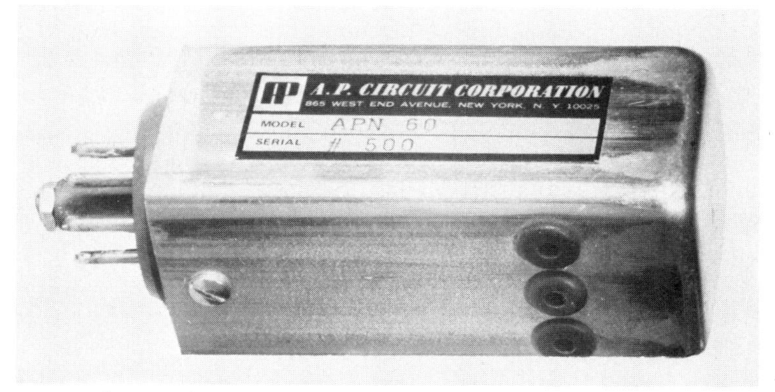

Fig. 4-20 High-Q notch-filter module with octal-base mounting. (A. P. Circuit Corp.)

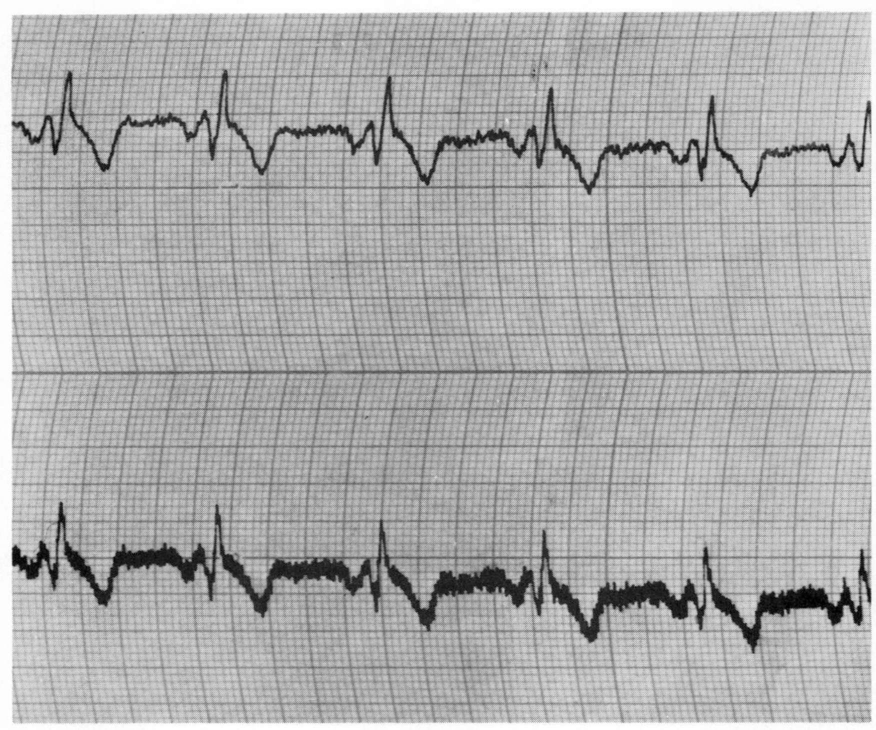

Fig. 4-21 Selective elimination of 60-Hz interference in electrocardiography with the aid of a Model APN60 Active 60 Cycle Noise Filter. Bottom tracing (lead 11): Note marked 60-Hz effect distorting physiologic patterns. Upper tracing: Same lead without 60-Hz interference. Note the preservation of muscle-tremor pattern in addition to the cardiac complexes. The APN60 Filter was connected after preamplification in the coupler of the Beckman, Offner Div., Type R Dyno Graph. (A. P. Circuit Corp.)

high-pass filter. These types are often referred to as *composite filters*. In the composite filters it is possible to set the upper frequency limit and the lower frequency limit independently. Any upper and lower cutoff frequency within the 0.02- to 2,000,000-Hz range can be selected, while the cutoff slope of 24 dB/octave is maintained at both ends. Several units can be cascaded to increase the cutoff slopes.

A type of variable-frequency bandpass filter (Fig. 4-22) is commercially available. This instrument is a two-pole device analogous to a resonant inductance-capacitance circuit. In this filter the center frequency can be swept continuously or set to any desired value. Both upper and lower cutoff frequencies are changed simultaneously when the bandwidth Q is adjusted. This type of filter is often referred to as a *tuned filter*.

A unique feature of this bandpass filter is that constant gain at the center frequency is preserved when the center frequency is varied over

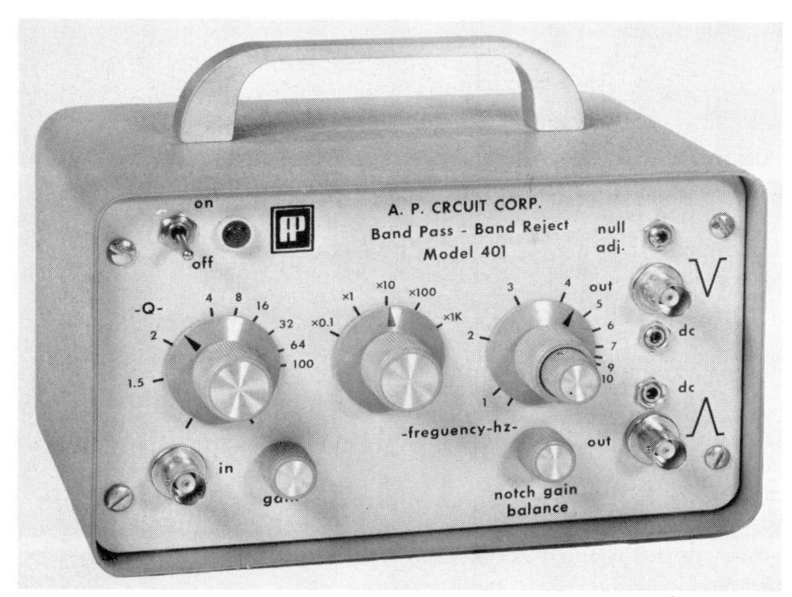

Fig. 4-22 Model 401 bandpass–band reject, variable-frequency, variable-bandwidth, variable-gain electronic filter.

the entire filter-frequency range. Similarly, constant gain at the center frequency is also maintained when the bandwidth Q is changed.

One potentiometer suffices for the continuous control of one frequency decade. The bandwidth is set by another potentiometer from 25 percent to 1 percent ($Q = 4$ to 100). Most variable-frequency two-pole devices require two ganged potentiometers for frequency control. In contrast, the filter shown in Fig. 4-22 requires only one potentiometer to adjust frequency. It is this "one-pot" approach which makes it possible to preserve constant filter gain in the passband throughout the filter range while the frequency is being varied.

Although this instrument has a noise level in the 100-μV range, a low-noise preamplification stage is incorporated to increase its dynamic range for low-level signals.

Low signal levels can be amplified up to 100 times or strong signals attenuated. It is this feature which assures that the typical dynamic range of 90 dB is available in all practical cases. Thus it is possible to detect signals in the low-microvolt region.

The tuning range of the Model 401 extends from 0.1 Hz into the audio-frequency spectrum. Thus it is well suited for biomedical work, especially in EEG frequency analysis where the waveform to be measured consists of a number of frequency components. Its frequency-sweeping capability makes it easy to single out such frequency components as the alpha or beta EEG waves. For example, it is possible to detect some unexpected EEG frequency components in response to repetitive visual stimulation when the filter frequency is swept and the output of the filter monitored.

In biomedical signal processing it is sometimes required to remove extraneous signals and to pass only specific frequency components. This type of filter will prevent the transmission of noisy or distorted waveshapes and assure that only the frequency component of interest is obtained. This type of filtering is often required prior to computer processing. In practice, this tuned-bandpass filter can be used in conjunction with a frequency counter to correctly measure a desired frequency of a compound waveform.

In another example, it is possible to clean up the output signal of an airflow transducer responding to a 3- to 6-Hz pressure excitation superimposed on the normal breathing process. The transducer signal is passed through the filter. When the center frequency of the filter is tuned exactly to the excitation frequency, the output is a clean and noiseless signal. Since this filter has no phase shift at the resonant center frequency, it is possible to tune the filter to the excitation frequency by sweeping the frequency knob until zero phase shift occurs between the excitation frequency and the output of the filter.

In general, two or more of these two-pole filters can be cascaded to form a multipole-filter characteristic.

Figure 4-23 compares the characteristic curve for the composite bandpass filter with a family of curves for the tuned-bandpass filter.

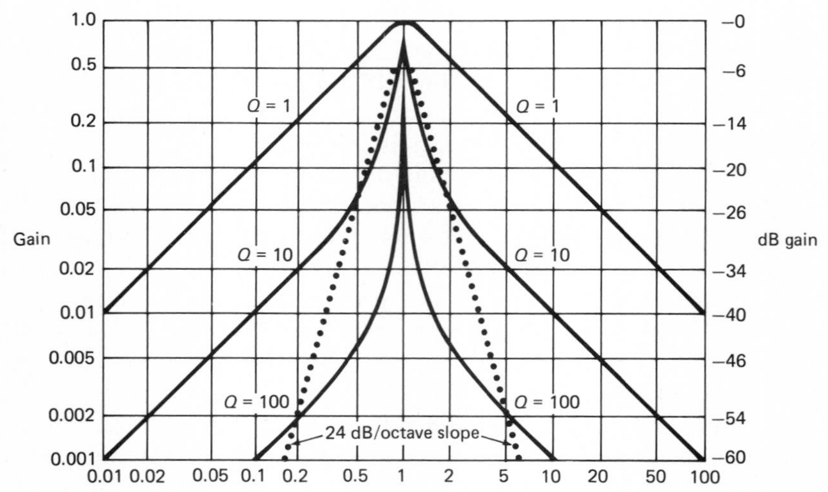

Fig. 4-23 The solid lines are universal resonance curves. These can be compared to the 24 dB/octave frequency cutoff rate of a composite high-pass–low-pass filter as shown by the dotted lines. (A. P. Circuit Corp.)

The composite filter is shown for the case where the high-pass cutoff and the low-pass cutoff frequencies are set to identical values. For frequency sweeping, the composite filter requires a simultaneous rotation of two knobs by the operator, with little chance of keeping the bandwidth constant. On the other hand, the variable-frequency tuned filter can be easily swept by the rotation of one single knob. This same argument also applies for the variable-frequency band-reject filters. The variable-frequency band-reject filter shown in Fig. 4-22 can be tuned from 0.1 to 6000 Hz to reject interfering signals within this part of the spectrum.

4-7 DETERMINING FREQUENCY OF INTERFERENCE

If the medical instrument has a CRT display with a time-calibrated base line, use this to determine the frequency of the interfering frequency. If not, connect an oscilloscope with a time-calibrated base line to the medical instrument one or two stages before the output to the recording or monitoring device. Using $F = 1/T$, the interfering frequency may be determined. If it falls below 10,000 Hz, the filters discussed here may be inserted in the medical instrument after the first or second stage of amplification. The filter should be adjusted so that its reject band is as sharp as possible so medical data close to the interfering signal are not lost. If the interfering signal is found to be in the high-frequency or RF part of the spectrum, then other techniques must be used, as we shall learn.

4-8 CARRIER CURRENT AND LINE NOISE

The corrective techniques thus far described will provide a solution if the interfering signals are entering the medical instrument or system through its data input terminals. To determine if this is so, short the input terminals together and ground the shorting wire. If the interference still persists, then it obviously is not coming in through the input terminals. It may on rare occasions be spurious radiations being generated by the instrument itself. More likely, however, it is being carried directly from the power line. The term *carrier current* has been used for years to describe the transmission of signals over the electric power lines, other than power itself. College radio stations use the power line to carry AM radio signals throughout the campus. More recently, wireless intercoms and computer terminals use the power line to carry voice and data. There is a carrier-current system in operation in Israel that sends voice signals over ordinary electric power lines for 200 mi.

Under the proper conditions, it can be seen that the power line makes a very efficient transmission line for medium-frequency signals.

Theoretically, any signals or noise on the power line should not create interference. The grounded core or frame of the instrument power transformer should stop all signals coming from the ac power line. Toroidal power transformers have excellent shielding properties, and little or no power-line noise will get through. However, most medical instruments use laminated "E"-type cores in their power transformers. High-frequency shielding is poor, especially for fast pulses which constitute much of the problem.

Even power-line distribution transformers, which theoretically should stop high-frequency signals, sometimes pass them. Not long ago, elevators, motors, air conditioners, and furnaces were the only sources of line noise. Today, because of the increased use of automatic solid-state switching circuits, almost any electric device can become an offender.

IDENTIFYING THE SOURCE

Identification involves two problems: discovering the location and determining the offending device. To do this effectively, a high-quality line-noise detector is needed. Once the input data terminals have been shorted, and interference remains, we are ready to hunt it down. In addition, line-noise detectors are valuable to determine whether newly installed hospital equipment is a source of line noise. Line-noise detectors allow the interference pattern to be seen on an oscilloscope to aid identification.

The Millen Type 71001 Line-Noise Detector is designed for application as a tool for determining the presence, type, and degree of interfering signals present in an ac power circuit. Its use should simplify the detection and elimination of "spike noise" in particular, an important consideration in the proper functioning of medical electronic devices.

LINE-NOISE GENERATORS. Typical noise-generating devices which are frequently connected to ac power circuits include the following:

1. Silicon controlled rectifiers (SCRs) and triacs (bidirectional SCRs)
2. Silicon power rectifiers
3. Germanium power rectifiers
4. Commutator motors (universal or ac-dc series-wound), repulsion-induction motors
5. Switch contacts associated with inductive or fairly high current loads
6. Ultrasonic washing machines, especially with improper installation (grounds)

7. Radio transmitting equipment
8. Pulse devices, including spot welders, pulse radar equipment, digital computing devices, digital counters, and experimental physics laboratory equipment (sometimes poorly isolated from the ac power line unless the experimenter is aware of this problem)
9. Slow-breaking switch contacts, such as bimetallic thermostats, motor-driven commutators, and similar devices

USING A LINE-NOISE DETECTOR

Each noise-generating device has some characteristics associated with that particular device. Use of the Millen 71001 Line-Noise Detector (see Fig. 4-24) with oscilloscope or radio receiver indicator will usually make it possible to locate the circuit carrying the interference, if such interference is of local origin, and to ascertain that the noise is conducted on the ac power leads. Further investigation may be necessary to determine the origin of the noise if the characteristics do not point to a recognized noise-generating device. In any case, noises detected by the Millen 71001 Line-Noise Detector are noises being carried on the power wires (conducted interference).

The Millen 71001 Line-Noise Detector incorporates two asymmetrical pi networks as filters, one in each side of the ac power circuit.

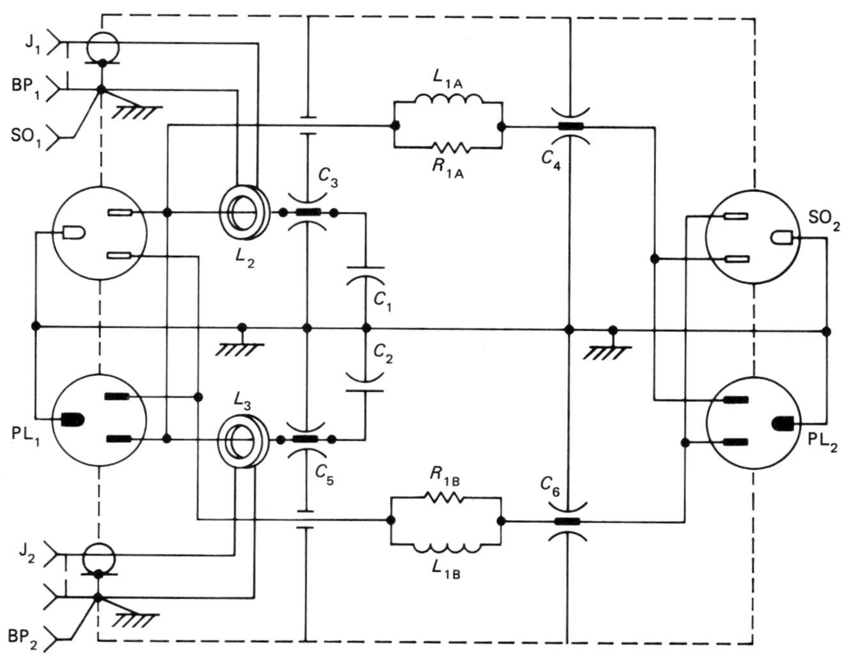

Fig. 4-24 Schematic diagram of the Millen Type 71001 Line-Noise Detector.

These filters separate the high-frequency noise currents on the line from the power currents and present the noise currents to detection devices for external display.

The detection circuit in each line can be considered to operate as shown in Fig. 4-25.

Power current, containing noise currents, is supplied from the ac line to point A in the filter. At point A, the currents divide according to the inverse ratio of the impedances presented by the inductive path L and the capacitive path C_1. The power frequencies (generally 60 Hz) will see a low reactance looking into L [370 microhenrys (μH)] of only 0.14 Ω, and the power current will then tend to flow mainly to the load Z_L. C_1 has a value of approximately 5.5 microfarads (μF), or about 500 Ω reactance at 60 Hz. At higher frequencies, the impedances change, giving a lower impedance to ground through C_1 than through L. At 6000 Hz, for example, C_1 should exhibit only 5 Ω reactance, whereas L now shows 14 Ω reactance.

This simplified view of the operation of the filter explains how the noise currents are extracted from the power lead and detected by the toroidal current transformer on the lead to the capacitor C_1. The separation of the power currents and the high-frequency noise currents is effective up to high radio frequencies as C_1 incorporates a feedthrough RF capacitor to keep the impedance low. Resonance in the leads reduces filter effectiveness as the noise frequencies become higher, but the detector is usable up to approximately 30 MHz. Above 30 MHz the

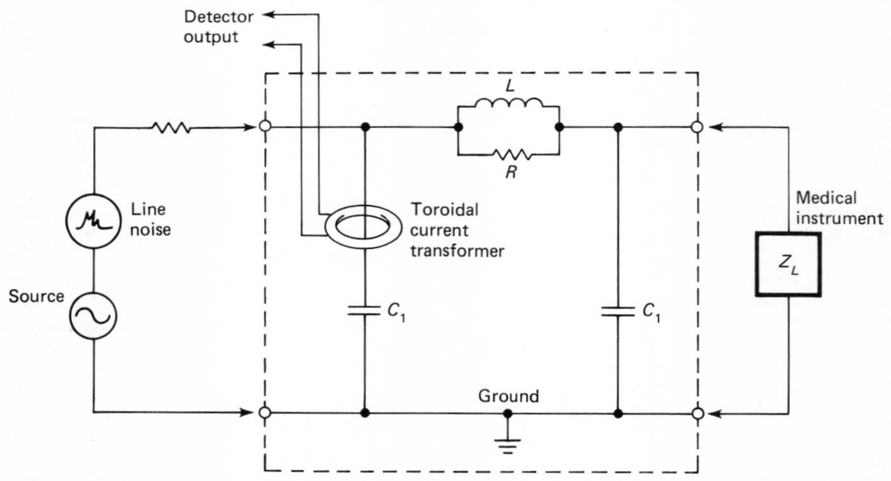

Fig. 4-25 The equivalent circuit of the Millen 71001 Line-Noise Detector connected to a typical electric power line. The source can be seen on the far left. The line noise has been imposed somewhere between the source and the detector. The instrument which has the interference is seen as Z_L at the far right. The noise filter, composed of L, C_1, and C_2 permits more of the line noise to be trapped in the detector before reaching the load.

distributed capacitance in the power line will effectively dampen or short out any noise.

SOLUTIONS

Having determined the type of noise, it can then be traced to its source. This is done by observing the noise amplitude while moving the noise detector to different locations along the power line. The higher-amplitude locations are closer to the source; the lower-amplitude locations are farther from the source. The pulse shape of the spike as observed can also give an indication as to the source. SCR and triac switches produce a very sharp spike, whereas heavy-current motors produce a pulse of wide duration. Careful inspection of the circuitry in the offending device will reveal how this noise is feeding back into the power line.

Once knowing this, we can proceed to purchase or build a tuned filter or to swamp out the noise with a low-impedance capacitor before it ever reaches the power line. The *LCXf* nomograph at the end of the book will provide the values for inductors and capacitances should we decide to build a resonant filter. However, in many cases, where the noise has a broad frequency spectrum, it can be "swamped" out at its source. Inductances and distributed capacitances at the noise source have created a medium- to high-impedance path, allowing the noise or spikes to propagate. High values of capacitance shunting the noise to a good ground from both sides of the power line will upset this path, thus killing the noise at its source of origin.

4-9
RFI

Only a few years ago, the AM radio band (0.5–1.5 MHz), the amateur radio bands (up to 220 MHz), the FM band (88–108 MHz), and TV were the only sources of radio-frequency interference (RFI) encountered when working with biomedical instrumentation. Today, the problem is compounded by the extensive use of biomedical telemetry (174–216 MHz), RF intrusion detection devices, radar intrusion alarms, citizens band radio (27 MHz), RF-operated garage door openers, FM wireless microphones, wireless TV cameras for surveillance, and, not to leave out an entirely new area of RFI, auditory training systems that send their signals to teaching machines through the airwaves. A simple way of illustrating the extent of this problem is to unplug your phonograph turntable from your hi-fi audio amplifier at home. Connect a 10-ft piece of wire to the microphone input of the hi-fi amplifier and turn the gain up. It will not be very long before you pick up a radio signal from a nearby transmitting device which is so strong that it has made your hi-fi amplifier into a short-wave receiver.

Intracellular recording, ECG, EEG, EMG, and nerve-conduction studies all fall within a part of the audio-frequency spectrum. Pickup leads from the patient act as an antenna, and strong RF signals are rectified into audio-frequency signals in the instrument itself. This takes place for two reasons. The interfering signal can be extremely strong, as, for example, a nearby transmitter or transmitting antenna or a passing vehicle. The extremely strong signal from a nearby transmitter is the easiest to solve. Simply find out the wavelength of the interfering transmitter and build or buy resonant filters to be inserted in the instrument lead near the patient. If you build a filter, the values of the inductance and capacitance can be determined from the *LCXf* nomograph. However, before buying or building a resonant filter, try, if possible, to move the equipment to another location to minimize the interference. Or try to have the patient leads placed in a position which will be parallel to the direction from which the interfering signal is originating. This will help to reduce pickup.

TUNED PATIENT LEADS

Figure 4-26 shows a simple patient-lead arrangement. The problem in this case is that our instrument often picks up citizens band radio signals. We have determined this by the dip technique, as we shall discuss later in Sec. 4-10. The citizens band is on 27 MHz. Our first thought is that the patient leads are tuned to this band because their length is a natural quarter wavelength at that frequency. Using the formula for the natural wavelength of a piece of straight wire,

$$\text{One-quarter wavelength} = \frac{246}{\text{frequency in megahertz}}$$

we find that one-quarter wavelength at 27 MHz is 9 ft. What is the significance of one-quarter wavelength?

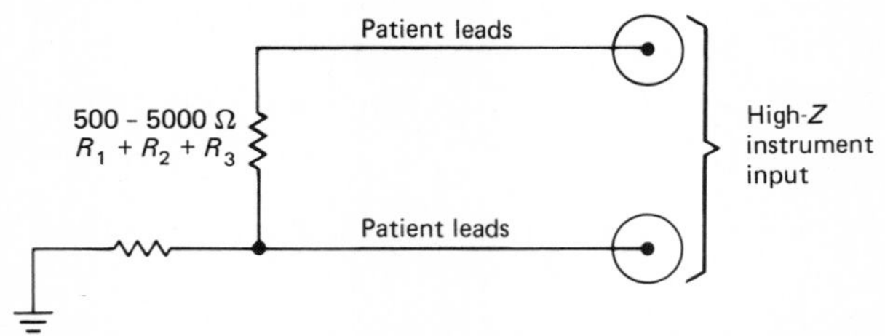

Fig. 4-26 Equivalent electric circuit representing the patient, the electrodes, the patient leads, and the instrument input terminals. The main point of this illustration is that a perfectly balanced ground is rarely possible because of the variation in lead capacitance or lead current.

The impedance the RF sees along a piece of wire reverses every quarter wavelength. For example, at 27 MHz, one end of a 9-ft wire will be extremely high impedance and the other end extremely low impedance. If we terminate such a wire in its natural impedance, we have an excellent receiving antenna for that particular wavelength. The biomedical instrument with the interference problem has extremely high input impedance, so the wire at the instrument end is terminated in a very high impedance. If the impedance 9 ft away is extremely low, then that wire will make an excellent receiving antenna for 27 MHz. A 9-ft wire we might say is cut for 27 MHz. In our case we have a 4-ft wire, so the first assumption is that we have been mistaken. This wire is not tuned to 27 MHz after all. However, investigating a little more, we find that the end of both wires at the patient side is not low impedance. R_1 and R_3 are the tissue-electrode impedance, and R_2 is the impedance between the electrodes. We find that the impedance of R_1, R_2, and R_3 can vary up to 500 Ω. If it turns out that this impedance is the proper terminating impedance for 27 MHz at the end of a 4-ft wire (opposite end is high impedance), then we do indeed have patient leads tuned to 27 MHz.

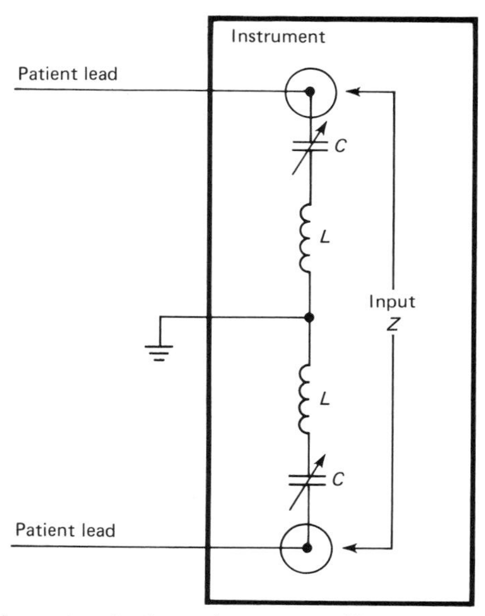

Fig. 4-27 Either of the patient leads can become an efficient RF antenna if it is properly matched to the instrument's input Z. These series resonant filters (wavetraps) can be used when there is no RF bypass capacitor across the instrument's input terminals. When there is an RF bypass capacitor, then use the circuit in Fig. 4-28. C can be 3 to 30 pF for frequencies from 35 to 300 MHz, and 10 to 120 pF for frequencies from 3 to 35 MHz. Consult the inductive reactance table to determine the inductance of L. Several companies manufacture these tunable filters.

This explains why citizens band radio stations are constantly being received on this particular medical monitoring system. Even though most manufacturers install an RF bypass capacitor at the instrument input, the interference still gets through because poor contacts, protective diodes, or other solid-state devices rectify the RF into audio. Also, the RF bypass capacitor helps to tune the patient lead (antenna) to the instrument (receiver), as has been described. Thus the input RF bypass capacitor has little effect.

RF FILTERS

A series resonant filter would pass only the interfering frequency. Figure 4-27 shows two series resonant filters inserted between the two differential inputs and ground. The natural RF high impedance across the input terminal is upset by the filters, and the citizens band signals are shunted to ground instead of being rectified inside the medical instrument. In Fig. 4-28 we find an example of parallel resonant filters which offer an extremely high impedance to the tuned frequency. To the interfering signal, the two patient leads are open at points X and Y. This results in the patient leads being detuned away from the interfering wavelength, which no longer sees a tuned antenna.

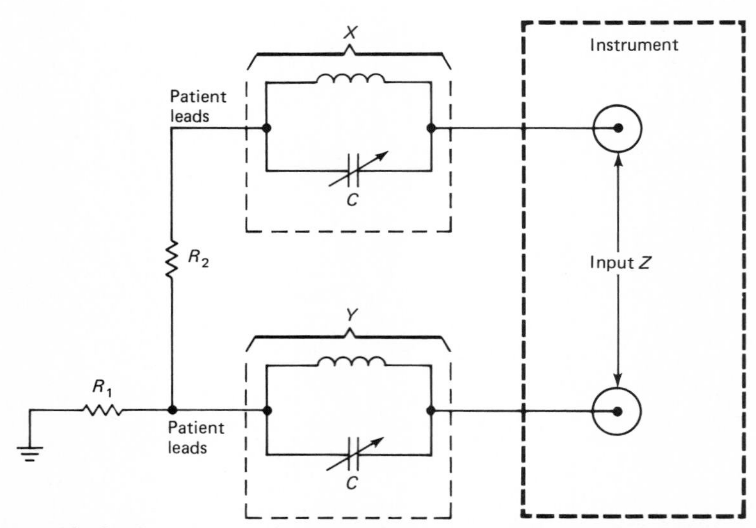

Fig. 4-28 The leads connect to the patient and are properly grounded. However, as the analogous circuit of R_1 and R_2 shows, an imbalance to ground is still created. In addition, either one of the leads may become an RF antenna. A parallel resonant filter (wavetrap) is shown in each lead. They should be close to the input terminals. If you decide to build your own, C should have the same values as in Fig. 4-27.

4-10
THE UNKNOWN FREQUENCY

Once the interfering frequency is known, 246 divided by the frequency in megahertz will give us the quarter wavelength natural length of wire. From there we can determine the tissue-electrode and patient impedances to find what frequency the leads are tuned to. There are several methods of determining the unknown interfering frequency. By far the best is the heterodyne method. To use this technique a high-quality dipper, or calibrated RF-tunable oscillator, will be required. The Millen No. 90652 (Fig. 4-29) is recommended. It is solid-state and battery-operated. This feature has many advantages besides safety, as shall be described later. This dipper can be used for a number of useful tests and measurements. First, the heterodyne test will be described.

Before the interfering signal can be eliminated, it is necessary to know its wavelength. The Millen dipper is supplied with a series of plug-in coils. Depending on the coil plugged in, the dipper will oscillate from 1.7 to 300 MHz. Hold the dipper in your hand, as shown in Fig. 4-30*i*. Connect a pair of earphones (through a coupling capacitor) to the output of the next-to-last amplifier stage before the recording de-

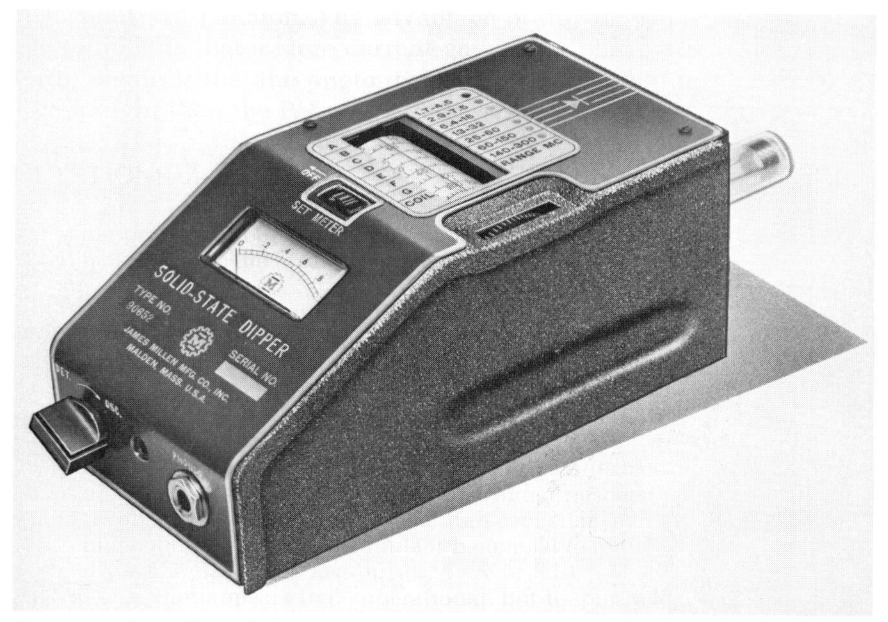

Fig. 4-29 The Millen solid-state dipper. This battery-operated device will determine the resonant frequency of any tuned circuit from 1.7 to 300 MHz. It will also detect small amounts of radiation over these same frequencies. (Courtesy James Millen Mfg. Co.)

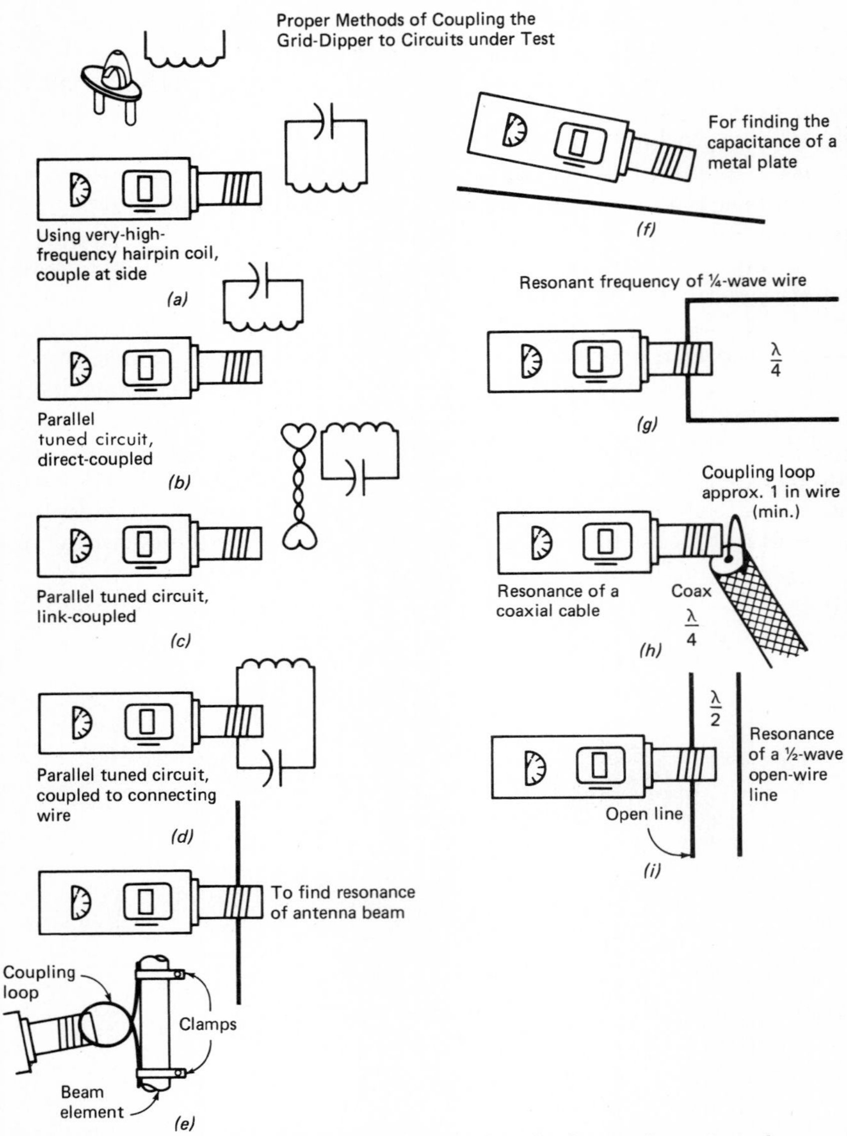

Fig. 4-30 Use of the dipper to determine the wavelength of a tuned circuit, or the wavelength of an antenna for medical telemetry, or to detect the presence of radiated energy in coaxial cable, a tuned circuit, or a wired lead. The angle at which the dipper is held relative to the circuit under test can be extremely critical. For best results, follow these illustrations carefully.

vice or monitoring device. Using the 300-MHz plug-in coil, tune the dipper through its entire frequency range. With the medical instrument on, listen to the earphones for a whistling or buzzing noise as the dipper is being tuned. If none is heard, plug in the next lower-frequency coil and repeat the procedure. Go from coil to coil until the "zero beat" or heterodyne is heard. Observe the frequency indicated on the dipper calibrated dial. This is the interfering frequency.

Series or parallel resonant filters (Figs. 4-27 and 4-28) must be tuned to this frequency to eliminate the interference. In Chap. 9, Troubleshooting Biomedical Components, various additional measurements using this dipper will be described.

4-11
BASE-LINE SHIFT

Except in the fields of electromyography and neurology, most of the physiological data the BMET encounters will have an extremely low-frequency component. Waveforms depicting pulmonary function, blood pressure, and ECG and EEG variations have components below 1 Hz. The need to observe these low-frequency data combined with the necessity of amplifying these data many times in our instrumentation often creates a severe problem known as *base-line shift*. The problem may be traced to the instrumentation or to variations originating prior to the instrumentation. Living organisms have a dc ionization potential which changes at various parts of the body and is constantly changing with respect to time. Whenever the patient moves, the tissue-electrode interface resistance changes. If that were not enough to create instability, human tissue itself goes through relatively large fluctuations in its electrical characteristics. It is true that some of these undesirable variations are direct current, and capacitors can be used in biomedical amplifiers to minimize these effects.

The problem is, however, that so much of the data we wish to recover are so close to direct current that the energy-coupling capacitors must be large enough to present an extremely low impedance (capacitive reactance) to these low frequencies. These large capacitors must have large amounts of dielectric material to store energy at large time constants. Although dielectric materials are insulators, they have an inherent leakage factor. To illustrate this point, tie a dry piece of paper between two terminals of a high-voltage power supply. Tape a thermometer or thermistor to the middle of the dry paper. After a few minutes the paper's temperature will rise as the high voltage succeeds in moving electrons from atom to atom within the so-called paper insulator. This leakage factor rises sharply as the capacitor (or its dielectric material) begins to age. Thus as any instrument ages, the leakage in each coupling capacitor from input to output increases. The net effect is cumulative, and the unavoidable result is base-line shift.

OSCILLOSCOPE BASE-LINE SHIFT

An electrostatically focused oscilloscope will have two vertical deflection plates (Fig. 4-31) to determine the vertical position of its horizontal base line. This base line is an electron spot which is swept or moved from left to right by the horizontal deflection plates. In Fig. 4-31*a*, the potentiometer arm represents a hypothetical power source, where the vertical deflection plates are given different voltages against ground, thus simulating an actual biopotential input. Biopotentials of both a positive value (shifting the spot upward) and of a negative value (shifting the spot downward) can easily be observed. Should the base

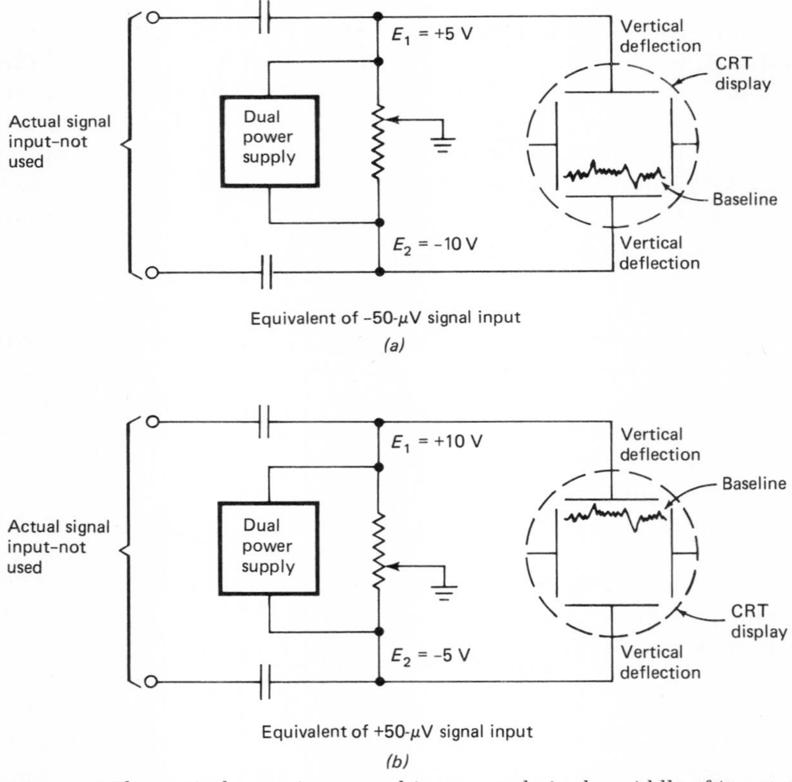

Fig. 4-31 (*a*) The vertical centering control is set exactly in the middle of its rotation. This is the equivalent of the absence of an input signal. The voltage on both CRT plates is equal. The base line appears across the middle of the display. (*b*) The centering control is reset. The lower plate is now more negative than the upper plate is positive. This pulls the base line to the bottom. (*c*) The centering control is again reset. This time the top plate is more positive than the lower plate is negative. The base line is pulled to the top.

line move to the bottom of the display, negative potentials would no longer be seen; should it move to the top of the display, positive potentials would no longer be seen.

The difference between Fig. 4-31*a* and *b* is a 10-V change on the vertical deflection plates. The bottom plate in Fig. 4-31*b* lost 5 V, while the top plate gained 5 V. A change of 100 μV at the oscilloscope input terminals created a change of 10 V on the vertical deflection plates. In other words, the oscilloscope amplified the input signal 100,000 times. At this high amplification factor, very fast changes in tissue characteristics, body movement potentials, patient ionization potentials, and so on, can create a situation through slowly charging capacitors or leaky capacitors that will move a centered base line to its position in Fig.4-31*a* or *b*. Worse than that, the base line can drift off the display completely.

REMEDIES

In Chap. 3 we learned that transducers are biased to produce a stable base line in the readout device. Now we discover that tissue variation, body movement, and other artifacts may upset this transducer bias and cause base-line shift. Also high-impedance surface electrodes are very vulnerable to large time constant and dc ionization changes in the body itself. Add this to the fact that components such as capacitors, resistors, tubes, and transistors change their specifications with age, and we are faced with a formidable base-line-shift problem.

One remedy is to examine crucial components in the instrument, such as all capacitors coupling the signal, as well as bypass capacitors. These should be checked for leakage on the highest ohms scale of the FET multimeter. Resistance values obtained should be referenced against a brand-new capacitor of the same capacitance value. A higher leakage will indicate a deteriorated dielectric. One capacitor lead should be removed from the circuit so that the associated circuitry does not produce a false reading on the ohmmeter. If leaky capacitors have been replaced and base-line shift persists, then compare all circuit voltages with those listed in the instrument's service manual. A discrepancy of over 5 percent is usually a clue that a resistor has changed value; locate and replace these.

If, after these procedures, there still is base-line shift, another remedy exists. Several home-brew circuits have been designed by biomedical engineers to solve this problem. In general, these devices can be called *self-balancing systems,* or SBS.

WHEN SBS IS MOST NEEDED. Keep in mind that if our monitor or recorder performs at direct current, then we must rebalance the base line manually during the monitoring. This is a nuisance and sometimes impossible. Yet in impedance pneumography, high-quality EEG, blood-pressure measurement, etc., our system must respond down to 6000 ms (6 s) or about 0.2 Hz. When collecting data from a sleeping but restless patient, body-movement artifact becomes a special problem. Also in recording data from subjects during exercise (without using telemetry) and in measuring long-term skin resistance, extreme base-line stability is essential. In ECG, poor base-line stability will cause the peak of the QRS complex to be lost. In EMG, high-amplitude fibrillations will also be lost as a result of severe base-line shift.

SELF-BALANCING SYSTEMS. Although there are many SBS concepts, the two systems discussed here are a general guide to SBS. Figure 4-32 is an SBS arrangement that will work with tape or chart recorders with input ranges of from 1 to 3 V. The system rebalances and brings the recording pen into the center line. Although chart recorders have self-balancing potentiometers, their response time is too slow for many momentary long-term constant disturbances. In Fig. 4-32, physiological input from the trigger controls the gate's ability to allow multivibrator (IC_3) pulses to reach the counter. When the trigger opens the gate, the counter output is multiplied by constants proportional to the weights of their digital positions, adding to the output of the "zero level" circuit. Set the output to zero when the binary count is 1000 (corresponding to a decimal count of 16), the midpoint of its range. As long as the gate is on, the binary count increases until it reaches its maximum count of 31. It then resets to zero and again increases to its maximum. The output corresponding to this counting is a sequence of staircase functions of steps when referred to the output. The output then always changes in the same direction whether the

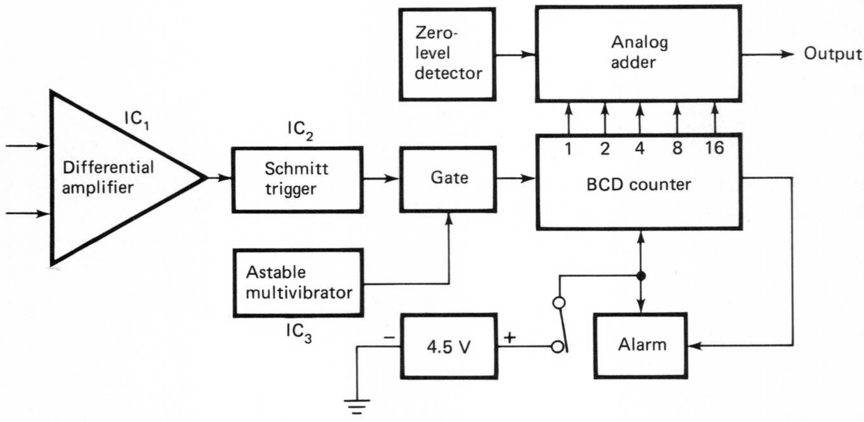

Fig. 4-32 Block diagram of a self-balancing system (SBS) with an automatic alarm triggered by an excess count or an overlimit condition.

input is too large or too small. If the shift is too great, the gate remains on and causes the output to cycle repeatedly. This situation is sensed by the alarm circuit and causes the alarm to lock "on" until the operator depresses the reset button, which shuts the alarm and resets the output to zero (binary count to 16).

While holding the reset button, the operator can manually rebalance the base line. When the reset button is released the system is again in operation. When low-priced integrated circuits (ICs) are used, the component cost of this system is about $30. This system rebalances in less than 1 ms, a negligible time compared to the typical period of slowly changing variables in the biomedical field. When used for respiration studies of sleeping persons, breathing patterns can be observed during and immediately following body movements. In Fig. 4-33*a*, without SBS, the base-line shift during body movement is so severe at point *X* that the respiratory data simply moved off the chart and were lost. In Fig. 4-33 a shift is observed at point *X* but it does not interfere with the recording.

Another SBS or automatic dc-level compensation circuit is based on feeding negative feedback to the input circuit to counteract a change in dc level. This compensation can be suspended when it is desired to record direct current. In this system as well as in the previous SBS arrangement the ICs (building blocks) are made by several manufacturers and are readily available. This SBS (Fig. 4-34) takes the input signal through a cathode follower to produce a low-impedance output. Compensation is achieved by integrating the cathode-follower output. The feedback network subtracts the integrated signal from the input to stabilize the preamp level at zero. The output of the two op amps is fed

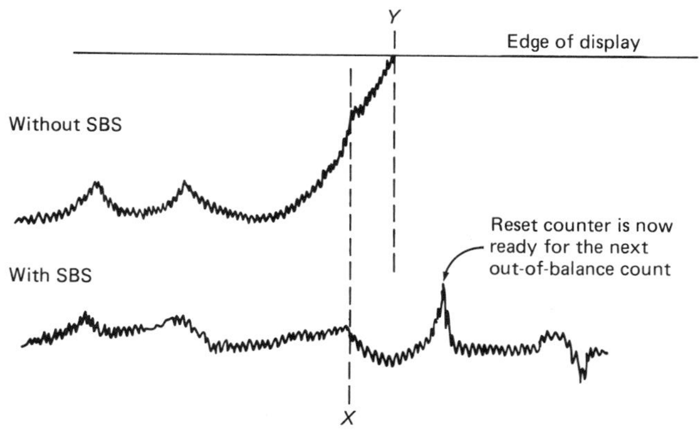

Fig. 4-33 Two base lines showing a thoracic respiratory test. (*a*) There is no SBS. An excessive bias causes the base line to begin to rise at *X*, and at *Y* it disappears off the display completely. (*b*) Self-balancing has been added to the system. At *X* the logic has determined that an out-of-balance condition exists, and the count begins.

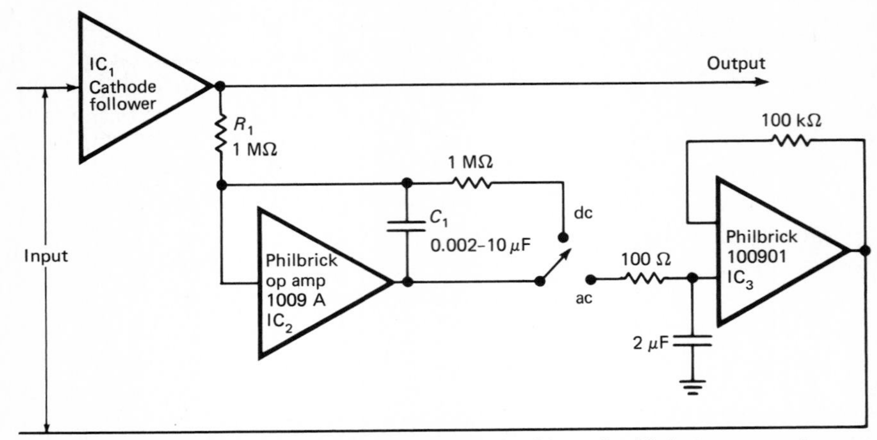

Fig. 4-34 A very simple SBS for those BMETs who like to build their own equipment. Three commonly available ICs and six discrete components constitute the entire system. The cathode follower may be any one of a number of ICs designed for this purpose. Different values of C_1 will change the time constant.

back to the cathode follower. IC_2 integrates and inverts the signal; IC_3 is also a cathode follower with unity gain. The compensating potential across the 2-mF capacitor decays very slowly because of the high impedance and low bias current of the cathode follower IC_3, which is an FET-input op amp. Varying C_1 between 0.002 and 10 μF will change the SBS low-frequency cutoff. Values between 80 and 0.02 Hz can be achieved depending on the R_1, C_1 time constant. The ICs in both systems are available from Philbrick, National, Signetics, or Burr-Brown.

THE IMPEDANCE CONVERTER. If you are measuring resistance, capacitance, or inductive changes and require good base-line stability down to direct current, there is an alternative to self-balancing systems. Rather than reproduce the actual physiological time constants directly, a high-frequency oscillator can be amplitude-modulated by the physiological data. The Biocom Model 991 impedance converter takes advantage of the fact that it is easier to stabilize a 50-kilohertz (kHz) oscillator than the data directly obtained. The subject becomes the oscillator load with a 1 percent impedance or load change producing a 10 percent (0.5 V) change in output voltage. This amplitude-modulated signal is demodulated in the AM detector (Fig. 4-35) and coupled to the output through an emitter follower.

The zero suppression circuit eliminates the dc bias (carrying the signal) but still retains dc signal response. This device has been used to measure respiration, pulse, volume changes (plethysmography), psychogalvanic response, peristaltic contractions, temperature, physical

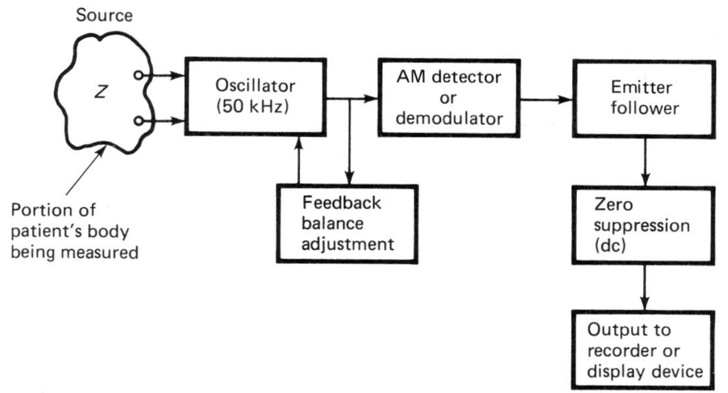

Fig. 4-35 The source acts as a load on the 50-kHz oscillator. The amount of feedback changes the oscillator's loading. This way a perfect match to the load impedance Z is achieved. The signal from the AM detector rides on a −5-V bias. The zero suppression circuit eliminates this bias so that only the data remain.

displacement (using a piezoelectric crystal pickup as a displacement transducer), and strain-gage variations.

QUESTIONS

1. Power-source energy (60 Hz) is a sine wave. Why does it appear on the ECG trace in Fig. 4-1 as a widening base line and not as a sine wave?
2. We wish to observe the following levels of biomedical data. In each case, give the approximate interference level that can be tolerated: 500 μV, 2 mV, 210 μV, 33 μV.
3. Making use of the magnetic field rule, specify the direction of a magnetic field in relation to the direction of electron flow through a wire.
4. A coil with 87 turns carries 5.2 A. What is the coil's magnetic flux?
5. What are two tests to determine if interference of the magnetic type originates from wire forming a loop?
6. What is the simplest way to eliminate magnetic-loop interference?
7. Flexing artifacts and distortion of very fast biomedical pulses could be a result of ________.
8. In Fig. 4-6, if the impedance from leads (across Z_0) to ground were equal, then there would be no interference. Explain the changes that result in a differential voltage or interference.
9. If the patient leads were picking up 20 nA of least-resistance current and electrode impedance imbalance was 5000 Ω, what would the interference voltage be?
10. Give two methods of reducing least-resistance currents in medical instrument leads.
11. In taking an ECG with the right leg grounded, what undesirable effect might occur?
12. Several instruments are used together. An abnormally high ac interference level is found. What is always the first condition to look for?
13. Describe the function of the buffer amplifier or cathode follower.
14. True or false: Active filters use inductors, resistors, and capacitors.

15. We need a filter to operate from 0.3 to 5 Hz. Would we use an active or a passive filter?
16. List the drawbacks of active filters.
17. Name the four basic types of filters.
18. In a notch filter, should the breakpoint be close to the frequency that you want to pass? Explain.
19. What problems can develop using a high-Q notch filter?
20. A medical instrument has interference from a TV station. When the input terminals are shorted, the interference disappears. Which method would be used to eliminate the TV interference?

chapter 5

The Readout

INTRODUCTION

By this time you should be familiar with the various techniques involved in changing biomedical data into electric signals. The causes and origins of interference have been covered, and techniques for eliminating them have been explored. After the signal has been "cleaned up," it is amplified and possibly processed. After processing, the data finally interface with the instrument operator in the form of a chart, a display, a digital readout, or some other device now on the drawing board.

In this chapter you will learn about pen recorders and how linearity (graphic fidelity) is a prime concern. There would be little value in taking intricate precautionary measures in the instrument circuitry to eliminate distortion if the readout defeated this effort. Poor chart or display fidelity could lead to a faulty medical interpretation, especially when the observed shape of data is critical.

Further along in the chapter, we will see how transducers and instrumentation systems can effectively capture very fast data (transients) but the readout will fail to store it for subsequent study. Thus special recording and memorization techniques are described that permit fast data to be retained. Not only do such systems keep the data alive, but they allow data processing equipment to examine this physiological material at any time.

One problem is to stretch out very fast data as an aid to readability. The opposite problem exists when very slow data are obtained over a long period of time. Here the clinical interpretation is often laborious at best, and incomplete at worst. For data having a long time period, processing involves time reduction or compression. As long as time compression must be performed, data can also be reprocessed or converted into more meaningful information. For example, raw multiple-channel data may be integrated into a single channel of comparative data, containing the most significant information. A typical system which accomplishes this is discussed.

5-1 PEN RECORDERS

Although pen recorders vary in construction, their mode of operation is basically the same. The following describes the theory of operation of a typical pen recorder of modular construction. Its basic essentials are a mainframe and analog recording channels. The block diagram in Fig. 5-1 shows a typical multichannel analog pen recorder.

THE MAINFRAME

The mainframe contains a switchboard, control board, control transformer, chart-drive motor, and transmission and event markers. On the switchboard are the operator controls: switches for power, chart-speed selection, and event-marker actuation. Indicators show when the power and the interlock are on.

THE CONTROL BOARD

Contained in the control board are the branch fuses, start-stop relay, power supplies, and timer. A relay controls power to the chart-drive motor. Ink solenoids, event markers, and optical couplers are located in the pen drive amplifiers. They receive power from the same relay which is energized when the chart STOP pushbutton is released. When energized, one set of contacts supplies power to the chart-drive motor and activates the ink-manifold solenoids. When deenergized, the other set of contacts inhibits the event markers and optical couplers in the pen drive amplifiers.

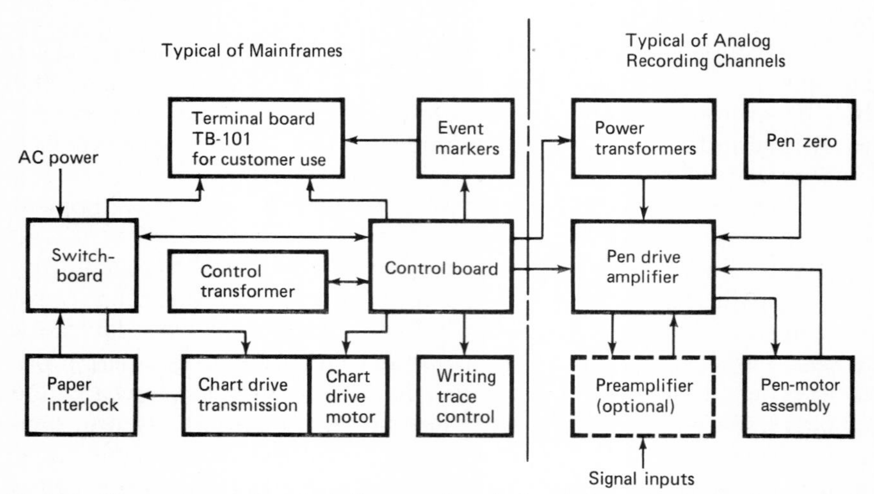

Fig. 5-1 The basic recorder block diagram. A typical mainframe is essentially a switchboard and a control board. A typical analog recording channel consists of a pen drive amplifier driven by the control board.

The unfiltered section of the power supply provides power to optional event-marker solenoids and the indicator lamps. The filtered section of the power supply provides power to the event markers to ensure accuracy when precise time events are required. Filtered power is provided for the pen-drive-amplifier optical couplers and timer.

Pulsating dc voltage is provided from a bridge rectifier to operate ink-supply solenoids. The timer operates as a function of the ac line frequency. The optical coupler shapes the sinusoidal wave into a square wave. Binary counters count each square-wave pulse. The output pulse then drives a monostable multivibrator, controlling the timer.

THE EVENT MARKERS

The event markers are activated by mark-event switches, optional timer, or remote application of transistor-transistor-logic (TTL) signals or contact closure. Depressing a mark-event switch permits current to flow through the mark-event solenoid, activating the event marker.

ANALOG RECORDING CHANNELS

These channels consist of a power transformer, pen drive amplifier, and pen motor. Channels are isolated from one another by separate transformer power supplies and optical couplers. The optical coupler disables the pen drive amplifier whenever a relay on the control board is deenergized.

Figure 5-2 shows a block diagram of an analog channel. The pen-motor drive amplifier is a complete servosystem. It uses a linear voltage-displacement transformer in the pen motor to develop position data and a velocity transducer to develop velocity data. These signals are summed up and added to the input signal in a dc error amplifier. After amplification, the output signal drives the pen motor.

THE SIGNAL LIMITER

The input signal enters the signal limiter and is summed with the pen zero signal. The summed signal is fed to a diode bridge circuit.

THE FREQUENCY-COMPENSATION CIRCUIT

Output from the signal limiter is fed to a frequency-compensation network. Here the signal's frequency response is adjusted to be flat within 2 percent from direct current to 30 Hz for 100-mm pen deflection. This curcuit also provides a gain change to allow use with either 50- or 100-mm pen motors. The frequency-compensated signal is then fed to a summing network, where it is combined with error and velocity signals.

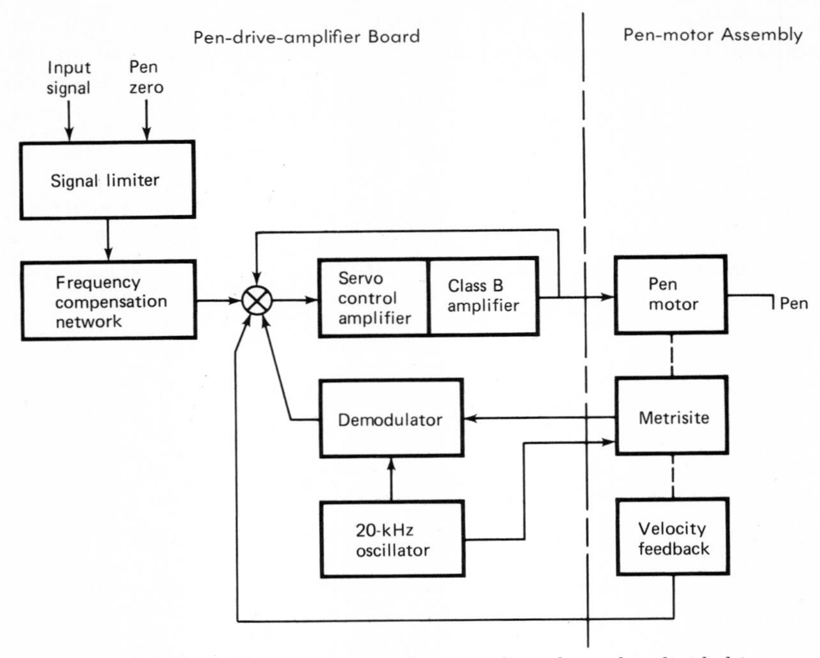

Fig. 5-2 Detailed block diagram of an analog recording channel is divided into a pen-drive-amplifier board (left and center) and a pen-motor assembly on the right. The velocity-feedback circuit is on the lower right. The signal-feedback loop starts at the class B amplifier output and goes back to the servocontrol amplifier input.

OBTAINING THE POSITION-FEEDBACK SIGNAL

Position feedback is obtained from a Wien-bridge oscillator. A demodulator attenuates this carrier. Output from the demodulator becomes the position-feedback signal. This signal is then fed to the servocontrol amplifier.

The compensated input signal, position-feedback data, and velocity data are summed at the input of the servoamplifier. The output of this stage drives a class B amplifier, which drives the pen to the proper position on the chart. This occurs when the summed signal is reduced to zero.

5-2 THERMAL RECORDERS

Several manufacturers are now producing thermal recorders because these have many advantages over the ink recorder. A thermal recorder using advanced concepts is the Gould Multipoint Thermal Recorder. A description of its operation will generally apply to all thermal recorders. The high-speed multipoint recorder permits high-resolution recording at high sampling rates. In the intensified mode, the recorder allows concentration of data on channels of greatest interest while also monitoring others. In the continuous mode, the recorder becomes a wide-chart, single-channel oscillograph for accurate monitoring at higher frequencies.

The recorder utilizes a single pen driven by a high-speed, feedback-controlled pen motor. In multipoint and intensified modes, the pen contacts the paper only as each channel is sampled. The value of the input signal, at the instant of sampling, is plotted by a discrete dot, resulting in traces for each channel made up of closely spaced dots. Sampling rate is infinitely variable from one sample every 2 s up to 16 samples per second. Channels not selected are not sampled; thus the sampling rate is distributed only on active channels.

Trace presentation is rectilinear. The paper is Z-folded and delivered to a catch drawer beneath the writing surface. Trace identification is performed. With the identification button depressed, each trace is interrupted briefly opposite a number printed on the chart margin corresponding to the channel interrupted. The resulting record is clear, easy to read, and uncluttered.

An accessory amplifier, with automatic thermocouple cold-junction compensation, gain adjustment, and zero suppression, plugs into the rear of the recorder. The amplifier, with a plug-in thermocouple compensator, provides a signal input sensitivity of 2 mV full scale into 1-kΩ impedance.

An optional event-marker kit may be installed and may be actuated by an optional internal timer that provides one pulse per minute.

A TYPICAL THERMAL RECORDER

The Gould 816 Multipoint Recorder is an eight-channel multiplex recording system consisting of four major groups: a commutator, a drive amplifier, a channel-identification circuit, and an optional multiplex signal conditioner. These groups are interconnected to synchronize an electromechanical pen lifter to a servocontrolled, position-feedback, high-torque pen motor. These are mounted on a 12-speed chart-drive assembly using prefolded Z-fold paper.

The function of the commutator is to sequentially scan the selected inputs and connect each input to a common signal line (see Fig. 5-3). The commutator consists of a solid-state shift register, a variable-frequency oscillator, a mode selector, and eight input reed relays (see Fig. 5-4). The rate of scanning is controlled by a variable-frequency oscillator which is continuously variable from approximately one sample every 2 s to 16 samples per second.

The mode selector is also an integral part of the commutator since it

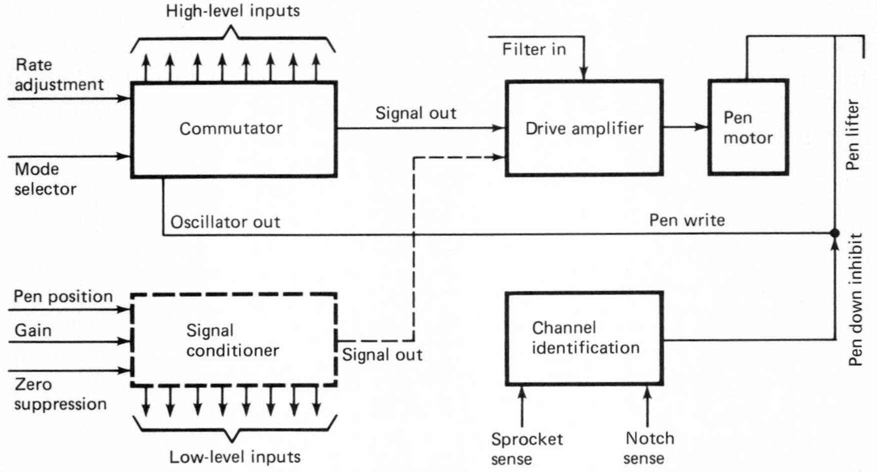

Fig. 5-3 Multipoint thermal-recorder block diagram. The commutator, drive amplifier, channel-identification circuit, and signal conditioner synchronize the pen lifter to the pen motor. The commutator scans the inputs, connecting them to a common signal line.

governs the type of scanning the commutator will perform. The mode selector is a multipole, multideck selector switch. The output of the oscillator is used to synchronize the pen lifting bar with the commutator so as to have the pen off the paper whenever the commutator is changing.

THE DRIVE AMPLIFIER. The function of a drive amplifier is to power the pen motor and position the pen at a point which represents the input signal. This circuit consists of the amplifier itself, a notch filter, and a summing network (see Fig. 5-4). The amplifier provides a ±2.5-V dc full-scale deflection with 50 kΩ input impedance. The notch filter is activated by the filter switch, injecting approximately 30 dB of 60-Hz filtering in series with the input signal. (Refer back to Sec. 4-6 for detailed information on notch filters.) When the filter switch is deactivated, the filter is bypassed. The filter and drive amplifier must have a constant input impedance. This is the function of the summing network circuitry.

IDENTIFYING THE VARIOUS CHANNELS. In Fig. 5-5, the channel-identification section generates trace interruptions. These interruptions are used for channel identification. This circuit consists of a sprocket-hole sensor, a notch sensor, a sprocket-hole counter, a binary-decimal decoder, a decimal comparator, and a pen-down inhibitor. Each page of the chart paper is notched so as to have the pen tip at the perforation when the notch is being sensed. This resets the counter

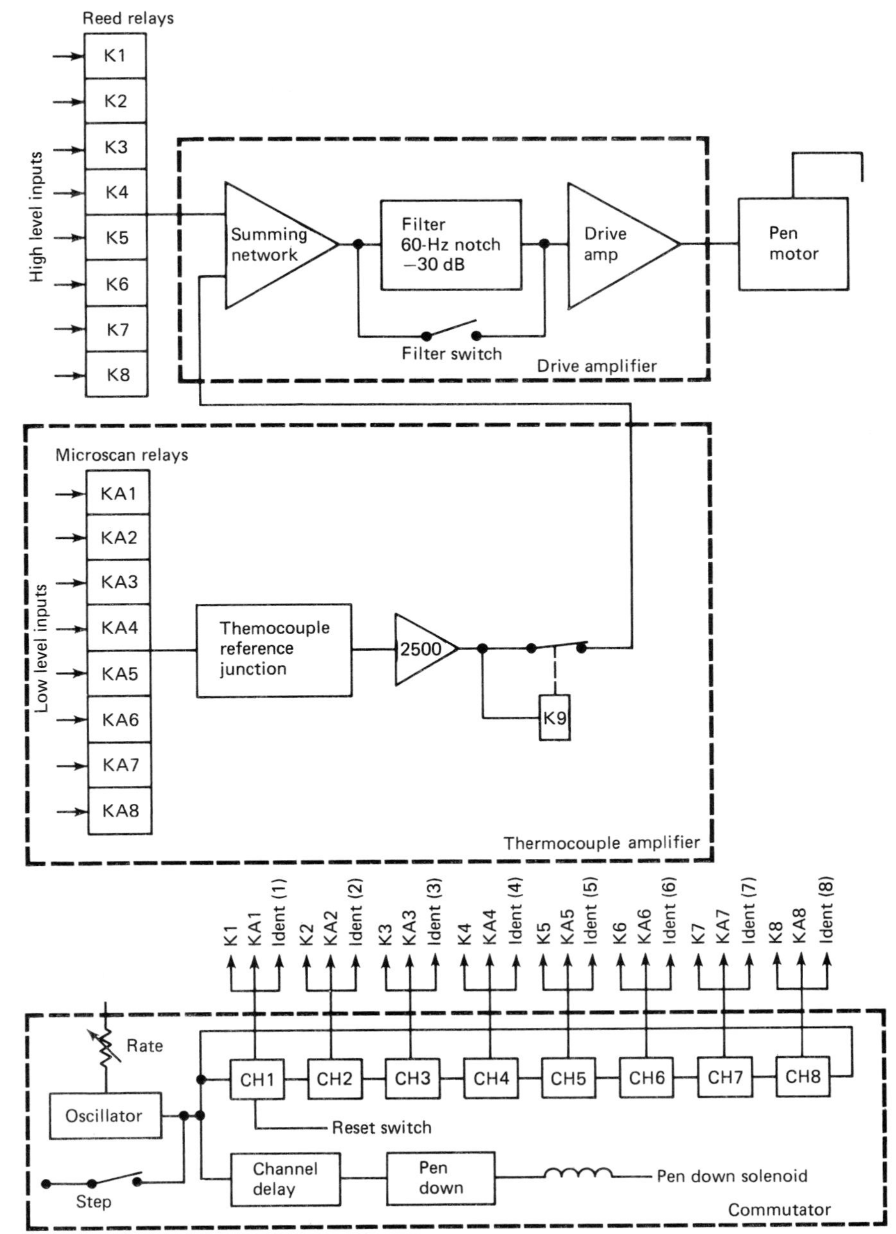

Fig. 5-4 In this multipoint signal-flow diagram the inputs (both high and low level) feed the drive amplifier which powers the pen motor.

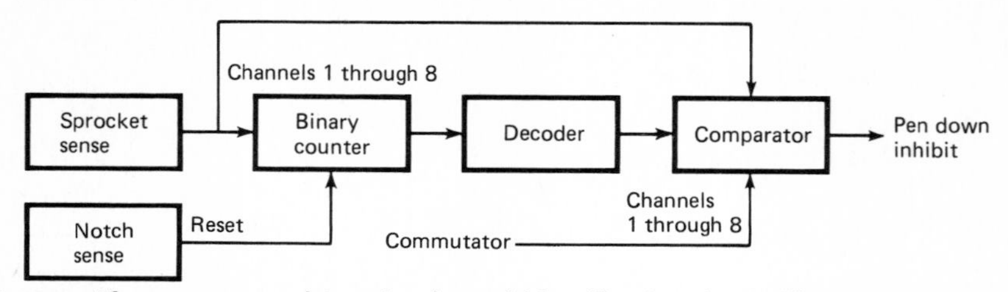

Fig. 5-5 The commutator drives the channel-identification circuit. The sensors, counter, decoder, and comparator synchronize the pen tip on the recording paper with the actual channel which is being sensed.

to zero. As each sprocket hole passes the sprocket-hole sensor, a count is put into the binary counter. This binary count is decoded into decimal information and compared with the commutator and the sprocket-hole sensor. When all three compare, i.e., when the count is 1 and the commutator is sampling channel 1 and the sprocket-hole sensor is sensing a sprocket hole, the pen will be prevented from writing. This process is repeated for all eight sprocket holes.

MULTIPLEXED SIGNAL CONDITIONING. The multipoint recording system provides the ability to add an optional multiplexed signal conditioner. This conditioner takes advantage of the commutating system employed by the recorder, thereby requiring only one conditioner for eight input channels.

The multiplex conditioner consists of eight low-level, special-purpose scanning relays, the signal-conditioning amplifier, a disconnect relay, and its plug-in enclosure. The eight relays are used to scan the low-level inputs in conjuncttion with the high-level commutator. These low-level signals are fed to a common line, properly conditioned, amplified, and summed with the high-level input. As previously mentioned, the summer is necessary for a constant input impedance to the filter. Since both the high- and low-level signals are summed, only one or the other in any particular channel can be used at any one time. That is, if channel 1 is being used for high-level signals, channel 1 in the conditioner cannot be used, and vice versa. The disconnect relay is necessary to ensure that the output of the conditioner is zero whenever no inputs are used.

HIGH FIDELITY. Whether the recording system is thermal, using heat-sensitive paper, or a pen recorder, the complex circuitry described here has one primary objective: to provide high-fidelity reproduction of the input physiological signal. Instruments vary widely in their degree of perfection. There is always a gap between the input waveshape and what is finally reproduced graphically. One of the major parameters in determining this gap is the degree of linearity achieved.

5-3
RECORDER LINEARITY

Some 50 years ago physiological data were recorded on paper with a heavy, crude stylus arrangement. The relationship between actual physiological data and the final ink impression on the recording paper was indeed poor. Although the electronics in those systems could be made to introduce little distortion, the main problem was the mechanical mechanism in the output. If a perfect triangular waveshape was fed into the pen recorder, the paper recording would show a pattern that would be far from the perfect triangle. A perfect recorded triangle would mean the recording system had excellent linearity. The degree to which the sides of the triangle were bent would indicate the degree or percentage of nonlinearity in our recording system.

TWO APPROACHES TO RECTILINEARITY

Figure 5-6 shows two types of rectilinear trace-writing systems used in direct-writing recorders. In Fig. 5-6*a*, an electrically heated stylus moves on an arc across a special heat-sensitive paper as the paper is drawn over a straight, fixed knife-edge. This system has no problem generating a perfectly straight line across the width of the paper when the paper is stationary. However, it is subject to a degree of geometric nonlinearity (described later) which may or may not be acceptable. Compounding the problem is the fact that nonlinearity may be specified in several ways, making evaluation and comparisons difficult.

The mechanism of Fig. 5-6*b* is part of a pressurized-ink system that writes on ordinary ruled chart paper. Deflection at the pen tip is a function of the angle of rotation of the pen motor, the ratio of the pulley

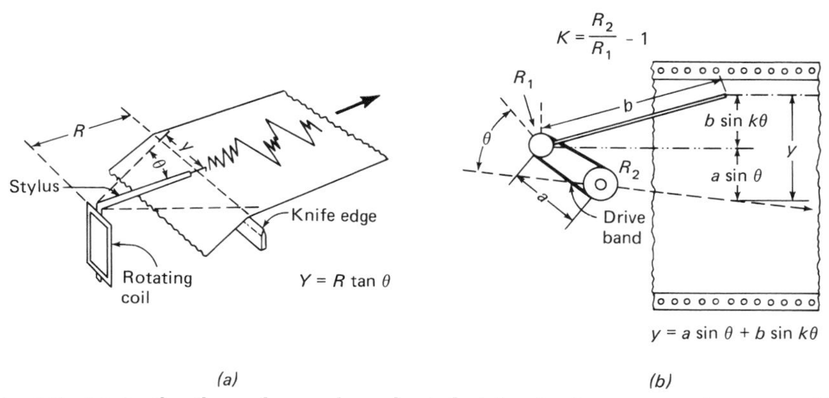

Fig. 5-6 (*a*) In the thermal recorder a heated stylus is shown sweeping across the thermal chart paper. The stylus is drawn over a knife-edge. (*b*) A parallel-motion mechanism keeps the pen tip nearly perpendicular to the direction of chart motion. In this case ordinary chart paper is used.

diameters connected by a drive band, and the ratio of pen length to drive-arm length. This mechanism generates a straight line within 0.0002 in across the width of a 40-mm channel and has relatively small geometric nonlinearity. This nonlinearity, incidentally, can be canceled electrically by a position-feedback system on the pen-motor shaft.

HOW STRAIGHT IS STRAIGHT?

A perfectly linear writing system would produce an output (pen deflection) that is directly proportional to the input (current to the pen motor). A corollary is that equal increments of input would cause equal changes in trace amplitude in any region on the chart.

The latter capability is especially important where trend curves or other traces span a major portion of the channel width. An example is the trace shown in Fig. 5-7, which depicts variations in tooth profile and eccentricity of a manufactured gear as checked against a master gear. An amplitude error anywhere on the chart gives an erroneous reading in that region. Geometric nonlinearity in writing systems can cause such errors.

Nonlinearity is measured in several ways. One method is maximum-deflection-based nonlinearity. This is the maximum departure of the calibration curve from a straight line drawn to give the most favorable accuracy. It is normally expressed as a percentage of full-scale deflection.

Another method is slope-based nonlinearity. This is the ratio of maximum slope error anywhere on the calibration curve to the slope of the nominal sensitivity line. It is usually expressed as a percentage of nominal slope.

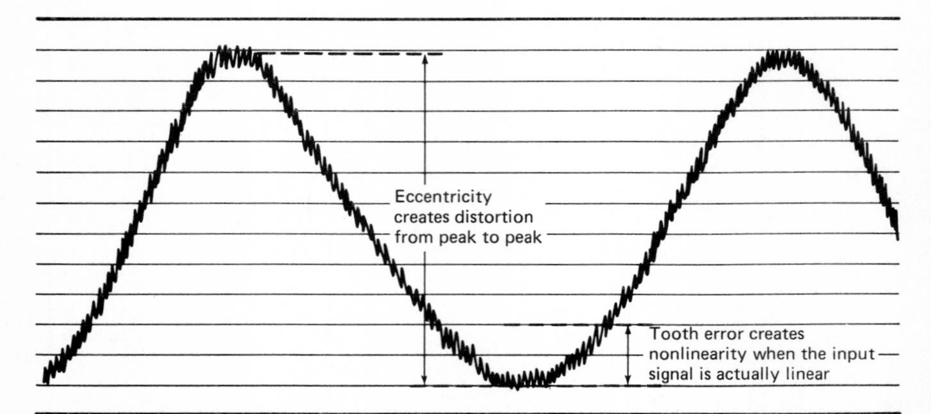

Fig. 5-7 Here we see nonlinear displacement only in specific chart areas. The input test signal was a perfect triangular wave with a sharp peak and a pointed bottom. Eccentricity creates unequal distances between peaks, caused by the eccentricity of a gear on the chart-paper roller mechanism. Also, tooth error rounds off peaks and troughs.

Within these two definitions there is leeway to position the straight lines in different ways. Thus, recorder manufacturers have an opportunity to practice nonlinearity "specmanship." In other words, not all nonlinearity specifications are alike, and some can actually mask design weaknesses or performance deficiencies.

SEEING THINGS STRAIGHT

Several valid ways of specifying writing-system nonlinearity can have different meanings to recorder users.

GEOMETRIC NONLINEARITY. The knife-edge thermal writing system has an input-output relationship, as seen in Fig. 5-6*a*. This is defined in terms of the relationship between the distance from the coil axis to the writing edge and the angular deflection of the coil from the channel center line.

Nonlinearity of this system can be determined by the slope-based method, Fig. 5-8*a*. This method uses a straight line with the same slope as that of the most linear portion of the input-output curve (near the channel center).

For small angles, θ in radians is approximately equal to tan θ, so that for up to about 6° of coil rotation the straight line coincides with the slope of the curve at channel center within $\frac{1}{2}$ percent.

When coil rotation gets up to about 18°, however, the deviation of the curve from the straight line (the error, or nonlinearity) becomes large. It is equal to

$$\frac{R \tan 18^\circ - R(18/57.3)}{R(18/57.3)} \times 100 = 3.4\%$$

This is the percentage of amplitude from channel center line to channel edge. If we consider full scale, the nonlinearity would be half this value, or ± 1.7 percent of full scale. No manufacturer uses this definition of nonlinearity because it looks so bad.

MAXIMUM DEVIATION. This is nonlinearity based on the maximum-deviation method and gives a more favorable specification. The system is calibrated at the channel edge, and deviations are measured between the curve and a straight line connecting the channel center and the calibration point, as seen in Fig. 5-8*b*. The maximum error occurs within the channel limits at a value where the curve and the straight line have the same slope (are parallel).

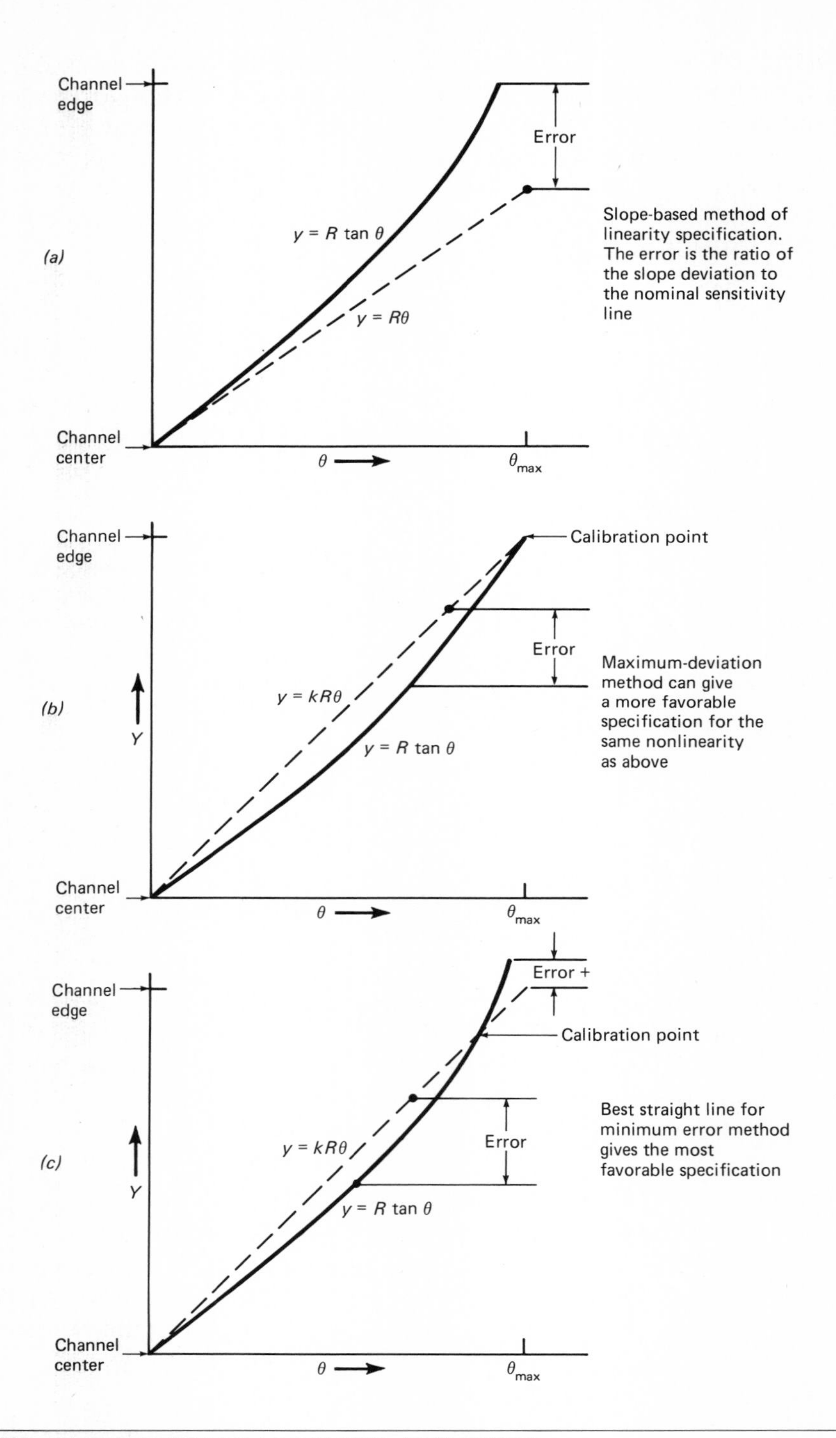
Channel edge
Error
Slope-based method of linearity specification. The error is the ratio of the slope deviation to the nominal sensitivity line
y = R tan θ
(a)
y = Rθ
Channel center
θ
θmax
Channel edge
Calibration point
Error
Maximum-deviation method can give a more favorable specification for the same nonlinearity as above
y = kRθ
(b)
Y
y = R tan θ
Channel center
θ
θmax
Error +
Channel edge
Calibration point
Best straight line for minimum error method gives the most favorable specification
Error
y = kRθ
(c)
Y
y = R tan θ
Channel center
θ
θmax

SPLIT DEVIATION. This method of calculating nonlinearity (Fig. 5-8*c*) gives an even better specification. It uses the best straight line for minimum error. Moving the calibration point inward from the channel edge splits the error found in the previous example into a plus and minus deviation. The error is not in one direction. This means that above the calibration point the deflection of the stylus is too great, and below the calibration point it falls short.

By proper positioning of the straight line (calibration), nonlinearity can be quoted as half that of the previous example. This is the way specifications are given by most recorder manufacturers. It is a legitimate method, but the BMET should not misinterpret it. For example, when a writing system has inherent geometric nonlinearity, small-signal errors can greatly exceed such a nonlinearity specification. This is illustrated by the following example.

PITFALLS: HOW TO AVOID THEM

The channel for the writing system in Fig. 5-6 has 50 equal divisions in 100 mm of chart width, and the distance from the coil axis to the writing edge is 15 cm. Coil rotation for this system for full-scale deflection and its input-output curve would correspond closely to the figures used to demonstrate the various ways of calculating nonlinearity (Fig. 5-8).

If the manufacturer uses the interpretation of nonlinearity developed in Fig. 5-8*c*, the most favorable, the specification could read: "Nonlinearity $\pm\frac{1}{3}$ percent full scale ($\pm\frac{1}{6}$ division)." To check this specification, a variable-voltage source and a good digital voltmeter would be used. You might find that the pen would be within $\frac{1}{4}$ division of where the voltmeter says it should be at all points along the channel. You might conclude from this test that all traces on the chart would be accurate with $\pm\frac{1}{4}$ division. Yet, you would be wrong!

To illustrate, suppose a 5-Hz ac signal (constant amplitude) is fed into the same recorder and the attenuator set to give a trace amplitude of five lines peak to peak near the center of the chart. By means of the pen-position control, the trace could be moved laterally on the chart while the input stays constant.

Figure 5-9*a* shows the trace that would result. Near the chart center the peak-to-peak amplitude of the trace is five divisions. Near either edge of the chart, however, it has become 5.4 divisions. It appears that

Fig. 5-8 (*page 156*) To become familiar with recording error caused by nonlinearity, you should know how nonlinearity is specified. There are three ways to specify nonlinearity: (*a*) the slope-based method; (*b*) the maximum-deviation method; (*c*) the best straight line for minimum error.

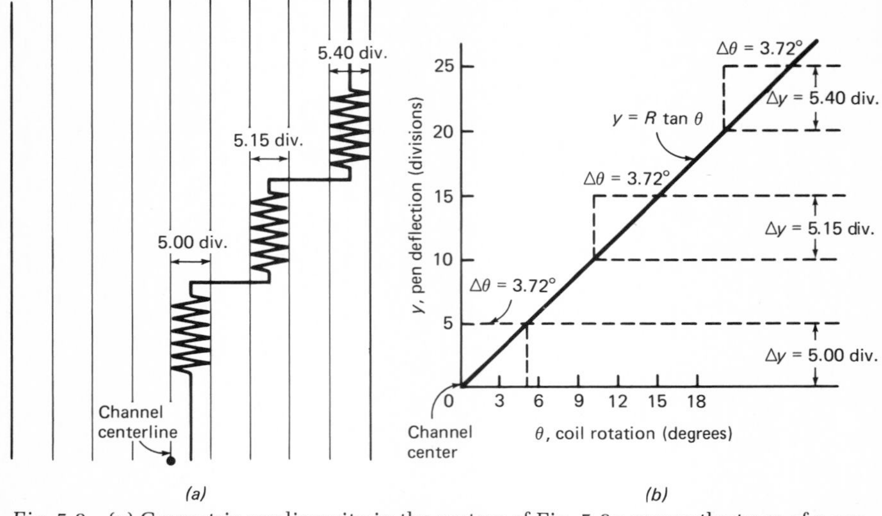

Fig. 5-9 (*a*) Geometric nonlinearity in the system of Fig. 5-6*a* causes the trace of a constant small-signal input to vary in amplitude at various positions across the width of the chart paper above. In (*b*) the coil rotation is in degrees vs. the pen deflection in divisions. The nonlinearity seen here creates the geometric nonlinearity seen in (*a*).

the signal has grown by 8 percent of its actual value. Is that nonlinearity of only $\pm\frac{1}{2}$ percent of full scale or $\pm\frac{1}{4}$ division?

The cause of this large error is explained in Fig. 5-9*b*. The geometry of this particular writing system is such that the slope of the pen deflection curve has changed a great deal near the chart edges. In other words, the slope, or scale factor, has increased at the channel edge due to the geometric nonlinearity of the writing system.

ELECTRONIC ERROR CORRECTION

The input-output curve for the rectilinear trace-writing mechanism of Fig. 5-6*b* is depicted in Fig. 5-10. This mechanism has about one-third the geometric nonlinearity of the previous device at a maximum deflection of $\pm 18°$. Nevertheless, it also produces small-signal errors in chart regions away from the channel center.

However, this mechanism is only a part of the complete writing system. The entire system includes a servoposition-feedback system and a noncontact position transducer which senses the angular position of the pen motor. The transducer output is an electric signal proportional to pen-motor coil rotation. Since the output of the position transducer appears to have the same error as the linkage, the apparent and real errors cancel one another, resulting in linear performance at the pen tip. This is shown in Fig. 5-11.

In practice, the output characteristic of the position transducer is

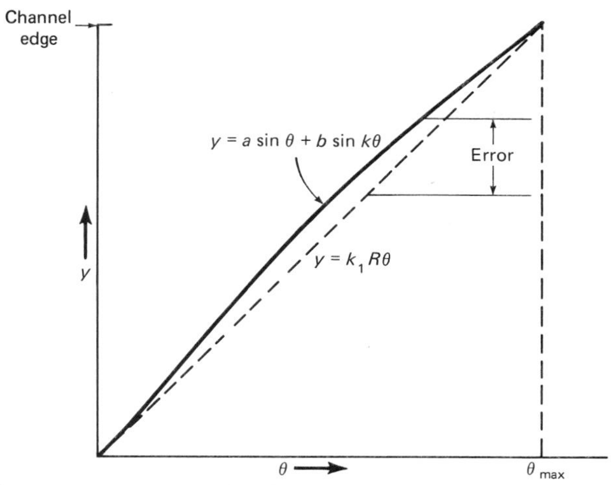

Fig. 5-10 This input-output curve for the system in Fig. 5-6*b* shows less inherent nonlinearity. However, some small-signal errors are seen in chart regions moving away from the channel center.

held within a tolerance of ±0.1 percent of the nominal linkage characteristic. Since the overall tolerance of the system is quoted as "nonlinearity ±½ percent of full scale," there is ample margin for differences in linkage that result from machining tolerances and eccentricities. A bonus benefit is obtained by including the drive amplifier and the coil of the pen motor in the feedback loop. Thus nonlinearity of the drive amplifier and of the magnetic field in the pen-motor structure are canceled as well.

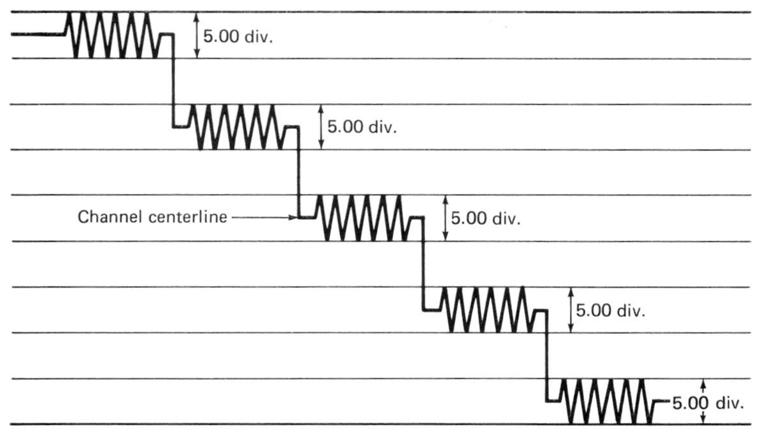

Fig. 5-11 Making use of servoposition-feedback control, the rectilinear trace-writing mechanism of Fig. 5-6*b* is now free from small-signal error. This fidelity is seen over the entire usable range of the recording paper, in contrast to (*a*), where different voltages show up as equal vertical divisions as a result of nonlinearity.

Most recorders using this system have nonlinearities of less than $\pm\frac{1}{4}$ percent, and some units have been measured to be linear within ± 0.1 percent of full scale. Of paramount importance is the fact that the amplitude of a small signal (or any part of a large signal) will be the same anywhere within the usable range of the instrument.

Thus most rectilinear trace-writing mechanisms have geometric nonlinearity. This can be greatly reduced, or totally canceled, by incorporating servoposition feedback in the writing system. The feedback loop can be extended back to the input side of the drive amplifier to cancel nonlinearity in that part of the system and to cancel nonlinearity contributed by nonuniformity of the magnetic field in the pen-motor structure.

The BMET must develop through experience a knowledge of the nonlinearity that can be tolerated. This will, of course, depend on how critical the medical application is. A good practice is to compare a questionable recorder with one whose linearity can be trusted. Should an intolerable difference be observed, check the servoposition-feedback circuitry in the recorder under test. Study of the recorder block diagram and schematic diagram will reveal the transducer which senses pen-motor coil rotation. Its amplifying circuitry then provides the servoposition-feedback signal. Feed a triangular wave into the recorder and adjust the feedback-amplifier gain for optimum linearity.

5-4 STORAGE AND RECALL

Pen and thermal chart recorders preserve data on paper. Once the data are recorded, the time base is fixed and the amplitude is fixed. In other words, it is impossible to vary the parameters for close examination. When a steady, recurring signal is observed on an oscilloscope, it can be squeezed, stretched, elongated, and shortened. In other words, it is live data.

Another problem with chart recorders is that they will not respond to what are considered very important data in the cell membrane, or to fast EMG (electromyogram) data and slow EEG (electroencephalogram) data. Muscle-fiber potentials, nerve-response potentials, and some EEG spikes are as short as a millisecond in duration. If they are not recurrent, they will pass so quickly that it would be impossible to study them on an oscilloscope. Tektronix, Hughes, and others manufacture a storage oscilloscope that allows chosen data to be frozen. Once the storage scope freezes the data, they are no longer alive—they cannot be altered. Another problem with the storage scope is that the scope must be activated at the very instant the elusive transient (desired data) appears. True, there are some medical specialists with nimble fingers who can catch a single pulse as it flashes by. However, these limitations discourage the widespread use of the storage scope in the medical field. In addition, today it is becoming more important to store live data for recall. This requires a digital format and some type of memory system. The marriage of data recording and computer techniques has created the need for two instruments which will now be discussed.

5-5
RECORDING TRANSIENTS

A transient recorder is an electronic instrument that uses digital techniques to record a preselected section of an analog signal as it varies with time. Thus the waveshape during the selected period of time is recorded and then held in the instrument's memory until a new recording is made or power is removed. While the information is stored in the memory, it can be (1) viewed as a reconstructed analog signal on an oscilloscope or *XY* display, (2) taken as a reconstructed analog signal for a strip-chart recorder to make a permanent record, (3) taken in digital form for a digital recorder, or (4) fed directly to a computer for signal analysis and processing.

The Biomation Model 802 Transient Recorder operates as shown in Fig. 5-12. A trigger to initiate the sweep is provided externally or can be derived from the input signal itself using trigger level and slope controls on the front panel. These controls are similar to their counterparts on better oscilloscopes.

The input signal is first amplified and then converted to its digital equivalent. The digital information is then stored in a semiconductor memory. The stored data output can be taken directly or can be processed through a digital-to-analog converter and smoothing circuit to reconstruct the analog input signal for presentation on an oscilloscope,

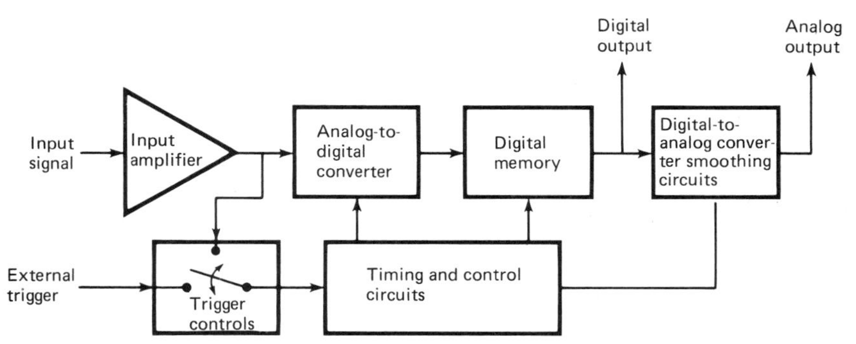

Fig. 5-12 Basic block diagram of the Biomation Model 802 Transient Recorder. The sweep is initiated by the input signal (or externally). The input signal is converted into digital form so that it can be stored in the memory. The stored data may be processed in the digital-to-analog converter for oscilloscope display.

strip chart, or YT recorder. Data in storage will remain there indefinitely until the instrument is instructed to make a new recording, when the new data will replace the old. Removing power from the instrument will erase the data from the memory.

TRIGGERING MODES

Triggering of the Model 802 Transient Recorder is accomplished in a manner identical to most modern oscilloscopes. The two basic types of triggering action are internal trigger or external trigger. The second choice is whether or not the trigger is obtained from the positive or negative slope of the signal. Finally, the trigger level determines the point on the waveshape at which the trigger or recording sweep is begun.

Aside from triggering internally or externally, there are three triggering modes: single, normal, and automatic.

In the single mode, the trigger circuit must be armed by pressing the ARM pushbutton or by applying a pulse. In this mode, the trigger circuit must be manually armed each time before new data will be stored in the memory. In the normal trigger mode, the trigger circuit will automatically be rearmed after each record and display cycle. In the automatic trigger mode, the trigger circuit is triggered at a fixed rate of every 0.1 s.

Figures 5-13 and 5-14 show typical input signals with the trigger levels indicated. Also shown in these figures are those portions of the input signals which would be stored in the transient recorder's memory.

TRANSIENT-RECORDER OPERATING MODES

The Biomation recorder has four different modes of storing data: trigger hold-off, delayed sweep, pretrigger recording, and switched time base.

In the trigger hold-off mode, dead time is added to the trigger circuit beyond the record time. Figure 5-15 illustrates a case where this mode would be used.

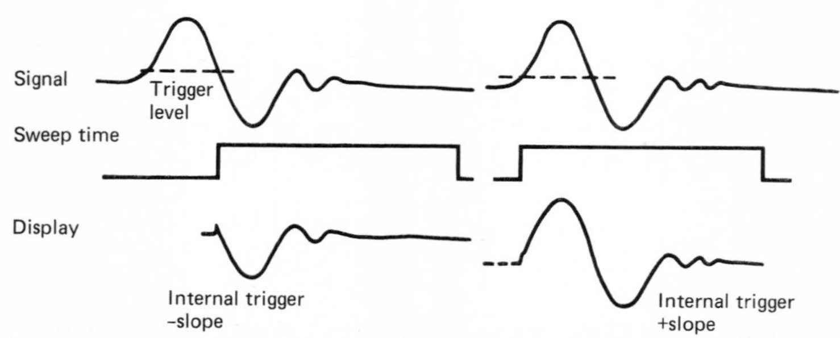

Fig. 5-13 Typical input signals with the internal trigger levels indicated. The horizontal dashed line denotes the trigger level. Portions of the input signal above this level will be stored in the memory.

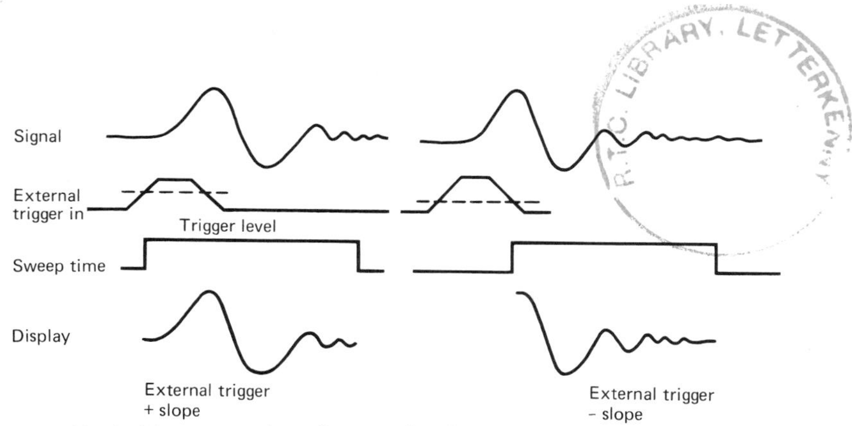

Fig. 5-14 Typical input signals and trigger levels. Again the signals above the trigger level will be stored. However, this time the sweep is initiated by an external trigger.

Let us suppose that we wish to examine a transient signal occurring at a low repetition rate. We wish to see how this signal changes over a period of time. "Normal" would be the selected trigger mode. Each signal is thus stored and displayed until the next signal comes along to replace it. If the desired signal is clean (amplitude disturbances are the object of investigation), there is no problem. However, following the desired signal there is often an unwanted amplitude disturbance which can trigger the instrument. In this case, the desired signal would be stored, but when the unwanted amplitude disturbance occurred, it would retrigger the recorder. The desired data would then be erased from the memory.

As shown in Fig. 5-15, the delay control can be used to "hold off" the

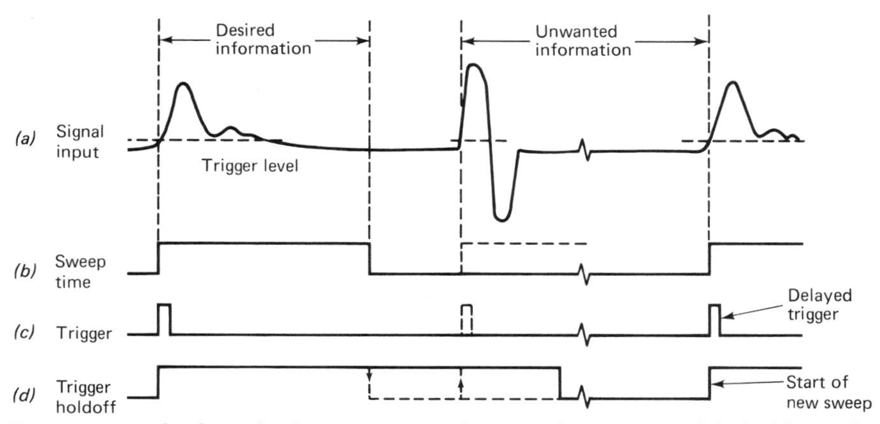

Fig. 5-15 (*a*) The desired information is seen between the two vertical dashed lines. (*b*) The new sweep would normally start at the third vertical dashed line and the unwanted information would be seen. (*c*) However, the trigger holdoff circuit has delayed the trigger. (*d*) The new sweep starts late, displaying only desired information.

trigger beyond the unwanted amplitude disturbance. This way, the desired data will not retrigger until the end of the delay period. Trigger hold-off delay time is adjustable to 10 times the sweep speed or 10 s, whichever is smaller.

The delayed sweep mode of operation is used in situations where the only good trigger signal precedes the data to be recorded. The delay between the trigger and the desired data may be greater than one sweep time. Thus the transient would not be captured with sufficient resolution to be useful. By delaying the sweep and operating at a faster sweep time, the data can be captured with good resolution.

Figure 5-16 shows a case where an external trigger is used, but the data to be captured are delayed from the trigger. The delay control in this mode of operation adjusts an internal delay so that the recording sweep will not start until the end of the delay period.

The pretrigger recording mode allows you to capture signals that you did not know you wanted to capture until after they had passed. This mode is also used when the only good trigger available follows the desired data (see Fig. 5-17).

In the two previous modes of operation, the memory is filled with new data when the trigger signal occurs. In the pretrigger recording mode, the memory is filled with data. However, these data are also being discarded at the same rate. When a trigger occurs, no further data are inserted in the memory; also no data are discarded. Thus the memory contains a block of information whose duration is equal to the sweep time. Since the memory is constantly storing and discarding data (stops on receipt of a trigger), the stored data are only of value in

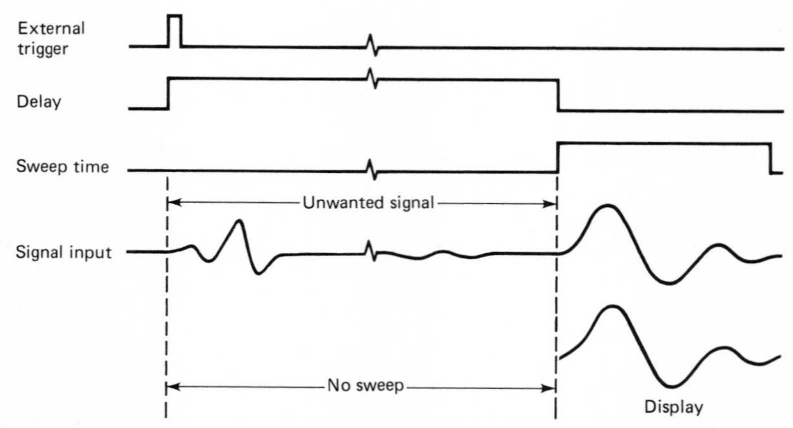

Fig. 5-16 By delaying the sweep and operating at a faster sweep time, the data can be captured with good resolution. The recorder is triggered externally, but the data to be captured are delayed from the trigger, and the unwanted signal is not displayed.

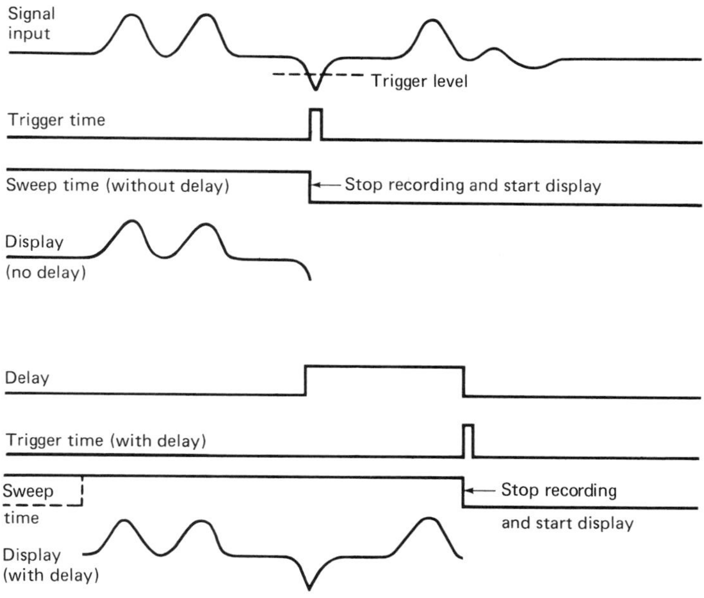

Fig. 5-17 Pretrigger recording. Here the only good trigger follows the transient or data we wish to capture. In this mode, information is not retained by the memory until a trigger occurs.

the single-sweep trigger mode. This mode can be put to good use when looking for an erratic cardiac pulse, muscle signal, or nerve impulse.

THE LIMITATIONS OF TRANSIENT RECORDERS

All instrument systems have their limitations. This is also true of transient-recording systems. These limitations should be carefully considered when deciding which type of storage system to use for biomedical data preservation or processing.

Let us start with the sampling rate. The sampling theorem states that the sampling rate must be at least twice the highest input frequency that we desire to measure. It is practical to have at least five data points with which to examine any complex waveform, such as a sine wave. If these data points occur within a cycle, some of the signal details can be observed. Sampling limitation can be seen when we operate a transient recorder at slow sweep speeds. The captured signal may have little or no relationship to the input signal. This limitation is avoided by using a higher sweep time or an external low-pass filter, limiting high-frequency input.

Another transient-recorder limitation is caused by output smoothing. The digital data leaving the recorder go through a smoothing digital-to-analog converter. This converter makes the output appear to be a somewhat continuous trace rather than the series of points normally expected from a digital instrument. However, the digital information in the memory might have a better risetime (pulse leading edge) than the visual presentation because of the smoothing circuit.

A third limitation in digital transient recorders is in amplitude resolution. For example, the Biomation Transient Recorder converts all analog input signals to an accuracy of 8 binary bits. This means that the resolution can be no better than 1 part in 256, or 0.4 percent accuracy.

The final transient-recorder limitation is time resolution. The Biomation's memory contains 1024 words of data. A word is a combination of bits and characters (refer to the glossary in Sec. 7-8). Normally only the first 1000 words are used on the CRT display. Any sweep time set on the front panel corresponds to the use of 1000 words of data. This means, with a sweep time of 500, a new data point is stored in the memory every 0.5 s, or 500 s/1000 words. This limitation in time resolution relates directly to the sampling-rate limitation as previously described.

5-6 THE NEUROGRAPH N-3

The Neurograph N-3 is an instrument which accepts high-frequency electric potentials from a physiological amplifier and places these potentials in a memory storage. It then automatically recalls these potentials from its memory. This happens slowly enough so that a chart recorder can produce a faithful representation of the high-frequency potentials over a longer time base.

To clarify this point, Fig. 5-18 illustrates a typical biomedical situation. In this stimulus-response setup, a stimulator excites some tissue by using a stimulating electrode. A synchronous output pulse from the stimulator triggers the Neurograph to store its input signals. These inputs originate in the excitable tissue and are detected by the recording electrodes connected to the input of a physiological amplifier. The output of the physiological amplifier provides the input signal for the Neurograph. The desired duration of the stored signal is determined by the record time base. This base can be controlled from 20 ms to 100 s.

Once the signal is in the memory storage, it can be recalled by using a time base of from 0.5 to 50 s. This feature allows the display of an action potential (or any other medical pulse) as short as 20 ms duration to be recalled on a time base of 50 s for display on a chart recorder. In its automatic mode, the Neurograph is ready to store after the memory has recalled the action potential. The entire sequence repeats automatically with the synchronous output pulse coming from the stimulator.

Figure 5-19 shows a record obtained from an intracellular electrode

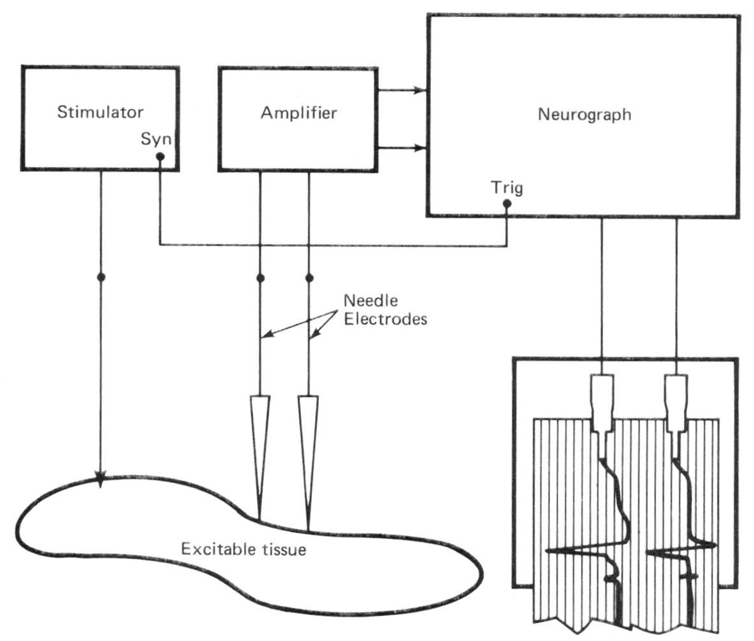

Fig. 5-18 A stimulator excites nerve tissue. A pulse from the stimulator triggers the Neurograph transient expander. Fast transients are recalled from the Neurograph's memory to be observed over a long time base.

in a muscle fiber. This record was obtained using the Neurograph in its scope mode with a nonstorage oscilloscope. The Neurograph repeatedly recalls the memory storage at a frequency of 50 Hz, so that the waveform is continuously displayed. Since the time base of the oscilloscope can be varied, a portion of the waveform can be examined in detail by increasing the sweep speed of the oscilloscope. Thus the need for a

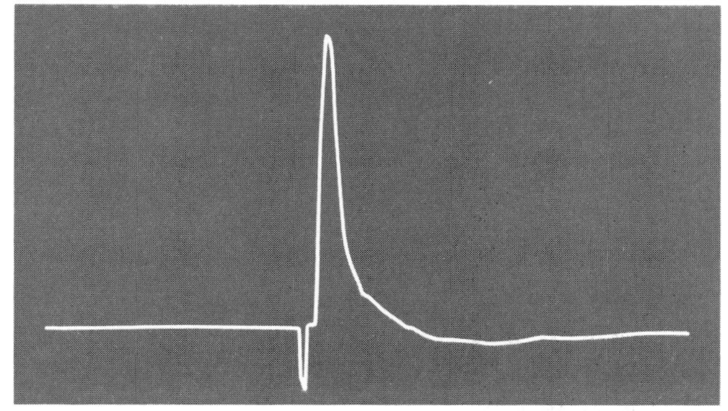

Fig. 5-19 A Neurograph recording of a muscle fiber obtained from an intracellular electrode. This transient waveshape was originally too fast to be seen by the naked eye. It is now continuously displayed as it was taken from the Neurograph's memory.

special storage oscilloscope is eliminated. Storage oscilloscopes cannot vary the time base once the event has been stored.

Furthermore, photography is simplified, since the Neurograph does not have the background haze from the flood guns that are used in the storage oscilloscope. The Neurograph permits an ordinary oscilloscope to do more than a storage oscilloscope, without the limitations of a storage oscilloscope.

5-7 TIME COMPRESSION

Thus far, the recording techniques discussed have either displayed the analog data in their actual "real time" form or expanded their time base so that very fast transients could be captured and slowed down for display on a chart recorder. In EEGs (and sometimes ECGs) there is exactly the opposite problem. A voluminous amount of data is obtained from the patient. A great deal of time-consuming interpretation by the physician is thus required. For example, an 8-hour EEG study of a sleeping patient presents a formidable problem in data reduction to obtain the necessary vital data. In this case, the vital data are the relative amplitudes of the various brain-wave components, for example, the relationship of the delta, theta, alpha, beta, and gamma waves to one another and to the overall raw data. In prolonged ECG studies, the averaged amplitude of the QRS complex might be the vital data. In both instances, some technique is called for to compress time. Thus only the vital data are taken from the voluminuous raw data.

5-8 THE MED EEG-5000

This system, made by Med Associates, is an EEG bandpass filter-integrator-multiplexer. It can accept the output of a standard EEG recorder or it can accept the output of an EEG tape recording. An 8-h EEG recording can be replayed at a playback-to-record ratio of 16 to 1 so that the vital data may be analyzed in 30 min. Five Butterworth active *RC* filters (with 30 dB/octave roll-off) discriminate between the delta, theta, alpha, beta, and gamma EEG components. Output from any of the five filters can be extracted individually. This might be done in an alpha-wave study.

Alpha-wave studies are now common in biofeedback and biorhythm research. Theta-wave studies are frequently undertaken in dream studies. Delta-wave analysis is common in epilepsy screening. Beta waves are important in determinations of hypertension. However, the key to conventional EEG clinical analysis is the relative comparison of the various EEG components.

Each filter in Fig. 5-20 is fed into individual integrators. Each of these integrators can sum its total input over a 5- or a 10-s period. Or the multiplexer can control the integrator period by its own reset pulse being fed back to reset each integrator. The multiplexed output is then applied to one EEG channel on an EEG recorder or to any single-channel chart recorder.

The result is a recording of the percentage of activity in each data band. Also, one integrator is used to measure the total amount of EEG activity, and this amplitude is then compared to the output of the inte-

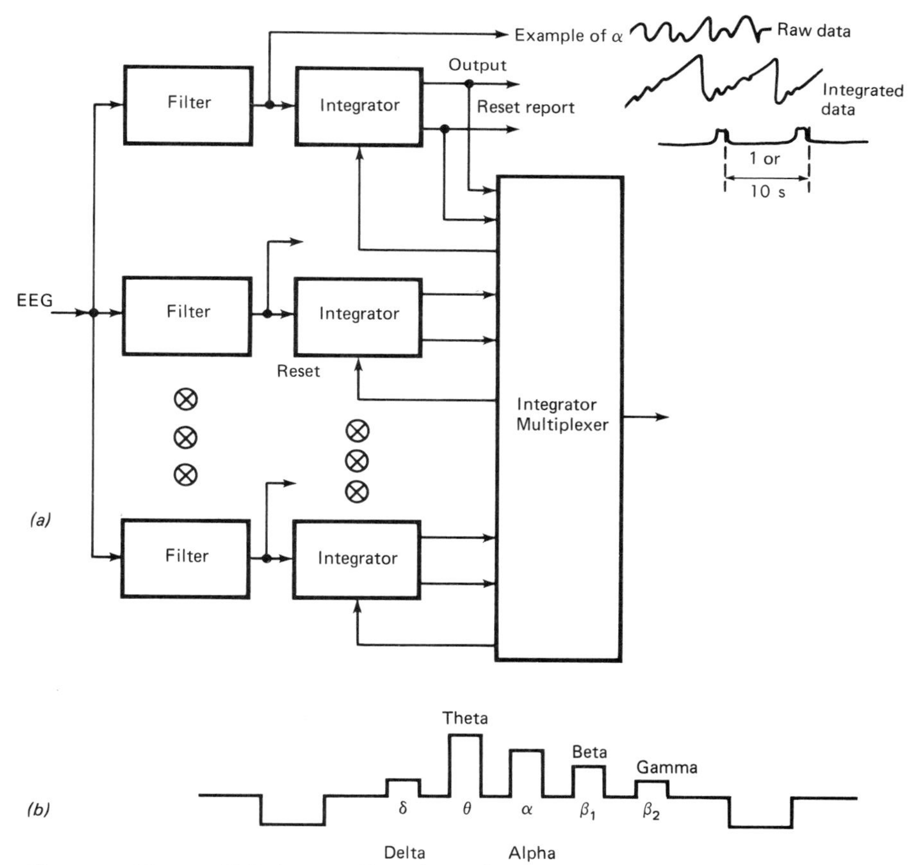

Fig. 5-20 The raw EEG data are filtered into their various component waves. The filter outputs are integrated over 10 s, then multiplied into single-channel data. On the right are shown examples of (a) the raw data, the integrated data, and (b) the final multiplexed data.

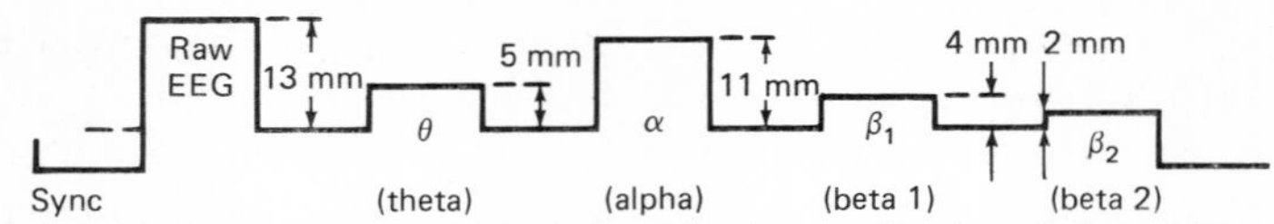

Fig. 5-21 A key parameter in EEG is the relative amplitudes of the various EEG frequency components. Here, the MED EEG-5000 shows the relative amplitudes of each EEG component and the intensity of each as compared to the raw data. The raw data and each of the components have been integrated over a 10-s period.

grators coupled to each filter. In Fig. 5-21, the following result is obtained:

$$\text{Total EEG} = 13 \text{ mm} \times 2 = 26 \text{ mm}$$

$$\% \text{ of } \theta = \frac{5 \text{ mm}}{26 \text{ mm}} \times 100 = 19.2\% \text{ theta}$$

$$\% \text{ of } \alpha = \frac{11 \text{ mm}}{26 \text{ mm}} \times 100 = 42.3\% \text{ alpha}$$

$$\% \text{ of } \beta_1 = \frac{4 \text{ mm}}{26 \text{ mm}} \times 100 = 15.4\% \text{ beta 1}$$

$$\% \text{ of } \beta_2 = \frac{2 \text{ mm}}{26 \text{ mm}} \times 100 = 7.7\% \text{ beta 2}$$

The total in these bands is 84.6 percent of all activity. The remaining 15.4 percent is contained in δ and frequencies beyond β_2. Time compression through filtering, integrating, and multiplexing has produced a readout displaying the vital data only. Studious interpretation by the medical specialist has been eliminated.

5-9 THE DIGITAL READOUT

The chart recorder and oscilloscope give us an analog waveshape. These data can then be interpreted by the specialist. The growing use of microprocessors allows us to process and interpret more data before they ever reach the readout. Thus the readout should appear in medically significant numerals. There are several devices that will produce a direct digital readout. There is the LED (light-emitting diode), the LCD (liquid crystal diode), and the electroluminescent display.

By adding a character generator and the proper synchronizing circuits to a CRT display, a digital CRT readout is produced. Alphanumeric printouts are produced by sending current through a tiny resistive element which becomes a segment of a letter or numeral. When this element is heated, it marks heat-sensitive chart paper. An alphanumeric printout results. Digital CRT displays (except for computer terminals) and alphanumeric printouts are not common in medical electronic instrumentation because of their high cost compared to the LED and LCD.

THE LED

With the LED we can obtain a direct readout of blood pressure, O_2 uptake, cardiac rate, or any other parameter that the instrument is programmed to analyze. An LED is a forward-biased semiconductor. The biasing of its PN junction creates carriers (electrons or holes) with excess energy. In the normal diode, this energy dissipates as heat. In the LED, this energy emerges as light.

Many of the semiconductors used to manufacture LEDs are made of gallium phosphide, which has a crystal structure like silicon. In 1955, the emission of red light from gallium phosphide was first discovered. Since then, growing crystals and PN junction formation has been found to be easier with gallium arsenide. This material is now used widely in LED manufacturing.

The color of the emitted light is determined by the band gap of the semiconductor and by the impurity levels in the band gap. Table 5-1 lists the band-gap energies of common semiconductor materials. The energies of photons giving the sensation of visible light are shown.

As Table 5-1 indicates, visible-light emission requires more energy than is available from gallium arsenide alone. Thus gallium arsenide is used with gallium phosphide and green is obtained. Nitrogen doping enhances this effect. Red and orange are obtained by doping with zinc and oxygen. LEDs are now used together with silicon photodiodes and phototransistors. These devices send and receive medical data via op-

Table 5-1 **Band-gap Energies of Common Semiconductor Materials**

Semiconductor	Band Gap, eV	Possible Emission Wavelengths, nm	Color
Silicon	1.1		
Gallium arsenide	1.41	900–950	Infrared
Gallium phosphide	2.33	560–570	Green
		575–585	Yellow
		590–600	Orange
		670–700	Red
Gallium arsenide phosphide:			
On GaAs substrates	2.00	650	Red
Nitrogen-doped on GaP substrates	2.0–2.20	625	Red
		590	Orange-yellow

tical coupling. When the small leakage currents found in electrical coupling are prohibitive, optical coupling is invaluable.

LCDS AND ELECTROLUMINESCENCE

The liquid crystal diode (LCD) is yet another device that gives an alphanumeric readout. The LCD uses a matrix of electrodes deposited under a thin layer of nematic liquid crystal. This matrix is then placed on a silicon wafer. The LCD consumes less power than the LED and has a wider viewing angle. Various colors are obtained with filters. LCD readouts are excellent for outpatient physiological monitors where battery drain must be kept at an absolute minimum.

Still another display device which holds great promise for the future is the electroluminescent display. An electroluminescent layer of material is driven by thin-film transistors deposited on a glass substrate. This device is more rugged than the LCD. A high voltage (200 V) is required for this type of display. A 6-in-square display of 12,000 elements contains 24,000 transistors overlaid by a phosphor layer of electroluminescent material. The same basic addressing technology (data reaching the proper element) is used for both electroluminescent displays and LCDs.

QUESTIONS

1. In a typical analog pen recorder, two signals are summed up with the input signal in a dc error amplifier. These signals are amplified to drive the pen motor. What are these two signals?
2. Describe the function of frequency conpensation in a typical pen recorder.
3. How is the position-feedback signal obtained?
4. What are the two advantages of the thermal recorder?
5. In the thermal recorder, what is the function of the commutator?
6. A multipole switch that governs the type of scanning done by the commutator is called the __________.
7. True or false: The drive amplifier powers the pen motor and also positions the pen.
8. Describe the output that a perfectly linear recording system produces as related to the input.
9. Maximum deflection nonlinearity is expressed as a percentage of what?
10. The ratio of maximum slope error (anywhere in the calibration curve) to the slope of the nominal sensitivity line is called what type of nonlinearity?
11. Briefly describe what instruments and test procedures would be used to test for recorder nonlinearity.
12. The position transducer output provides an electric signal which corresponds to the rotation of the __________.
13. The drive amplifier and the pen-motor coil are essential parts of the feedback loop. Describe the prime function of this loop.
14. Is it possible for a feedback loop to cancel nonlinearity at the input side of

the drive amplifier and also in the magnetic field of the pen-motor structure? Explain your answer.

15. What are two disadvantages of recording data on chart paper?

16. What are the major advantages of oscilloscope recording?

17. Would a standard oscilloscope be the best instrument to use to observe a very fast pulse which is not recurrent? Explain your answer.

18. To observe the data in Question 17, specify one advantage and one disadvantage of the storage oscilloscope.

19. On a digital transient recorder, why is the pretrigger feature so valuable?

20. You wish to record a frequency range from 5 to 120 Hz. According to the sampling theorem, what is the minimum sampling rate that may be used? Explain the consequence of using too low a sampling rate.

chapter 6

Ultrasonics and Telemetry

PART 1: ULTRASONICS

INTRODUCTION

Electromagnetic radiation in the audio part of the spectrum is not normally audible. However, acoustic radiation creates a disturbance in air pressure and becomes sound. We can increase the frequency of acoustic radiation to well beyond 10 MHz, and it becomes ultrasound. Ultrasound radiation can penetrate human tissue. It is reflected and refracted from acoustic interfaces. The changes in the direction of these sound waves can be compared to the bends that light makes while passing through a semitransparent material. This analogy should not be taken too seriously, however, for surfaces that reflect sound waves are not the same as those that reflect light or absorb x-rays. Diagnostic ultrasound is noninvasive. In the past, similar diagnoses could only be performed by an operation or an autopsy.

Within the past decade, ultrasound has gained tremendous popularity because it has no side effects, does not produce radiation damage, and causes no patient discomfort. The only connection between ultrasound and radiology is that they both develop an image of critical areas.

6-1 THEORY OF REFLECTANCE

Ultrasonic diagnostic technique is based on the theory of the reflection coefficient. This phenomenon depends on the specific acoustic impedance mismatch at a physical junction between two homogeneous media. In a simplified analogy, the transmitted ultrasonic wave flows like water along a straight, open gully. Suddenly the water (wave) encounters a large hill (impedance). It is then reflected or diverted away from its straight path.

In the body, acoustic impedance is seldom constant over any volume large enough to allow simple reflection theory to be used. In optics, the term *reflectance* is used to describe the expected, relative intensity of a wave which has been scattered from inhomogeneous structures. In ultrasonics, reflectance is the expected value of energy of a pulse reflected from a small volume of tissue back to the source transducer. Some arbitrary standard is used, and the ultrasonic-beam parameters are always constant. By far the largest single factor that affects reflectance is the angle of incidence. Another factor, relative reflectance, is a function of the time and space parameters of an ultrasonic beam. The relative reflectance of a small volume in space is proportional to the square of the relative amplitude of the reflected echo.

In ultrasonics, the propagated wave is said to be longitudinal. That is, the wave particles move in the same direction as the flow of energy. The particle oscillates around its mean position. This movement permits energy to flow through the medium. The velocity of energy transmission depends on the delay which occurs between this energy and the adjacent particles. The density and elasticity of the medium being penetrated determine the propagation velocity. This parameter, expressed in milliseconds, varies for different materials, as can be seen in Table 6-1. A given relationship exists between the wave velocity V and the characteristic impedance of the medium Z in determining the particle pressure P. This relationship can be represented as $P = VZ$.

When a wave meets the boundary between two different media, it may be partially reflected. The laws of optics determine the relative direction of the reflected wave. If the transmitted energy is interfered with by a reflected wave, then a standing wave is said to exist. The thickness of the medium at each plane, where the ultrasonic energy encounters resistance, affects transmission. If the thickness of the mate-

Table 6-1 **Average Values of Characteristic Impedances, Propagation Velocities, and Absorption Coefficients of Common Biomedical Material**

Material	Propagation Velocity, ms^{-1}	Characteristic Impedance Z, $(kg \cdot s/m^2) \times 10^{-6}$	Absorption Coefficient at 1 MHz, dB/cm
Air at STP	331	0.0004	12
Blood	1570	1.61	0.18
Brain	1541	1.58	0.85
Fat	1450	1.38	0.63
Kidney	1561	1.62	1.0
Liver	1549	1.65	0.94
Muscle	1585	1.70	1.3 (along fibers) 3.3 (across fibers)
Skull bone	4080	7.80	13
Water	1480	1.48	0.0022

rial is less than one-quarter wave, or an integral number of half-waves, the material does not affect transmission. However, the medium promotes complete energy transmission when its thickness is an odd integral number of one-quarter wavelengths.

6-2 ABSORPTION

Absorption in the medium is due to the relaxation mechanism. Energy exists between molecular, lattice, and vibrational relationships. The movement of ultrasound disturbs the equilibrium between these energy forms. The energy-phase difference results from varying equilibrium times. This phase delay increases with frequency. Thus, absorption goes up with increased frequency. From 1 to 10 MHz, the absorption coefficient is proportional to frequency. Absorption is determined by the total protein content. The ratio of blood absorption increases up to 10 MHz. In the bones of the skull, it increases up to 2 MHz. Below 2 MHz, absorption is proportional to the square of frequency. For lung tissue at 1 MHz, absorption has been found to be 41 dB/cm.

This relatively high absorption is thought to be due to the radiation of energy by pulsating gaseous structures. An ultrasonic wave may be attenuated during propagation by being diverted from a parallel beam, or it can be scattered by small discontinuities in characteristic impedance. Convergence of the ultrasonic beam is a result of an increase in intensity as the wave moves closer to a focal point. When a wave is totally absorbed, then all the ultrasonic energy is converted into heat. In the 1- to 5-MHz range, the absorption coefficient of soft tissue is expressed in decibels per centimeter. It is proportional to frequency.

REFRACTION AT BOUNDARIES

In Fig. 6-1*a* the transmitted ultrasonic wave encounters the boundary between two media. The angle of incidence is not oblique, so there is no refraction. Propagation takes place with no deviation in the receptive medium. However, in Fig. 6-1*b*, the ultrasonic wave encounters the boundary at an oblique angle. As the angle is oblique, refraction takes place (unless the initial medium and the receptive medium both have equal velocities). Only a fraction of the transmitted wave may be reflected at the boundary when the angle of incidence is not oblique, or is extremely small. This type of reflection is called *specular*. The instantaneous values of velocity and particle pressure are always constant. The velocity and density determine the medium's characteristic impedance Z. As a wave moves across the boundary between two media, the particle velocity and the pressure remain continuous. In each medium, the

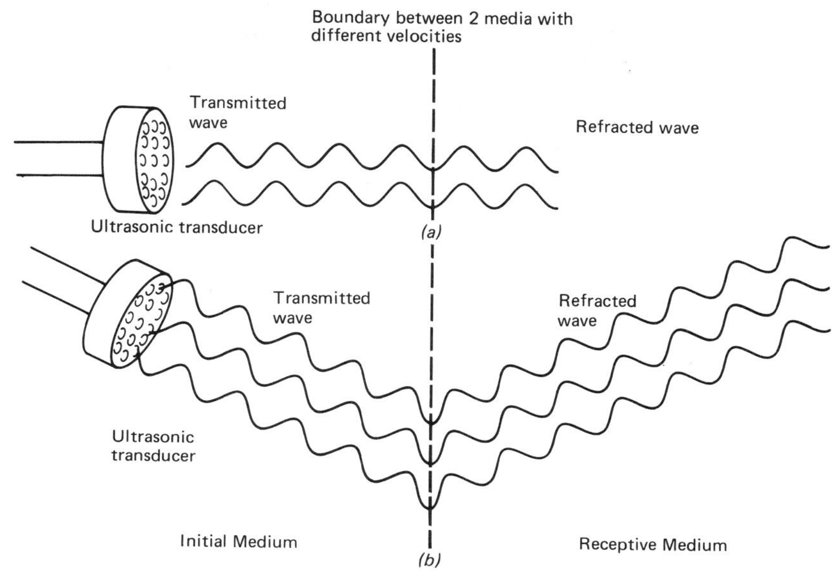

Fig. 6-1 As we see in (*a*), when the incident angle of the transmitted wave and the media boundary is 90°, there is practically no reflection from the media boundary. In (*b*), however, a sharp angle of incidence produces a similar angle between the reflected wave and the media boundary.

ratio of particle pressure to velocity is fixed, determining the characteristic impedance.

6-3 THE DOPPLER EFFECT

In Fig. 6-2*a*, the transmitted ultrasonic wave encounters a stationary reflector. The returning, or reflected wave, has the same frequency as the transmitted wave. In Fig. 6-2*b*, the reflecting boundary is moving toward the transmitting source. The result is a compression of the reflected wave. In Fig. 6-2*c* the reflecting boundary is receding. This time, the wavelength of the reflected wave is expanded. Wavelength and frequency have a reciprocal relationship. This frequency shift (for both advancing and receding reflectors) is known as the *Doppler effect*.

DETERMINING DOPPLER SHIFT

Where F_s is the source frequency and F_r (Fig. 6-2) is the reflected frequency, we may call the Doppler shift F_c. Then the frequency change $F_c = F_r - F_s$. If it is possible to determine the velocity of the moving boundary barrier, then we measure Doppler shift as

$$F_c \times \text{speed of sound} = \text{velocity} \times \text{transmitting frequency}$$

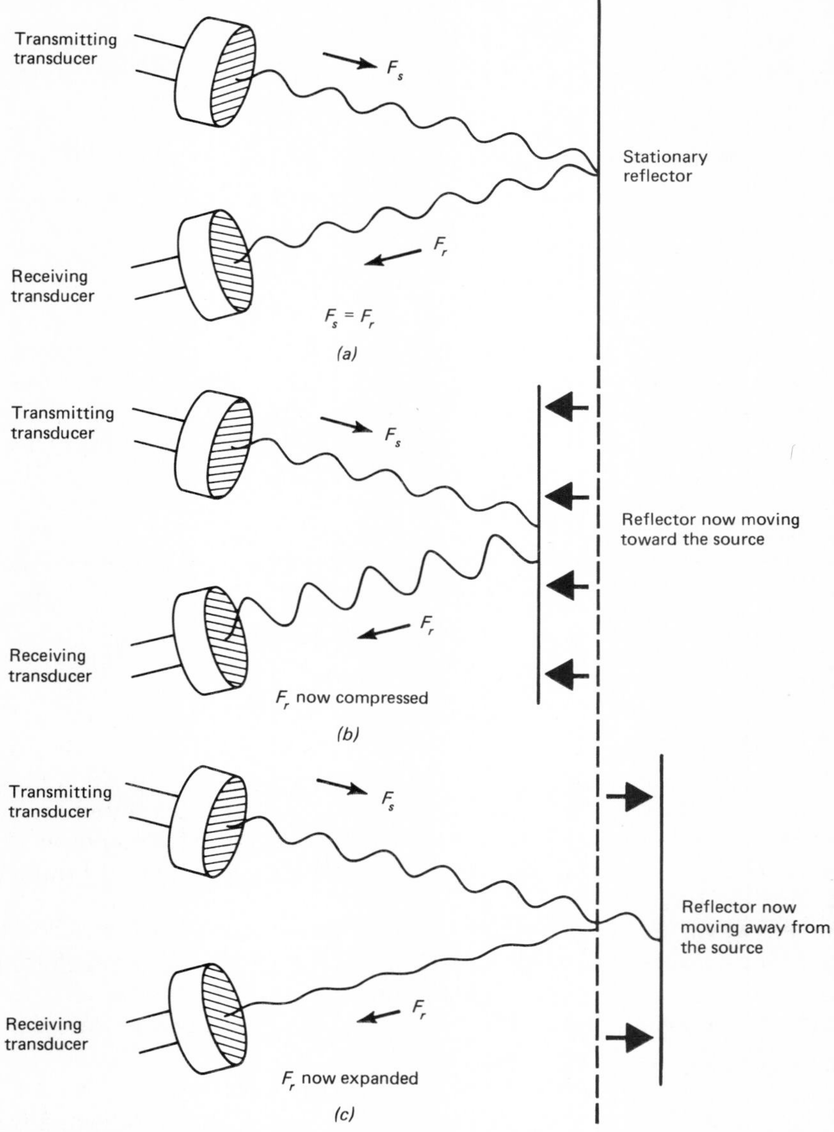

Fig. 6-2 Understanding the Doppler effect is simplified by examining the frequencies of the radiated wave (F_s) and the reflected wave (F_r). (*a*) When the reflector is stationary, both waves are equal in frequency. (*b*) The reflecting surface (or body) is moving toward the source. F_r is now compressed, or is lower in frequency. (*c*) The reflective surface moves away from the source, F_r is expanded in time, or rises in frequency.

When the transmitting frequency is known, the factor then becomes the boundary's velocity. Where the velocity of the boundary is known, then the Doppler shift can be calculated by

$$F_c = \frac{\text{velocity} \times \text{freq. of transmitted wave}}{\text{speed of sound}}$$

where the velocity is expressed in seconds and the frequency in hertz.

6-4 DOPPLER ARTERIOGRAPHY

Ultrasonic arteriography is used to define the geometry of the interface between flowing blood and the artery wall. A relatively high-frequency ultrasonic wave of 5 MHz is used to produce an extremely high resolution system. Using pulse-echo ultrasound imaging, it has been discovered that large, clearly visible echoes are produced from healthy arterial walls. These healthy arterial walls are used as references. They have reflectance levels of 0 dB. Blood itself has a reflectance level of −20 dB. Calcified deposits or plaques with flakes (or lumps) have a reflectance level of 0 to +10 dB. Hard calcified shells in the arterial wall may have a reflectance level of up to +20 dB. Atherosclerotic plaques (the worst condition) have reflectance values of about +40 dB.

The tubular channel (lumen) of a healthy blood vessel appears as a dark hole due to the very low backscattering from blood. Arterial lesions that are atherosclerotic also produce very low backscattering from blood. Such lesions can be confused with blood. Doppler blood-flow detection differentiates between normal flowing blood and nonscattering occlusions. Arteriography can map the blood vessel channel or lumen just as the imaging of static tissue is developed by using the ultrasonic B-mode technique. B-mode imaging will outline the region through which flow is occurring; however, it cannot identify the arterial walls or even show areas that are calcified. By identifying the arterial wall, the arterial constituents, and their dimensions, we have a valuable tool to study the progress of atherosclerosis.

6-5 B-MODE DOPPLER SCANNING

When ultrasound is scattered back from tissue, the relative measured power is proportional to the relative reflectance of the tissue at the corresponding depth. Of course, the propagation losses in the tissue attenuate the transmitted signal. Using the amplitude of the envelope of the echo to intensity modulate an oscilloscope, one line of a conventional

B-mode image is produced. When multiple lines are displayed, a full image is created.

The reflectance of blood is low, but its high velocity will produce a Doppler shift. As we have seen, the Doppler frequency F_c is the difference between the transmitted frequency F_s and the echo. F_c can be calculated by

$$F_c = \frac{2 \times \text{blood-flow speed}}{\text{speed of sound}} F_s \sin \phi$$

where F_s = transmitting frequency or source frequency
ϕ = Doppler angle between transducer beam and normal flow

The phase of each returned echo is sampled at a point which corresponds to the particular depth which the transmitting signal traveled.

In ultrasonics, as in radar, the number of pulses transmitted over a given time determines the rate of sampling. That is, the more returning pulses or echoes we have, the more information is obtained. The number of pulses is called the *pulse-repetition frequency* (PRF). The time rate of change of the sampled pulse is equal to the Doppler audio

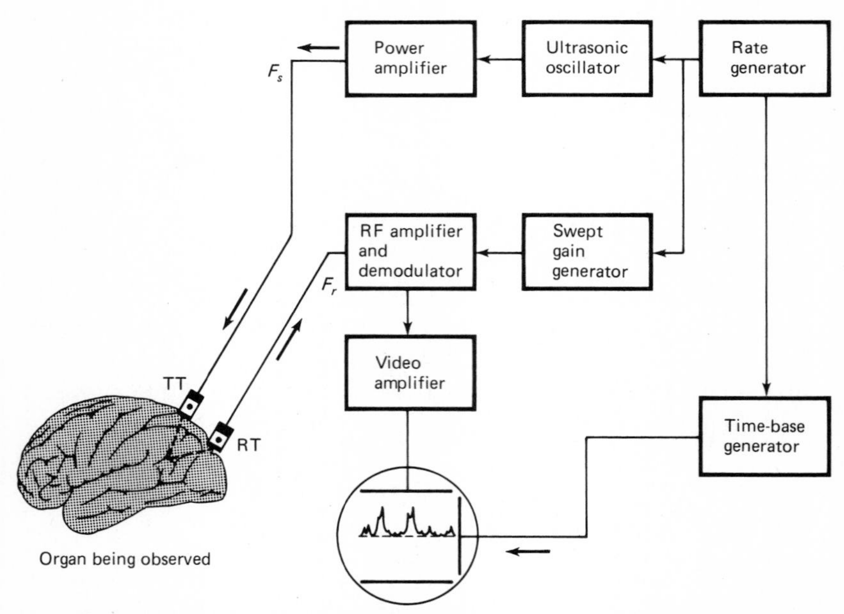

Fig. 6-3 The transmitting transducer (TT) sends the radiated ultrasonic wave (F_s) into the human brain. The receiving transducer (RT) receives the reflected wave (F_r). This wave is amplified, then displayed on a CRT. The rate generator (upper right) triggers the time base so that the time between TT and RT can be measured. The rate generator also controls the amplification of the signal from RT.

frequency. The returning echo is fed to a circuit which changes the minute Doppler frequency change into a particular voltage. This voltage is used to vary the brightness (intensity modulate) of an oscilloscope. A threshold detector is used to produce a white spot on the CRT when any flow is discernable. The total image is created by questioning enough points in the artery to cover the anticipated flow.

A cross section of the carotid artery is shown in Fig. 6-4. The Doppler angle is developed, giving the complete image of the arterial channel. Several repetitions of sampling take place over one cardiac cycle to yield about 10 points of Doppler data. The echo scan produces several complete two-dimensional images per second, whereas only 10 points of Doppler information are obtained each second.

6-6 ECHO-TONE

Doppler oscilloscope displays are extremely accurate, but they can also be expensive. In Doppler applications such as the detection of a fetal pulse, low-cost instruments are necessary. The Echo-tone technique allows a low-cost instrument to detect the fetal pulse as early as the tenth week of pregnancy and to localize the placenta since maternal

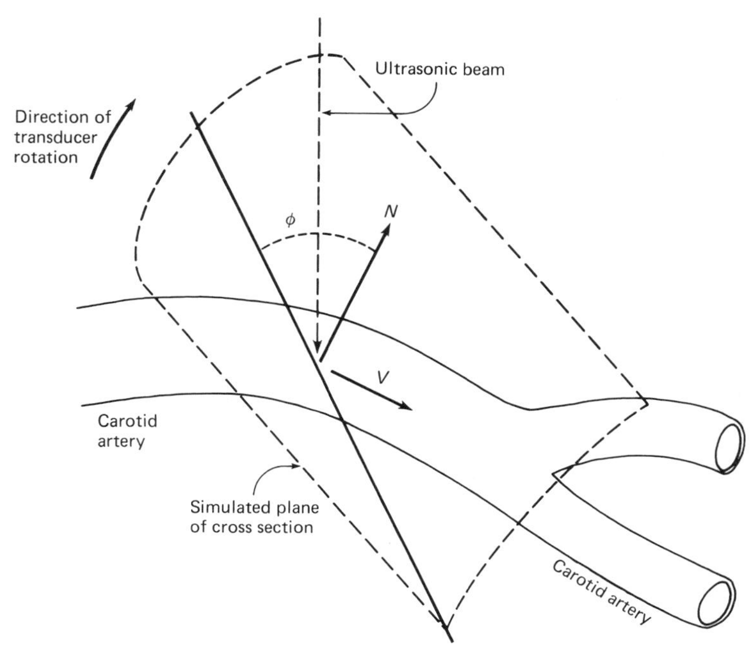

Fig. 6-4 Cross section of a carotid artery. V is the direction of blood-flow velocity, N is a vector normal to V and in a plane normal to the image plane, and ϕ is the Doppler angle.

arterial and venous blood flow have different velocities. A piezoelectric transducer converts the reflected Doppler frequency change into an audible tone. The pitch of this tone is then proportional to the velocity of blood or tissue movement. Although not shown in Fig. 6-5, the Echo-tone's output may be connected to a tape recorder, oscilloscope, or a fast chart recorder.

6-7 OBSTETRICS

Medical ultrasound is the child of sonar techniques used to detect ships and schools of fish. A professor of obstetrics (H. Donald) once observed that the fetus in the uterus and ships are both surrounded by fluid. He described how the placenta might be located by ultrasound. In this way, multiple pregnancies and fetal anomalies such as hydrocephalus could be detected. Precise measurements of the biparietal diameter in the fetus have become an important medical technique. The B-scan ultrasound examination during pregnancy has become as commonplace as the chest x-ray when the hospital patient is admitted. B-scan ultrasound permits the fetus to be dated, indicates twins, and outlines the placenta. The fetal heart motion can also be visualized. A B-scan display shows the orientation of the fetal head by scanning longitudinally and transversely, then observing the intracranial echoes. The diameter is then measured by switching to A-scan display. Even when the embryo skull is membranous, and the fetal brain mostly fluid, the sound velocity is not affected enough to destroy the accuracy of the results. With these techniques, the fetal skull is measured as early as the fourteenth week.

Accurate placenta localization is urgent when there is hemorrhaging or when amniocentesis is planned. If nuclear radiation were used, the mother would be exposed to approximately 500 millirems of radiation. Even radioisotope scanning involves some irradiation. The accuracy of ultrasonic placenta localization has been confirmed by cesarean section and by uterine exploration during delivery.

6-8 ECHOENCEPHALOGRAPHY

In this ultrasonic technique, a single wave of pulsed energy is transmitted through the head. The bony skull transmits sound so poorly that only intracranial structures such as the lateral ventricles and the midline can cause a sizable reflection. The reflected echo is then seen on an oscilloscope. The midline echo display is known as an A-scan display. Echoencephalography is used to select appropriate sites for an operation. It is also used to diagnose primary brain tumor, metastatic brain tumors, intracerebral hematoma, and intracerebral abscesses. Transdural echoencephalography is used to find cerebral infarctions, foreign bodies, and embedded bone fragments, and to guide a biopsy needle. The results of these examinations can determine the extent and depth of brain lesions and can select the site of a cortical incision.

THE ECHO-TRACE

In echoencephalography, ventricular measurements, breast exams, and pericardial effusion, a popular instrument is the Echo-trace. This instrument displays the reflected echo on a 5-in oscilloscope. The trace may then be photographed with a Polaroid camera. In Fig. 6-6 we see the strong reflected midline echo of the brain. This A-scope procedure shows the echo from the third ventricle. This echo has a high amplitude and appears in the middle portion of the trace. If a midline echo "complex" were seen, it would have a broad base with pulse-synchronous amplitude pulsations. If the strong, middle-area echo does not appear, we are alerted to an obstruction or other midline defect.

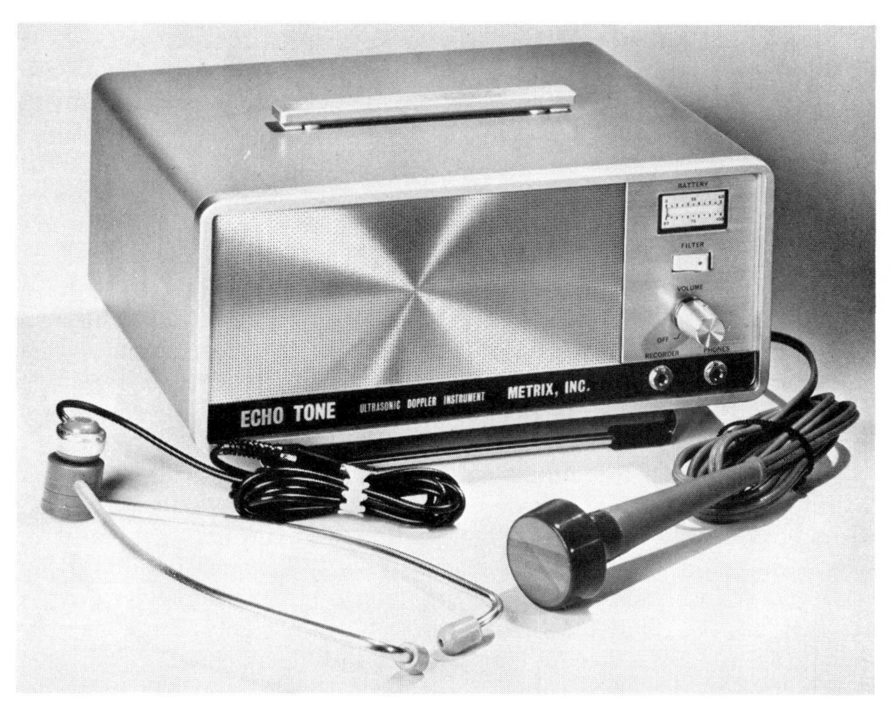

Fig. 6-5 The Metrix Echo-tone can detect the fetal heart in the tenth week of pregnancy. It can also localize the placenta and detect multiple pregnancies. (*Courtesy of Metrix Ultrasound*)

6-9
THE A-SCAN TECHNIQUE

When an ultrasound technique is based on the averaged amplitude of returning echoes, it functions in the A-scan mode. The depth of tissue is shown by the horizontal base line. The relative strength of the echo is represented by the vertical deflection from the base line. The strength of the returning echo can easily be measured on the vertical graticules of the CRT display. What is missing is the anatomical orientation. In other words, the lateral relationship of one echo to another is unknown. The anatomical orientation is essential if we are to correctly evaluate the amplitude data. The amplitude data (echo strength) are largely determined by the angle of incidence and the absorption of the overlying tissue. The details of this phenomenon were explored earlier in Sec. 6-1.

6-10
THE B-SCAN TECHNIQUE

Here we have an ultrasonic technique that gives us excellent anatomical and lateral orientation data. However, there is almost no contrast gradient, so that it is difficult to distinguish amplitude differences with the naked eye. The B mode is based on an entire plane being scanned. The reflection amplitude-modulates the intensity of a two-dimensional raster. Each echo becomes one dot. While the strength of that echo is lost (except for the intensity-modulation feature), a composite picture of many echoes is being built. In the B-mode technique, many waves are entering the body from many angles. The composite total of these is placed on the oscilloscope display simultaneously. In this way a cross-sectional or longitudinal (sagittal or coronal) view is built up. In a variation of the B-mode technique, a single beam of ultrasound is displayed in the B-mode form. This is called the M mode. In both B mode and M mode, the array of discrete bright spots on the screen corresponds to points of flow in the image plane.

It is important to remember that A scan is essentially a sampling technique. As much as 50 or 60 percent of the data may be lost. Although B scan with intensity modulation has a low contrast gradient, a video-inverted display can compensate for this. An area with edema can be seen with the naked eye. This inverted light intensity manages the gray scale so that the high-contrast portion of the available gray scale presents only a limited part of the amplitude data, and compression is used to accent amplitude changes.

Another ultrasonic technique makes use of the quantized image. An ultrasonic display containing a tumor has obvious geometric distortion. However, whether the displaced tissue is fat, optic nerve, or tumor tissue cannot be determined. By quantizing or repeatedly building the same echo, the details of the geometric distortion are developed so that a high-resolution acoustic profile appears. The shadow that is cast can then be identified as a tumor.

6-11
CARDIOLOGY

Ultrasonic techniques in this area have only begun to scratch the surface. The measurement and examination of all parts of the heart in motion is now feasible, including valve action, wall thickness, and stroke volumes. Any part of the heart cycle may be seen live, in a display similar to a movie stop-action scene. Atrial myxomas and congenital lesions in the heart can be observed. Mitral-valve lesions can be diagnosed. An ultrasonic system with 20 transducers located around the heart has displayed the detailed movement of all the cardiac chambers and valves as the motion occurred.

Pericardial effusion can be visualized by combining angiocardiography and echocardiography. Adding the ultrasonic technique eliminates the possibility of false negative-isotope indications. The angiocardiography eliminates the possibility of false echoes.

Ultrasonics allows the visualization of a ventricular profile within seconds. Only the first echo is used. A sharp outline of the ventricle is plotted by the echo's location along its time base. The amplitude or strength of the echo is not a factor. Local composite contours develop models of cardiac pumping performance. Visualizing of ventricular contours has previously been limited by the extent of catheter miniaturization. Catheter orientation has been greatly advanced by the use of ultrasonic echoes which program a computer. This computer then becomes the guidance system which steers the automated catheter along its route. Thus new techniques are made possible by the combining of technologies.

6-12
INTERNAL MEDICINE

Ultrasonics is used to visualize organs with a wide gray scale to bring out detail. The thyroid, gall bladder, and knee pathology can be diagnosed. By combining radioisotope aortography and ultrasonic nephrosonography, high accuracy is achieved in differentiating cystic from solid renal masses. The need for surgery can be determined by these techniques.

As we have seen, an ultrasonic wave passing through a fluid without interfaces produces no echo. This same effect is observed in a homogenous solid tumor. Two lesions can be discriminated ultrasonically by the degree of "through transmission." When the posterior wall of the lesion gives a strong echo, the lesion is probably cystic. On the other hand, if the posterior-wall echo is feeble, a diagnosis of a solid tumor can be made. In gynecology this ability to discriminate between solid and cystic tumors has been used to distinguish between fibroids and ovarian cysts. Ultrasonics is now used to discriminate between lesions in the liver and kidney. Excretory urograms are sometimes inconclusive or cannot be obtained because of poor renal function. Ultrasonics has been especially helpful in patients with chronic renal disease to rule out hydronephrosis and in the evaluation of patients who are allergic to contrast media or who cannot tolerate arteriography. Biopsy of the liver was once blind; it is now done under ultrasonic guidance. All renal tissue and kidney stone examinations are now being done with ultrasonic techniques.

6-13 SIMPLIFIED A-SCOPE CIRCUIT

Figure 6-3 shows a block diagram of an A-scope Doppler system. The term A scope was taken from the early days of radar when the radar field was an A-scope display. The rate generator triggers the time base, transmitter, and swept-gain generator simultaneously. The oscillator generates the ultrasonic wave, which is amplified by the power amplifier. The amplified output is then the source frequency F_s.

The ultrasonic pulse is delayed by about 13 μs/cm through the soft tissue of the organ under study. The reflected wave F_r is received by the

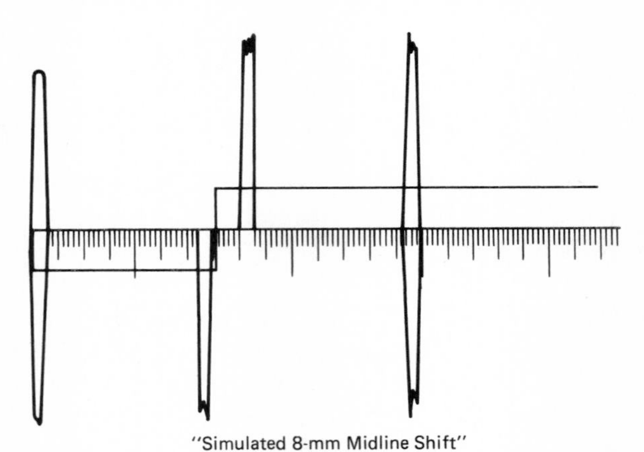

Fig. 6-6 The Metrix Echo-trace display. A strong midline reflection without other reflections indicates a normal patient. (*Courtesy of Metrix Ultrasound*)

receiving transducer (RT) and amplified. The swept-gain generator increases this amplification according to the energy absorption that takes place. The swept-gain generator is adjusted so that a given interface boundary produces a consistent appearance of the A-scan display, independent of the depth of the boundary. The demodulated video feeds the Y deflection plates of the CRT, giving vertical deflection. A variable delay might be added between the rate generator and the time base. That would allow reflections from distant interface boundaries to be observed on a very fast time base. In such a system, a typical rate generator would operate between 50 and 1000 Hz and might be synced to the 60-Hz power line or to a multivibrator. The time base usually runs about 25 μs for small organs such as the eye. However, the time base would be slowed down to 1 ms when examining a large organ (echoes from relatively large depth) like the stomach. Inexpensive systems using this principle would eliminate the oscillator and power amplifier. Instead, an SCR (silicon controlled rectifier) would discharge a capacitor through TT, the transmitting transducer. In order to observe very weak and very strong echoes, a typical system would have a dynamic range of 100 dB.

6-14 CRITERIA FOR CLINICAL ECHO SCANNING

Although no ultrasonic instrument can be optimal for all applications, instruments for universal application have been developed. In cardiovascular studies a live moving picture introduces a new dimension. The emphasis is on structure identification and speed of response. However, in organ imaging and obstetrics, picture detail is most important. To image the soft tissues of the brain through the intact skull, a relatively low frequency, of the order of 1 to 2 MHz, must be used. Because of the consequently longer wavelength, the resolution is limited to approximately 1 mm. Therefore a balance must be realized between penetration and resolution.

One of the key criteria of a live imaging system is that visual surveys of large regions can be made very rapidly. Detailed examinations can then be directed to selected areas. The resulting increase in the efficiency with which routine procedures can be performed is an important step toward achieving widespread clinical use of ultrasound. In addition to the many practical features inherent in a good clinical instrument, the following general criteria describe a versatile ultrasonic system.

1. *Real-time imaging* with response fast enough to follow the motion of any structure of the body. This should include the capability for

stop-action image storage as well as provision for dynamic recording.

2. *Hand-held contact probe* with a very small transmit-receive aperture for application to any point of the body at any angle.
3. *Wide-angle field* of view with provisions for magnification and minification in a large-screen format.
4. *Image-quality properties* such as resolution and gray scale should permit general clinical use, including intracranial procedures.

6-15 THE ECHOSTAT

The Echostat is one instrument system used in cardiology, neurology, obstetrics, and general organ imaging which embodies the features mentioned above. It is a wide-angle electronic sector scanner based on the original work of Somer, which began in 1967 and resulted in the clinical neurological use of prototypes in Holland and Germany.

The principle of operation of the Echostat (made by Diagnostic Electronics Corp.) is the electronic phasing of a small ($\frac{1}{2}$ by $\frac{1}{2}$ in) array of crystals (Fig. 6-7). Because the radiating-receiving surface consists of many small elements, it can be electronically controlled not only to generate and steer a beam of ultrasound but also to focus it. In essence, it can simulate a single, large curved crystal with an electronically variable focal point (Fig. 6-8).

The field of examination can be electronically varied in depth, width, and direction (Fig. 6-9). The origin of the display sweep can be oriented to agree with the position of the probe on the patient for a particular clinical measurement. The scale of the display can be 0.5, 1.0, 1.15, or

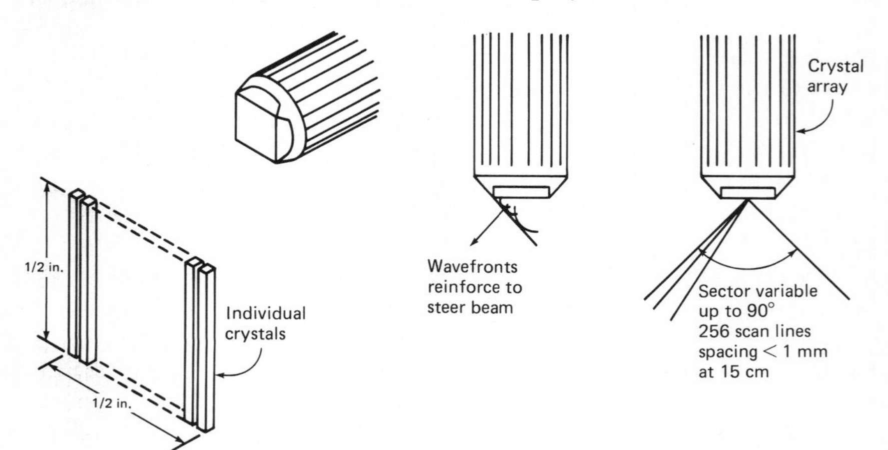

Fig. 6-7 Principles of electronic sector scanning. Multiple crystals placed in an array steer and focus ultrasonic waves.

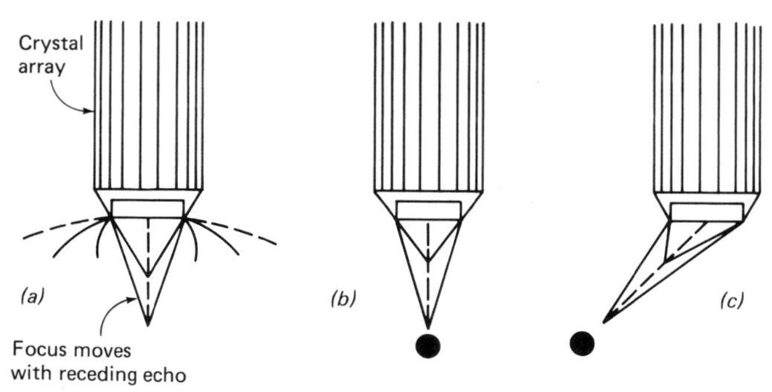

Fig. 6-8 Dynamic electronic focusing of phased array. In the receiving array (*a*), the phasing is continuously focused on the receding echo point. In (*b*) and (*c*), transmitting arrays focus on the target or dot.

2.0. The 1.15 scale approximates standard x-ray magnification. The width of the field can be varied from a sector of 0 to 90°, the depth from 3 to 30 cm, and the direction of the sector to any part of the full 90°.

The image quality (Fig. 6-10) can be optimized independently by controlling the signal sensitivity for tissues at different depths in the body. Several signal-processing modes may be chosen, including gray scale and edge detection. Dynamic focusing may be used during transmission and reception.

Interstructure distances (Fig. 6-11) in millimeters can be indicated automatically on the digital panel display by manually setting arc and radial cursors at any point along the field. Centimeter depth markers can be displayed, and any one of 256 radial scan lines can be selected for external A-mode display. This radial may be used to produce a

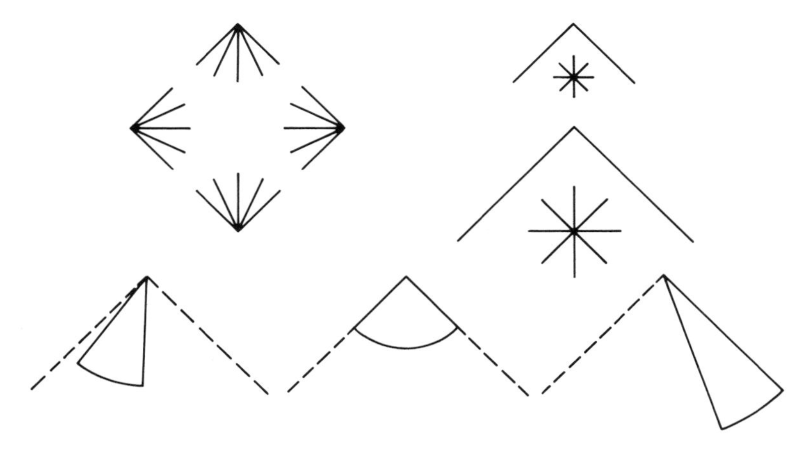

Altered phase vector here results in focusing patterns seen above.

Fig. 6-9 Orientation, scale, and field size when the dynamic electronic-focusing, phased-array method of scanning is used.

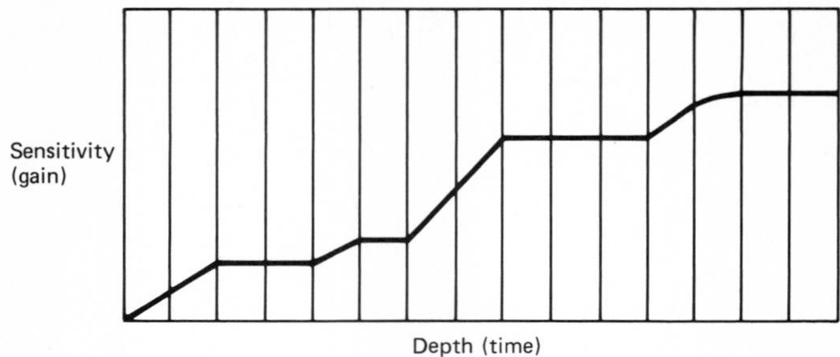

Fig. 6-10 Image sensitivity in electronic sector scanning. It can be seen that sensitivity (gain) increases in a nonlinear manner as the depth (time) increases.

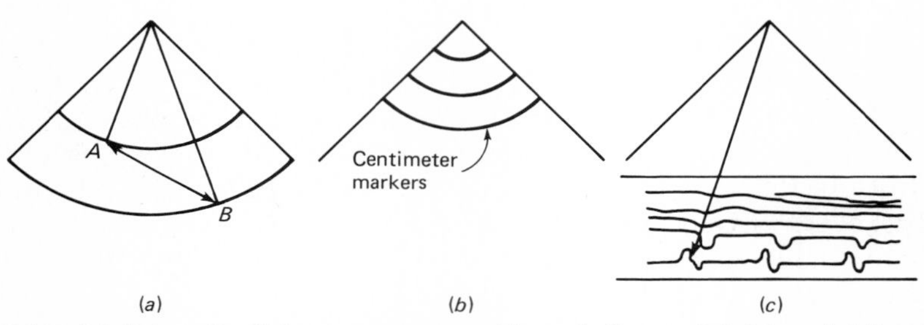

Fig. 6-11 (*a*) Automatic distance measurement is made from point *A* to point *B* on this scan using a phased array. (*b*) To calibrate automatic distance measurements, centimeter depth markers can be displayed. (*c*) A radial is selected for automatic distance measurement from the source.

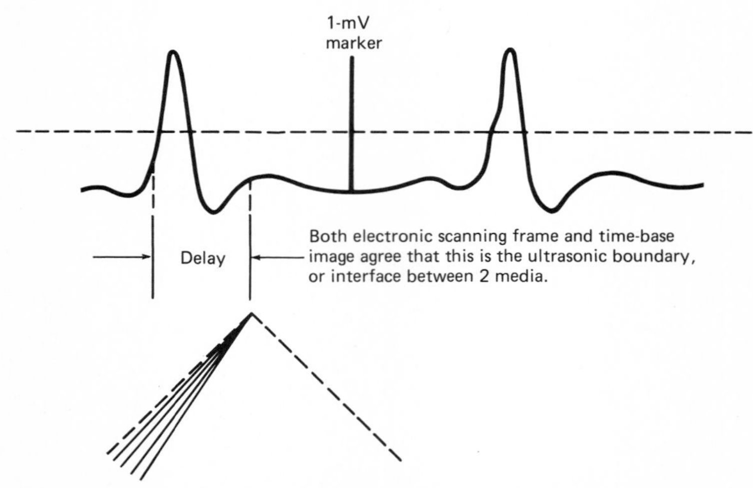

Fig. 6-12 Here, two image frames are synchronized. The electronic distance frame is shown below; the time vs. amplitude image frame is shown above.

simultaneous time-motion recording of moving structures such as valves and arteries.

Cardiac synchronization is provided by a built-in diagnostic-grade ECG channel (Fig. 6-12) to permit triggering of single frames from the R wave, or farther along in the cardiac cycle. Single- or multiple-frame scans may also be triggered manually or from an external source.

6-16 THE MIDLINER ECHOENCEPHALOGRAPH

The Midliner echoencephalograph, shown in Fig. 6-13, determines the location of the midline structures in the brain. A built-in digital computer performs all calculations, enabling nontechnical personnel to make rapid, accurate, and objective midline measurements.

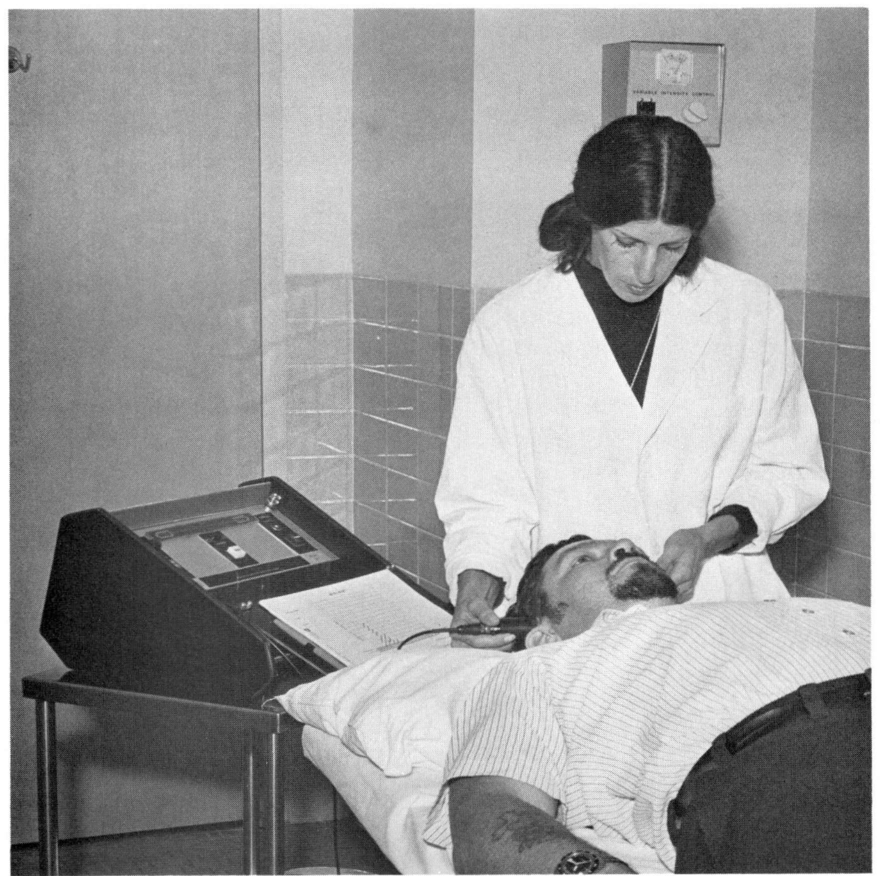

Fig. 6-13 The Midliner echoencephalograph in use in the emergency ward of Norwood Hospital, Massachusetts. (*Courtesy Diagnostic Electronics Co.*)

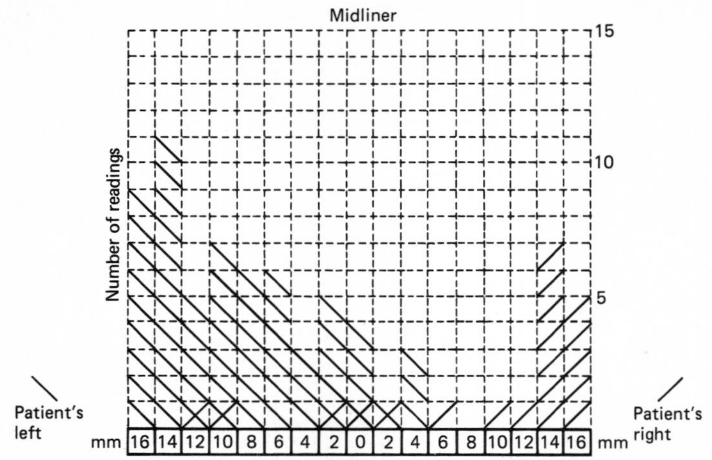

Fig. 6-14 A Midliner echoencephalograph bar chart is shown. From the nature of the echo, it was concluded that there was a possible space-occupying lesion on the right side that could indicate probable intracranial disease. Other tests verified these conclusions. The actual diagnosis was of a congenital hemicerebral atrophy.

In actual operation, a transducer which transmits and receives ultrasonic pulses is positioned against the patient's head. The Midliner automatically computes the true center line of the head, locates a major midline echo, and produces a readout of its location directly in millimeters of shift from the center line. Simultaneous audio signals indicate successful determinations and calculations. The operator is thus free to concentrate visual attention on probe positioning. Statistical accuracy is achieved by manually recording a number of successive readings on a simple bar graph which serves as a permanent patient record. Such a bar graph is shown in Fig. 6-14. Evidence of lesions indicating congenital hemicerebral atrophy are seen on the right side. Figure 6-15 shows three typical summarized bar graphs. The Midliner is accurate to ± 1 mm. The built-in digital clocks time echoes to within microseconds. An independent reference standard checks the system's accuracy.

6-17 THE UNIRAD ECHOENCEPHALOGRAPH

The Unirad Sonograph echoencephalograph seen in Fig. 6-16 is a complete ultrasound system with a Greatone and zoom display feature. The design is modular so that it can be expanded to satisfy future clinical needs. The Greatone process allows the full dynamic range of ultra-

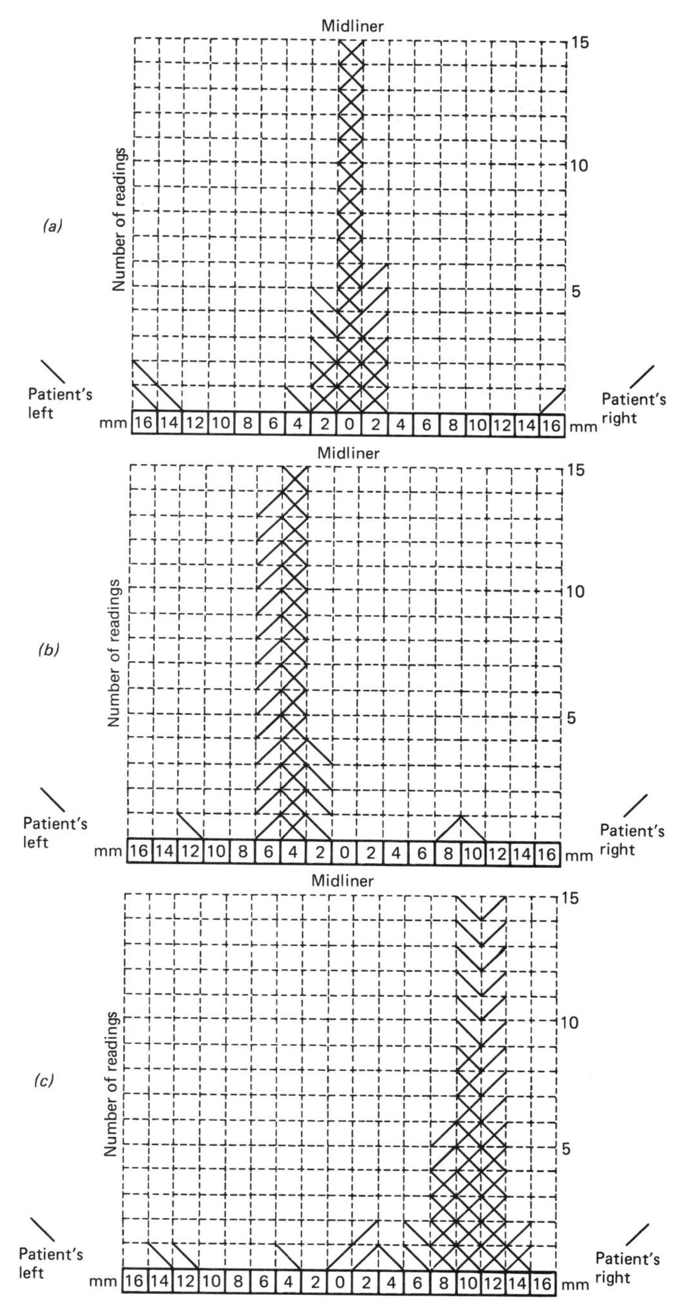

Fig. 6-15 (*a*) The normal adult pattern reveals no abnormal reflections over a number of readings. (*b*) We see a midline shift to the left of approximately 4 mm. As this is not a normal pattern, other tests will have to be made to verify this finding. (*c*) Again we discover an abnormal pattern. This time the midline shift is in the patient's right hemisphere. An actual shift of approximately 10 mm is observed.

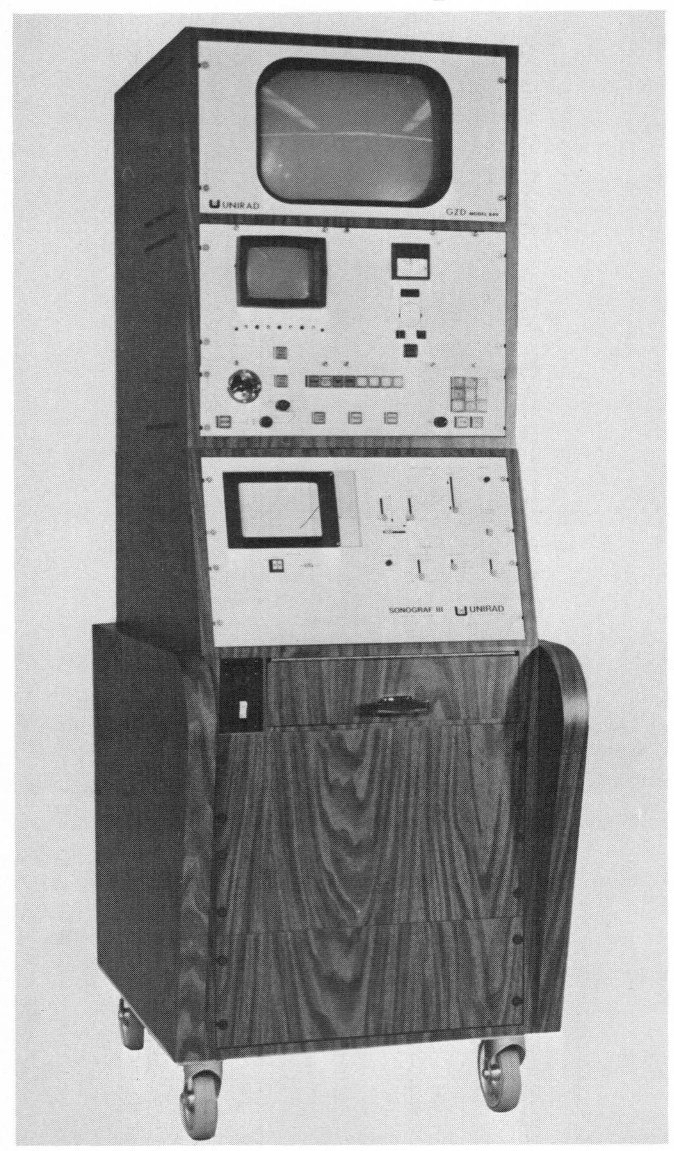

Fig. 6-16 The Unirad Sonograph is a complete ultrasound diagnostic center with a Greatone feature and a zoom display feature. The design is modular to make it possible to expand to satisfy future clinical needs. The Greatone process allows the full dynamic range of ultrasound images to be optimally displayed as shades of gray. Thus detailed scans are possible.

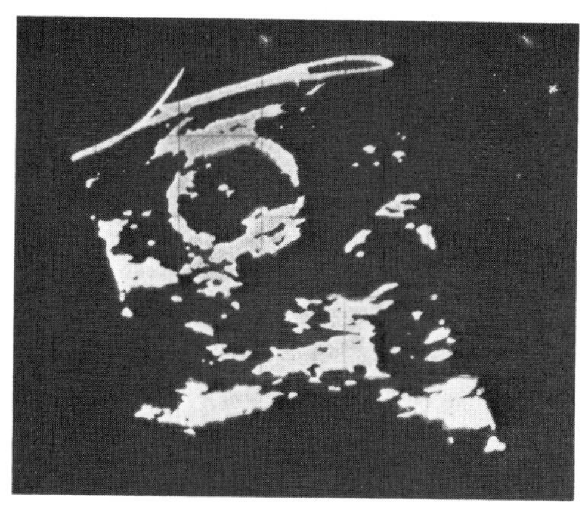

Fig. 6-17 Typical ultrasonic scan of a pregnant uterus.

sound images to be optimally displayed as shades of gray. Thus a great amount of detail can be observed in the various scans. The Sonograph has stop-action imaging of the heart and cine display of the heart in slow motion, real time, or accelerated motion.

The Unirad Sonograph has three recording modes. The scan mode is used to record B-scan data. The scan image can occupy the full screen or one-ninth of the screen depending on the setting of the display group controls. The Cardioniner mode makes use of an ECG-triggered technique to simultaneously record nine images of the heart, where each image is a different phase of the cardiac cycle. This technique has the advantage over the multiple-transducer real-time imaging approach because proper transducer angulation for optimum viewing angle and focus is obtained. The Cardioniner mode allows for "still" frames and dynamic visualization in pseudo-real-time display. In the third recording mode, the time-motion mode, TV pictures are generated. Their format is similar to strip-chart recordings but with immediate viewing and Greatone processing.

The Sonograph Niner Display allows storage of up to nine separate images. Any one of these images can be blown up to full size. The sequence feature causes the nine stored images to be stepped through in sequence at a rate from $\frac{1}{16}$ to 1 s per image. The first image, however, will be read out for twice the duration of the other eight images to allow the observer to determine the reference location of the first image during the sequence operation.

PART 2: TELEMETRY

INTRODUCTION

Telemetry systems transmit continuously or at recurrent intervals. Medical telemetry systems measure a variable which is displayed, recorded, or used to activate a control mechanism or alarm circuitry. The measurement may be used for several purposes. For example, it may activate alarm circuits, and, at the same time, update patient medical history and generate research data.

Telemetry was not always wireless. The first published record of telemetry was that of P. L. Shilling, a Russian who exploded mines by telemetry when the French were advancing during the War of 1812. Today's medical telemetry may be a combination of wired and wireless. For example, a wireless system may send data from the patient to the hospital-ward console. Then at the console, the data may continue their trip over the telephone lines.

6-18 WHAT CAN BE TELEMETERED

From deep within the body, pressure, pH, or temperature can be telemetered. Telemetry can be used to detect intracranial pressure, EMG, EEG, ECG, or respiratory ventilation. Oxygen analysis, breathing analysis, or the localization of bleeding may be telemetered. Examples of slowly changing parameters that can be telemetered are blood pH; digestive tract and pH; P_{O_2} in blood, expired air, or the digestive tract. In phonocardiography studies, the various sounds may be difficult to pick up from moving objects. When recording respiratory ventilation, care must be taken that motion artifacts are not confused with respiratory movements. Likewise, EMG potentials may be actual muscle action or may be artifacts from subcutaneous movements.

6-19 DECIDING WHETHER TO USE TELEMETRY

In making this difficult decision, a primary consideration is whether the system is to be operational or experimental. Experimental systems provide a broad spectrum of data. All data, no matter how detailed, might be of major importance once the system goes operational. Thus all data must be collated and computed. On the other hand, in the operational system, the warning of danger is primary. Data collection is secondary. Data must be presented in a way that affords fast, correct decisions. Therefore an operational system based on highly selected, critical data is better suited to telemetry. The experimental system with its exhaustive data requires numerous channels and may not be a practical telemetry system.

Another factor in deciding whether to use telemetry is the way in which medical monitoring attendants make decisions. Usually, available data are used to make trend projections. In other words, for a straight-line extrapolation, at least two points are necessary, one point being the present and the other taken from the past. From these two basic bits of data, some assessment of the future can be made. Increasing the number of data points gives us more knowledge of past situations. The accuracy of a prediction is thus increased. Whether we are evaluating our bank account, sailing our boat, or monitoring critical patients, we unconsciously use this approach. However, when several parameters must be correlated simultaneously, decision making becomes more difficult. It becomes almost impossible for paramedical personnel to make decisions when additional patients are added to the system.

Especially in times of stress, personnel cannot keep track of numbers or transient displays. A cardioscope display shows the patient's present status but does not show past history. Also, numerical or digital displays relate to present status but must be converted into a graph to aid decision making.

Thus two different types of displays are needed by the medical team: present status and past history. This data-display requirement influences the overall system design. For example, if there is only one primary display, and we wish to switch the system rapidly from one patient to the next, the sampling rate of the system will become important.

A human monitor requires a finite time to see and to digest data. A 15-s viewing period might be sufficient. This means that if there are four patients, each patient will be surveyed by the machine every minute. If there are 12 patients in the system, each one will be surveyed every 3 min. In this type of application, the system might automatically home in on the patient who exhibits an alarm situation. If heart rate were the critical parameter, one heart-rate meter (with alarms) would be used for each patient. One scope and recorder could be used which would be switched to the patient in the alarm condition. Consideration of how many channels of data are needed and the sampling rate can influence the decision whether or not to telemeter data.

6-20 THE BEST WAY TO ACQUIRE TELEMETERED DATA

The type of physiological data required will determine the kind of transducer to be used. A review of Chap. 3 will help in making this decision. The transducer table (Table 3-1) shows us transducer output levels. With this information, we can determine the type of signal conditioning or amplifier required.

If telemetry is used, all transducers or sensors, amplifiers, and the carrier generator must be attached to the patient. In addition, they must have the required encoding circuitry to put data on the radio carrier. The transmitter and its batteries must also be attached to the patient. Remember that if telemetry is not used, only the transducer itself must be attached to the patient. Everything else is in a more permanent location, such as at the bedside or at the ward office.

The essential arguments for telemetry center around the small size of the sensors and transducers. What we must realize is that there is nothing preventing us from using these same miniature devices with an ordinary wired system. Some people exclaim over the clarity of signals received over a telemetry system. By using the same care in attaching electrodes, tracings can be just as clean in a hard-wired system.

The important question is: "What premium do we wish to pay to eliminate wiring from the patient?" If patients are ambulatory and critically ill, then telemetry is a must. If you want to have any of the hospital's beds a potential coronary-care station but cannot afford the wiring and switching networks, then telemetry is a useful and successful solution. If you are concerned about the hazards of multiple ground-path leakage and possible harm to the patient, then telemetry (by virtue of its isolation from the ac line) is a reasonable answer. If you have trouble with ac interference that cannot be overcome, then again telemetry might be a solution. If it is necessary to monitor the patient from more than one fixed location, telemetry will be helpful. If the patient is hyperactive or is exercising, then telemetry is useful. If you are in limbo between old and new facilities (and do not wish to install wires in both buildings), telemetry can fill in during the interim. A more satisfactory solution might be to use existing intercom wires and multiplex the various channels onto one set of wires. This can be done with pulse-width modulation, which will be discussed shortly.

Telemetry may have its greatest value when the distances involved are large, when environments are hostile to wires, or when the subject must have a high degree of mobility. It has often been said that telemetry is invaluable in impressing hospital donors, boards of directors, and naive members of the uninformed press. In any event, the freedom of wireless monitoring often means a somewhat lower level of dependability for the overall system. The low-power signal from the patient transmitter is subject to reflection and interruption by walls, metal surfaces, objects, and people in hallways. Careful placement of the antenna, knowledge of the desired range, and other technical factors should precede the decision to use telemetry in place of hard-wired systems.

6-21 MODULATION AND MULTIPLEXING

In wireless telemetry, the carrier is the signal which carries the data through the body or through the air. The data themselves modulate this carrier. Modulation refers to a nonlinear operation in which message data are used to modify some characteristic of the carrier. The carrier is usually sinusoidal or a periodic sequence of pulses. If it uses pulses, then the operation is called *pulse coding*.

In FM, or frequency modulation, the carrier frequency remains constant over the long term. However, it is temporarily shifted or deviated in accordance with the audio or data imposed upon it. If we impress a 1000-Hz tone on the carrier which "pulls" it 3000 Hz away from the carrier, then we have an FM rate of 1000 Hz with a deviation of ±3 kHz. In frequency modulation, the average transmitted power is not changed when modulation occurs. Hence the average unmodulated power and the average signal power are both given by

$$P_C = P_S = \tfrac{1}{2}C^2$$

where P_C = average unmodulated carrier power
P_S = average signal power
C = carrier amplitude

Multiplexing refers to a sharing operation. This permits a telemetry system to transmit data from many different patient transducers simultaneously. Multiplexing of data can be on a time-shared or a frequency-shared basis. When the various types of modulation are considered and the possibility of multiplexing is considered, the following must be evaluated:

1. The frequency spectrum occupied by the telemetry transmission
2. The transmitted power as a function of the signal-to-noise ratio required
3. The critical threshold above which the system must operate
4. How efficiently the system must utilize the data capacity of each channel

PULSE MODULATION

The carrier in a pulse-modulated system consists of a periodic sequence of identical pulses. These pulses are rectangular in some systems, but they may have any shape. Their shape is determined by the bandpass characteristics of the system. For a single channel, the pulse rate corresponds to the sampling rate required to describe the data sent. Each sample of data is then used to modify some characteristic of one pulse. The most common pulse characteristics that are modified are (1) amplitude, (2) duration, and (3) position.

FREQUENCY-DIVISION MULTIPLEXING

A sinusoidal carrier is modulated by one channel of data at only one frequency. If three channels of data are used, then three frequencies would be required. The required modulating frequencies are called subcarriers. They each modulate a much higher frequency, which is the RF carrier. A common telemetry problem is *crosstalk* from one channel to another. In a frequency-division system, crosstalk results from the modulation products of one data channel having frequency components falling within the frequency region assigned to a second data channel. The amount of crosstalk depends on nonlinearities in the system, bandwidths of the individual channels, and the choice of subcarrier frequencies.

TIME-DIVISION MULTIPLEXING (TDM)

TDM is accomplished by sampling the different data channels at slightly different times and using these samples for one of the pulse-modulation methods described. Crosstalk is also present in time-division systems and arises from pulse widening due to restricted bandwidth or from poor time synchronizing. In TDM systems, synchronization is achieved by a precision clock (oscillator). This clock generates the sync pulses for the entire system. Therefore the clock and the phase of its various outputs become extremely critical.

6-22
TELEMETRY SYSTEMS

All telemetry systems (wired or wireless) need both transmitter and receiver. In multiplexing, several signals are placed on one carrier. Signal conditioners convert and amplify raw data and also match the incoming signal to the multiplexer or transmitter. A block diagram of a typical single-channel system is shown in Fig. 6-18.

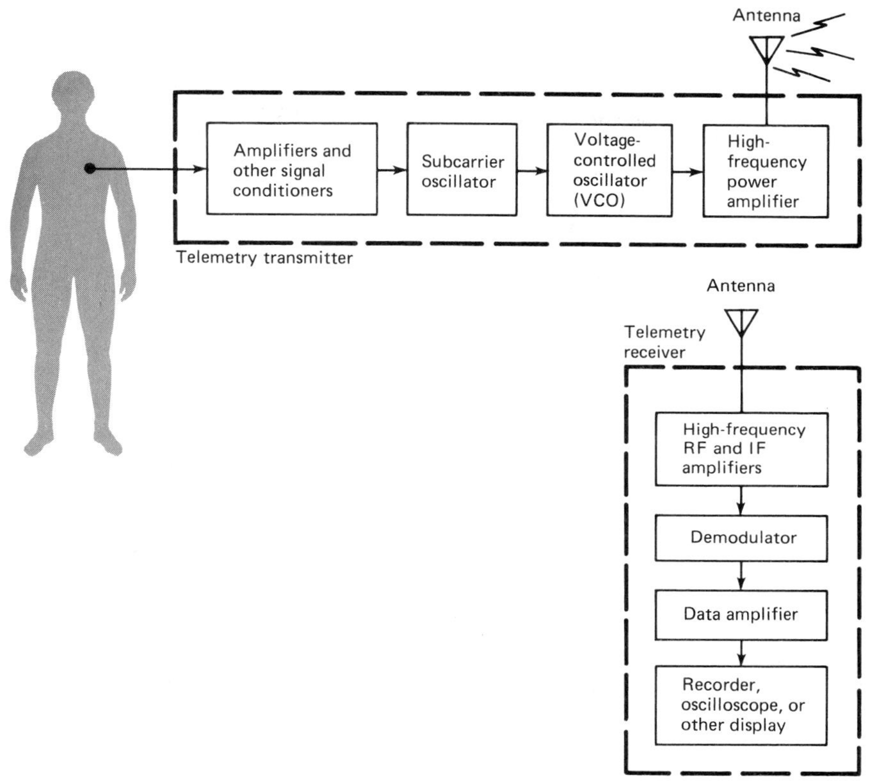

Fig. 6-18 Typical single-channel telemetry system. Electrodes or a transducer feed the medical data to the signal conditioners, which modulate a subcarrier oscillator. Its output can be a variable voltage which supplies data to the high-frequency signal or the transmitter voltage-controlled oscillator. The receiver detects or demodulates these data and drives the readout devices.

TRANSMITTER

The transmitter may operate in the standard 88- to 108-MHz range or the FM broadcast band. If many data channels are required, or the hospital is located in an FM-congested urban area, then 88 to 108 MHz might be impractical. In that case, 206 to 225 MHz could be used. In this band there are 62 channels set aside for telemetry. Between each channel is a 500-kHz spacing with an allowable tolerance of 0.01 percent around the carrier frequency. The bandwidth allowed for each channel is 3 kHz.

Some telemetry transmitters have a defibrillation protection circuit which protects the transmitter from high external shocks. Other telemetry transmitters have a slew-rate limiter which cuts down artifacts from an implanted pacemaker. A slew-rate limiter will discriminate against the large-amplitude, short-duration pulses of a pacemaker, leaving the cardiac input data unaffected. A typical battery-powered telemetry transmitter will operate from 3 to 22 days continuously without a battery change. When selecting a particular transmitter, take special notice of its power consumption or battery-drain current.

It is a simple process to calculate the anticipated operating time of a telemetry transmitter. Let us assume the transmitter has a drain current of 600 μA and the battery has a rating of 0.3 A·h. Thus, if our battery drain is 0.3 A (300 mA), the battery would last 1 h. However, in this case, the battery drain is 600 μA, or 0.6 mA, thus

$$\frac{300 \text{ mA}}{0.6 \text{ mA}} = \text{hours of battery life} = 500 \text{ h}$$

This particular battery would last not quite 21 days. Knowing this, we can mark our calendar to denote the nineteenth or twentieth day (depending on how critical the application is). This reminder tells us when to change the battery. In this way, a disastrous situation is avoided. The nurse on duty might lose the patient's telemetered signal and be unable to locate the BMET.

Always store the transmitter without its battery. When using the transmitter after a long storage period, always check the battery *under load*. When using single-channel equipment, always determine if the transmitter channel number is the same as the receiver channel number. If you are putting different components of a system together yourself, make certain that the signal sensors are capable of fully modulating the transmitter. This means that the transmitter input impedance must match the transducer or source impedance and that the transmitter's modulation sensitivity is high enough. A typical FM sensitivity may be 15 kHz/mV. This means that 1 mV of audio modulation is required to produce full RF modulation (FM deviation) of 15 kHz. If 1 mV is not available at the transmitter's modulation input terminals, then low modulation can be anticipated.

SUBCARRIER OSCILLATORS (SCO)

Not only are most biological signals of low signal level, but they are also in the low-frequency range of direct current to 100 Hz. While it is not impossible to transmit these frequencies directly, it is more reliable to first superimpose the data on a more easily handled, higher-frequency audio signal. This is the function of the subcarrier oscillator (SCO). The subcarrier in a single-channel system varies its frequency as a function of applied voltage (frequency modulation). Since this subcarrier is superimposed upon an FM frequency, the system is called an

FM/FM system. This subcarrier can be a changing audio tone which is used to tune up the transmitter or to monitor the received signal. Using this technique, a variation in distance (within range) will not affect the signal being recorded. Another benefit of FM/FM is that it allows the user to record the audio signal directly from the receiver on any home-type tape recorder. Playback of this recording through the demodulator (built into the receiver) yields the original data as transmitted.

RECEIVER AND DEMODULATOR

The receiver may have a tape recorder, strip-chart recorder, or other form of display attached to its output. Some telemetry receivers have electrode-failure lamp indicators to indicate if the patient electrode is loose or has fallen off. A good receiver will often have an indicator to reveal when the transmitter battery is low or when the patient is outside the receiver's range.

A single-channel receiver uses a demodulator or discriminator to convert the varying frequency into the original modulating voltage. A multichannel receiver will require several subcarrier demodulators, each one being sensitive to only one subcarrier. Thus only one particular subcarrier signal is fed into the discriminator.

Typical modulator output is approximately 0.5 to 1.0 V for full-scale modulation. This signal may be recorded on any direct writer, displayed on an oscilloscope, or both. If the receiver output is stored on a recorder, it may later be played back through the FM subcarrier demodulator.

ANTENNAS

Telemetry range is usually specified by the manufacturer. This range is probably based on a nondirectional one-quarter wavelength rod for both transmitter and receiver. Either transmitter or receiver can be given the advantage of a multielement directive antenna. If both receiver and transmitter have an efficient, high-gain directive-antenna system, a system gain approaching 40 dB can be achieved.

To calculate the meaning of a 40-dB system gain, let us suppose that 1000 yd from the transmitter a 0.1-μV signal exists at the receiver input. Our hypothetical receiver needs 1 μV or more to produce a good signal-to-noise ratio at its demodulated output. Obviously then, our telemetry system will not function, for we need a minimum of 10 times more signal than is available.

Suppose we installed a directive antenna at the transmitter with 20-dB forward gain. If the receiving antenna is directly in the path of the maximum forward lobe of the beam antenna, we would now have 100 times the 0.1 μV previously available. With 10 μV now at the receiver's input terminals, our telemetry system would certainly function well.

How would we achieve a system gain of 40 dB? Let us suppose we install another another high-gain directive antenna, this time on the receiver. This will give us an additional 20-dB forward gain. Once again the voltage gain can be multiplied 100 times. By adding the two antennas to the system, we have a voltage gain of $100 \times 100 = 10{,}000$. Without directive antennas we had 0.1 μV at the receiver; now we have 1 mV. If the telemetry system operates in the 88- to 108-MHz band, commercial FM directive antennas may be used with modifications. However, extreme care should be taken to match antenna impedance to either receiver input or transmitter output.

Using such a highly directional antenna system, researchers at one institution achieved a distance of 1 mi when monitoring the ECG of racehorses. The antenna was mounted at the top of the stadium in the press box, a better than "ideal" situation. The dramatic results obtained by NASA in telemetering the astronauts' biomedical parameters are primarily due to high-gain parabolic antenna arrays.

OTHER TELEMETRY PROBLEMS

There are two major areas of difficulty which usually arise in biotelemetry. The first is the interface between the biological system and the electric system. Electrodes and transducers must be put on with great care. The other major area of difficulty is the interface between transmitter and receiver. It is not wise to squeeze the last bit of range out of the system. Fringe-area reception is likely to be noisy. In telemetry, the system with the smallest volume and weight and with the greatest range usually has the most appeal. In electronics, as in other areas, it is unusual to get something for nothing. Small size and volume come at the sacrifice of other features: battery life, range, flexibility, repairability, ease of finding replacement batteries, etc.

MULTICHANNEL SYSTEMS

When it is desired to broadcast more than one channel of data over the same transmitter, the task gets more complicated. The conventional approach has been to use a separate subcarrier frequency for each data channel. The cost of these systems is high, and the modulation sensitivity of the subcarrier oscillators has been low (1 to 5 V). In addition there is often a problem with crosstalk between channels. Expensive and complex filters are used to reduce crosstalk. A technique known as pulse-width modulation (PWM) is now used for multichannel systems. PWM has high modulation sensitivity, extreme simplicity in both modulation and demodulation, minimal crosstalk between channels, small size, and low power requirements.

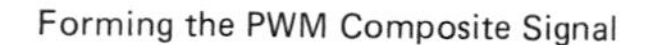

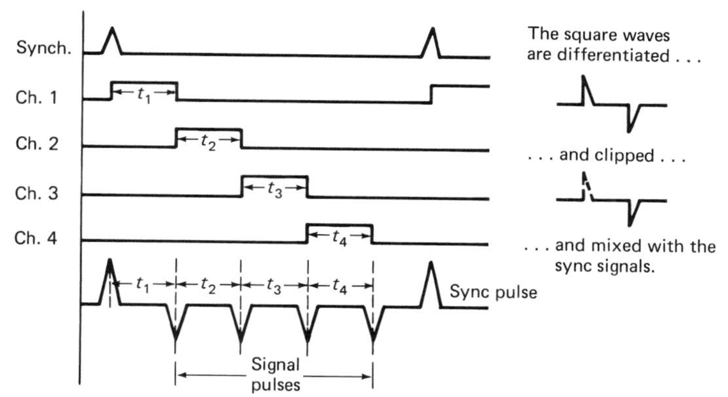

Fig. 6-19 In the pulse-width-modulation technique, sync pulses are positive, and medical data or signal pulses are negative. After mixing, the sync pulse determines the beginning and end of each run of medical data. The medical data themselves determine the time position (width) of pulses.

THE PWM SYSTEM. The transmitted signal in the PWM system is a composite of positive synchronizing (sync) pulses and negative "signal" pulses. The data to be telemetered cause the signal pulses to move back and forth in time (t_1, t_2, t_3, t_4), as shown in Fig. 6-19. This method is also called pulse-position modulation (PPM), since the relative position of one pulse to another carries the data. Referring to the functional block diagram of the transmitting system in Fig. 6-20, it will be seen that the sync generator begins the action. Its pulse turns the first channel one-shot multivibrator ON. How long it remains ON depends on the level of the data being fed into it at that instant of time. Its return to the OFF position triggers the next channel, and so on down

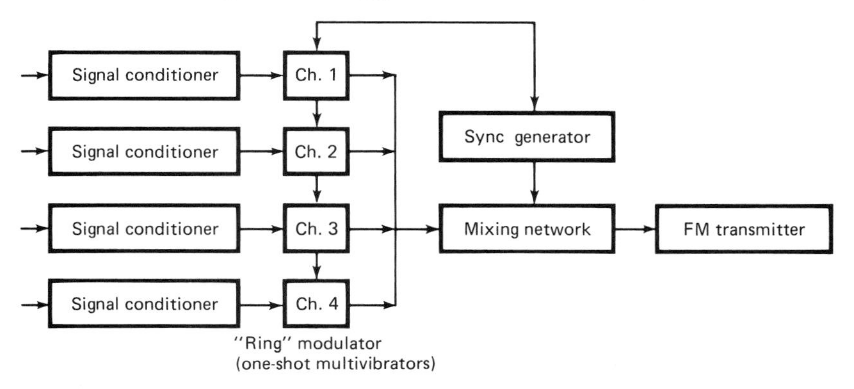

Biolink PWM Transmitting System

Fig. 6-20 In the PWM transmitting system, the outputs from the various channels are mixed to form negative pulses which determine pulse position. The sync generator initiates the start of a new "data run."

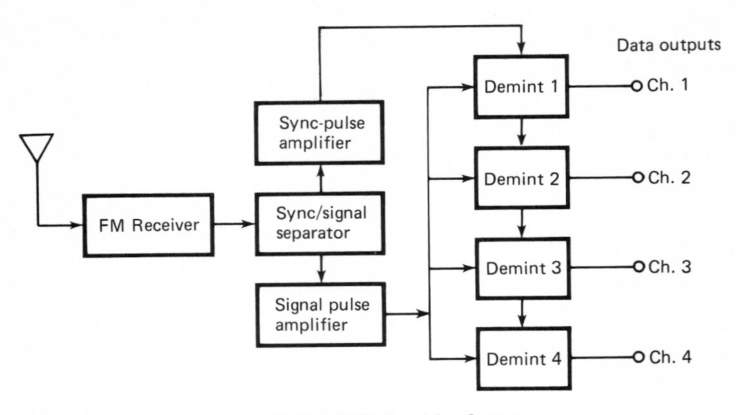

Fig. 6-21 The sync pulse turns on the first demint. After separation from the sync, the medical data control all demints (flip-flops), determining their ON-OFF duration. Thus the square-wave output corresponds to the square waves that modulated the transmitter.

the line. The resultant square waves are thus width-modulated by the data.

DEMODULATION. After reception, the composite signal must be separated and re-formed to be properly demodulated. The sync-signal separator and amplifiers perform this function. Each "demint" in Fig. 6-21 consists of a flip-flop multivibrator and an integrating network. (The name demint comes from DEModulator-INTegrator.) Signal pulses are fed through a suitable diode network to all demints. The sync pulse is fed to the first-channel demint only.

In operation, the sync pulse turns the first flip-flop ON. The first signal pulse comes in and would turn any ON flip-flops OFF. Since channel 1 is the only unit which is ON, it is turned OFF. When it returns to the OFF position, it automatically triggers the channel 2 flip-flop ON. The second signal pulses are used to turn off (or gate) each demint after it has been turned on. The resulting square wave out of each flip-flop varies in width exactly like the original square wave in the transmitter. Simple integration yields the original data.

6-23 TELEMETRY ELECTRODES

The biological-electronic interface is the major source of difficulty in securing reliable results from telemetered subjects. Here is a basic guide to good telemetry electrode procedure, to eliminate noise and interference:

1. Skin resistance must be as low as possible—5000 Ω or below is ideal; 10,000 Ω will work but can give rise to trouble. Light abrasion is the best way to minimize skin resistance. The outer layer of skin is not an electrical conductor. This layer *must* be removed to properly record data from the active subject. Use Scotchbrite, a nylon-mesh abrasive material made by Minnesota Mining and Manufacturing Co. The dark maroon Scotchbrite (grade 7447) is preferable for telemetry applications. Several light swipes across the skin will suffice Examine the Scotchbrite material for the presence of a light powder. This residue on the pad is dead tissue and indicates that the abrasion was effective. Elderly patients will generally exhibit a higher resistance, since their layers of dead tissue are thicker, requiring more abrasion. Do not draw blood, as this can lead to infection. Some of the electrode jellies, especially the bentonite clay compounds, can cause extremely severe reactions which are difficult to heal and may leave permanent scars. Electrode jellies often are good mediums for sustaining bacterial growth. Some of these compounds contain bacteriostatic agents, but some do not and can cause infections.

2. Electrodes should have small mass and low intertia so that they will not cause artifacts due to their own motion relative to the skin. Connecting wires should be durable, yet very flexible, for both patient comfort and minimal injection of noise into the system.

3. Electrode jelly (in a fluid column) should couple the electrode to the skin. The metal electrode should be a silver–silver chloride mixture, semiporous, yet very rigid. Electrodes should be held in a fixed position and should *never* be allowed to touch the skin. Dissimilar metal (solder joints, etc) cannot be exposed and cannot contact the fluid column. Some metals can migrate out of an alloy and be deposited on the skin, causing severe allergenic reactions. Copper and lead can do this.

4. Avoid sharp edges. Any material which creases, indents, or wrinkles the skin can cause itching. The electrode base or rim should be fairly wide (at least $\frac{1}{4}$ in), thus affording a wide distribution of the pressure over the contact area.

5. Many of the jellies designed for ECG will be highly irritating in long-term telemetry application. Lanolin-base creams or "sols" have a high resistance and do not work well for active subjects. They are too greasy and melt into the skin. The Biocom 1090 Biogel was originally formulated by NASA for long-term use on Apollo astronauts. It has a pH of 7.0 and a relatively high viscosity, making it easy to work with in the electrode holder.

6. The skin is not a pure resistance. It often behaves like a semiconductor or piezoelectric device. Try to prevent pressure from the tape from interacting with the subject's musculature, causing a shifting base line and other artifacts.

7. Measuring electrode resistance. The purist will tell you that electrode resistance measured with a dc ohmmeter is not correct.

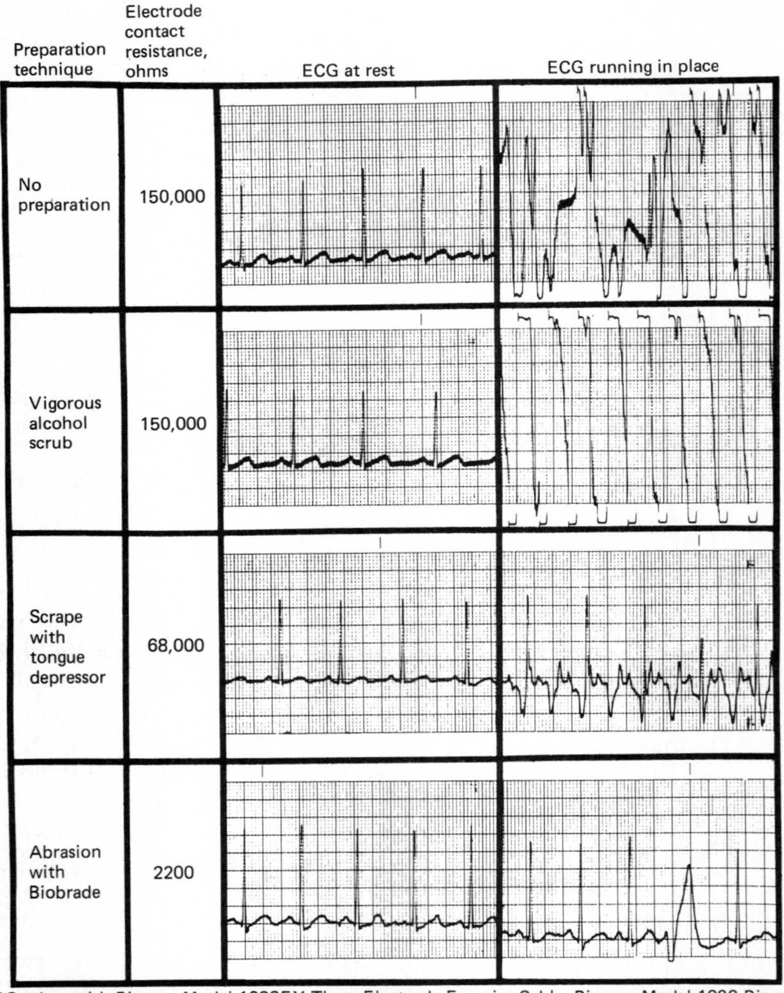

Preparation technique
Electrode contact resistance, ohms
ECG at rest
ECG running in place
No preparation
150,000
Vigorous alcohol scrub
150,000
Scrape with tongue depressor
68,000
Abrasion with Biobrade
2200
ECG taken with Biocom Model 1083EX Three-Electrode Exercise Cable, Biocom Model 1090 Biogel Biopotential Contact Medium, and Biocom Model 2122 Bioamplifier. Electrode/subject contact resistance measured with Biocom Model 1089 Bootest Electrode Tester. Test current 25 μA.

Fig. 6-22 Comparison of electrode resistance and ECG patterns for various techniques of electrode site preparation. Electrode location: manubrium to V5. Reference electrode location: V5R. Note PVC (premature ventricular contraction) in bottom-right trace.

Although this is somewhat true, the values obtained using direct current will indicate contact integrity. A 30-μA constant-current source is the quickest way to check electrode resistance. Exercise cardiologists who encounter poor ECGs often find that the electrode tester usually shows poor electrode application technique.

8. Location of electrodes is important. Avoid placing them near a large muscle mass unless you are trying to pick up muscle potentials. The most reliable electrode placement for ECG is the M-X lead (manubrium-xiphoid process). Place the electrodes on the sternum at the midline, separated by 3 or 4 in. Exercise cardiologists do not like this location and instead prefer a sternum to V5 location. With good electrode application this position serves admirably for exercise ECG work (Fig. 6-22).

9. If the trace is noisy and filled with artifacts as soon as the patient starts to move, then the source of the problem is poor electrode contact. Do not try to abrade the skin with a paper towel or a gauze pad. The fact that the skin turns red as a result of this abrasion does not mean that you have removed the horny layer of insulating dead tissue. If your electrode application is poor, remove the electrode and start all over.

6-24 APPLICATIONS INVOLVING THE ACTIVE SUBJECT

Single-channel ECG telemetry is useful in occupational hygiene, sports medicine, and cardiac diagnosis. ECG rate is important when investigating workloads. The bicycle ergometer tests the relationship between heart rate and energy expenditure. A cardiotachometer will record this relationship. Oxygen consumption from one heartbeat to the next is also valuable information in analyzing work-related problems. In industry, finding the right person for the right job means testing the applicant's work capacity. Figure 6-23 shows a telemetered cardiotachogram (CTG) of a factory worker lifting a heavy crate. The CTG shows S-T depression while the worker is lifting the third crate. Thus a heart defect was revealed. This defect might have gone unnoticed until a heart attack occurred, bringing with it severe heart damage.

Epileptic seizures often do not show up while the subject is at rest. Using a multichannel telemetery system, various EEG waves can be explored during work or sports activities. A latent epileptic subject might be uncovered in this manner. In electromyography as well as ECG and EEG, there are times when exercise is required to reveal an otherwise hidden problem. A muscle disease might not show up while the

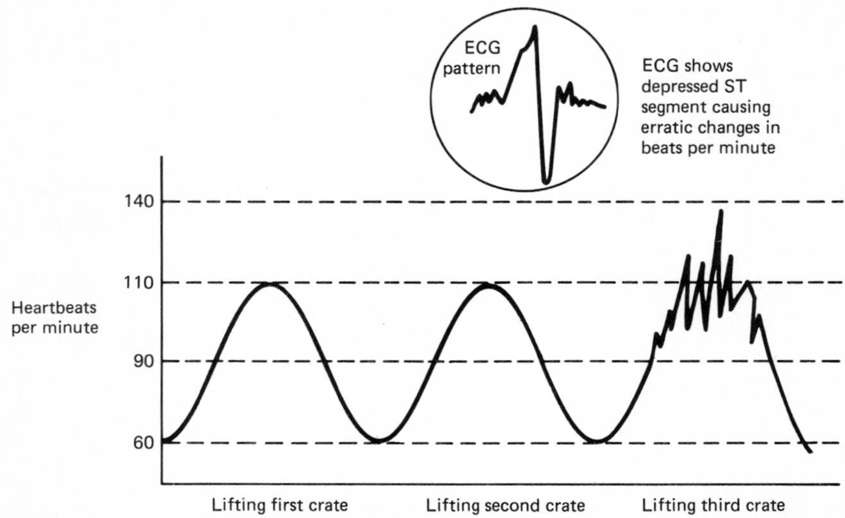

Fig. 6-23 Cardiac beats per minute (BPM) while worker is lifting a heavy crate. BPM rate increased evenly and decreased evenly when worker lifted the first and second crate. However, on lifting the third crate, both the ECG (inset) and the BPM rate showed an abnormal pattern.

muscle is at rest, but revealing "fibs" might appear when the same muscle is active.

6-25 THE BIO-PHONE

When a fire department heart rescue unit is called to an emergency, ECG data must be telemetered instantly and accurately. In a real-life drama which transpired in Los Angeles, a fire department heart rescue unit associated with Harbor General Hospital responded to a call from a local restaurant. They found a 48-year-old woman in acute distress.

The heart rescue unit had with them a self-contained emergency medical communication system called *Bio-Phone*. The Bio-Phone, pictured in Fig. 6-24, is a radio transmitter-receiver (transceiver) which allows two-way voice communication and ECG telemetry. Its frequency range is 450 to 470 MHz, and transmitter power is 12 W. The transmitter can be modulated by biological signals from 0.1 to 100 Hz, with a 90-dB common-mode rejection. Full 12-lead ECG transmission is possible.

Paramedics with the fire department rescue unit applied the Bio-Phone electrodes to the distressed woman. Twenty-five miles away, at Harbor General Hospital, cardiologists were able to see the ECG pattern shown in Fig. 6-25*a*. Upon instructions from the cardiologists, the paramedics defibrillated the distressed woman. After defibrillation, the

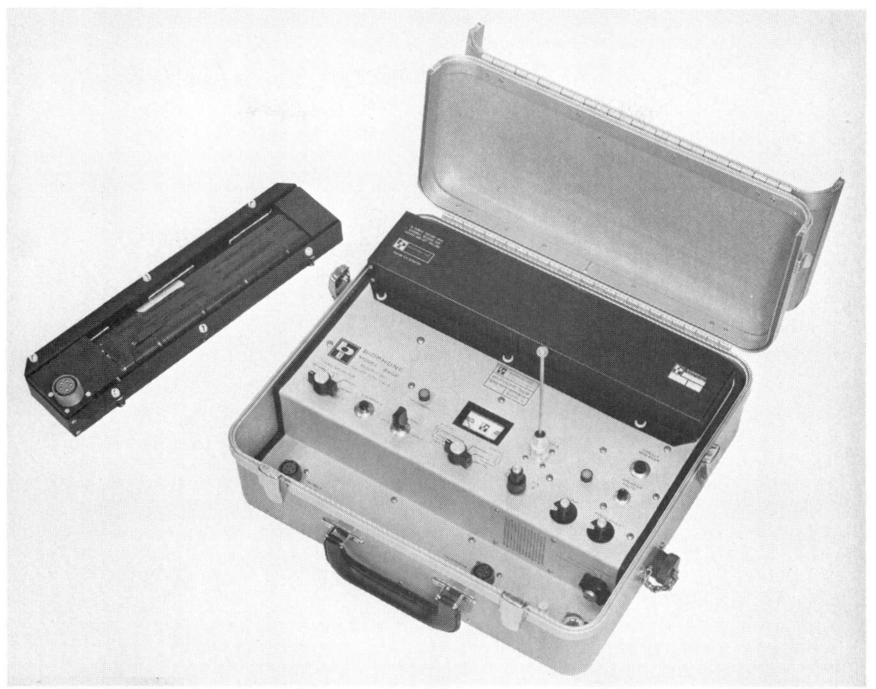

Fig. 6-24 Bio-Phone transceiver operates at 450 MHz. The lead connection switch on the left permits 12-lead ECG data to be transmitted over one channel. The battery pack is seen on the far left. The antenna is seen to the right of the modulation meter.

first appearance of pulsatile cardiac activity became evident, as seen in Fig. 6-25*b*. Again, upon instructions from the hospital, atropine was administered intravenously and the third waveform (Fig. 6-25*c*) was recorded. Because of the increased heart rate, lidocaine was prescribed. The subsequent ECG, recorded after lidocaine was administered intravenously, is shown in Fig. 6-25*e*. This pattern now shows a more stable rate with a stronger QRS complex. Upon arrival at the hospital, her lungs were suctioned and all the foreign material was removed. Finally, after 48 h, a normal sinus rhythm was recorded (Fig. 6-25*f*). The woman subsequently recovered.

6-26 WIRED TELEMETRY

The earliest telemetry experiments, over 150 years ago, were not able to take advantage of wireless technique. Connecting wires conveyed data from one point to another, just as telephone lines convey voices from one point to another. Wireless telemetry is useful where distances are

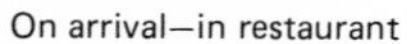

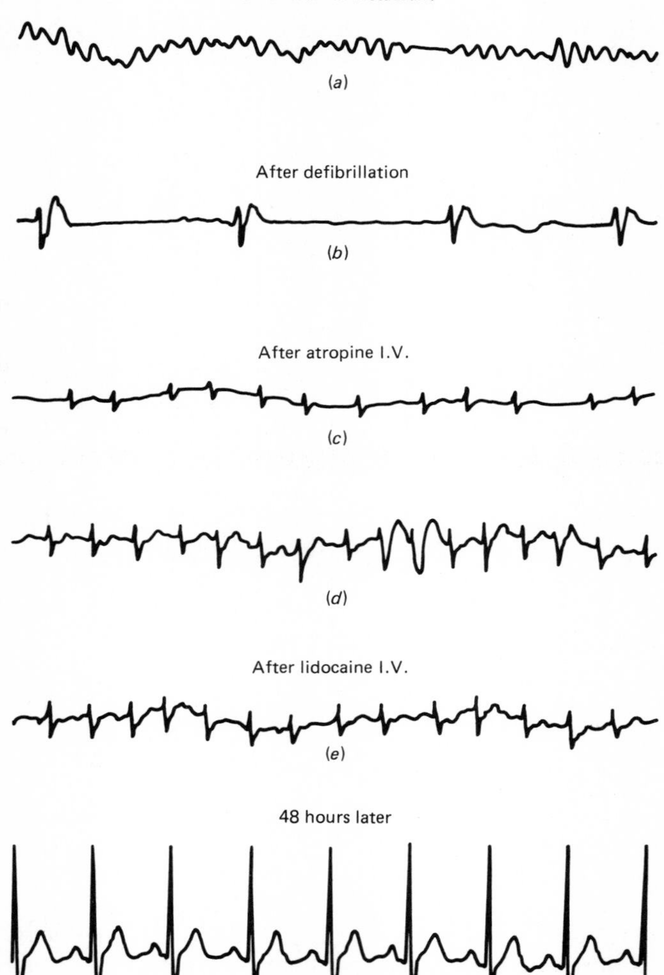

Fig. 6-25 Fire department paramedics transmitted these ECG patterns over the Bio-Phone transceiver to Harbor General Hospital. In pattern (*a*) the patient did not show pulsatile cardiac activity. In pattern (*f*), taken at the hospital, a normal ECG pattern is finally observed.

relatively short. However, where long distances are involved, reliable radio communication equipment becomes bulky and expensive.

The high frequencies used in medical telemetry are in the "line of sight" part of the spectrum. That is, the distance covered would typically be limited to the 20- to 40-mi range, the higher distances being feasible only over ideal terrain and where extremely high transmitting power is used. One solution to this problem is an orbiting satellite. Ham radio operators trigger a satellite named Oscar to send messages around the world. It is only a matter of time before a medical data Oscar is launched. In the meantime, long-distance medical data transmission is accomplished over ordinary telephone lines.

6-27
THE BIOTONE

By far, the most urgent application of telephone telemetry is the immediate monitoring of an unstable coronary condition upon the onset of distress symptoms. A specialist in the same city, or on the other side of the earth, can make an immediate assessment of the onset of myocardial infarction. Most myocardial-infarction patients experience either bradycardia, tachycardia, heart block, or excessive premature ventricular contractions before reaching the hospital. These arrythmias precede cardiac arrest, killing 60 percent of heart attack victims before they reach the hospital.

The Biotone, made by Biocom, is a battery-operated, pocket-sized tone generator. Its tone is frequency-modulated in accordance with the patient's ECG data. With the Biotone placed near a telephone handset, the patient's ECG can be heard around the world.

At the other end of the telephone line, a Biocom receiver demodulates the modulated tone. These ECG data can then be fed to a conventional ECG recorder in the physician's office, hospital coronary-care unit, or any coronary diagnostic center. For circuit data on FM modulators and demodulators, refer to Chap. 8, Common Biomedical Circuits.

6-28
OUTPATIENT MONITORING

When a patient has a pacemaker installed, has cardiovascular surgery or treatment, or has a chronic cardiac problem, there is often a need for frequent outpatient ECG data retrieval. Normally, this application requires that ECG data be transmitted from the patient's home to the doctor's office or to the hospital. The long distances involved make radio a questionable solution. It is an ideal application for telemetry by telephone.

The patient connects two limb bands to the ECG transmitter shown in Fig. 6-26*a*. A standard telephone handset is placed on the Tel-e-Mitter. Only a single lead is sufficient to determine spike-to-spike interval and capture. The same transmitter can, however, transmit a standard 12-lead ECG and pacemaker signal over the conventional telephone line. A visiting paramedic on call can connect the patient's leads

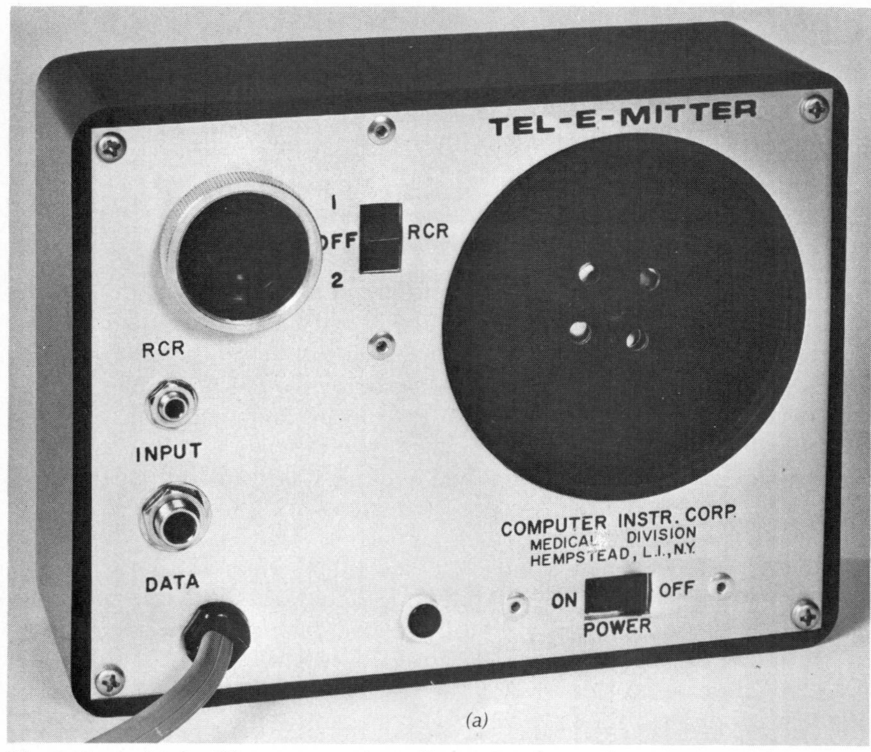

Fig. 6-26 In (*a*) the Biotone transmitter allows ECG data to frequency-modulate an audible tone. Its companion piece in (*b*) is held close to a telephone receiver. The ECG MIN-E-C'VER then demodulates the ECG data sent over the telephone line. The MIN-E-C'VER output can be fed to any standard ECG recording or storage device.

for a 12-lead ECG. These data can then be sent to the doctor's office, hospital, or home.

Battery operation of both the transmitter and receiver eliminates shock and leakage problems. Battery life is approximately 350 transmissions. The transmitter amplifies the ECG signal, sending it to an FM modulator. This modulator changes the frequency of an audio tone in accordance with the amplitude variations of the patient's ECG. At the other end of the telephone line a standard handset in the hospital or doctor's office is placed on a data-receiver terminal which demodulates the frequency-modulated tone sent over the telephone line. A counter, external to the receiver, displays the pacemaker spike-to-spike interval or spikes per minute.

A reverse channel-recognition option permits the receiver to signal the transmitter with instructions. For example, the receiver may signal the person at the transmitter to pick up the phone. The receiver can also receive data from a Bell Telephone 603 Dataphone, or the equivalent.

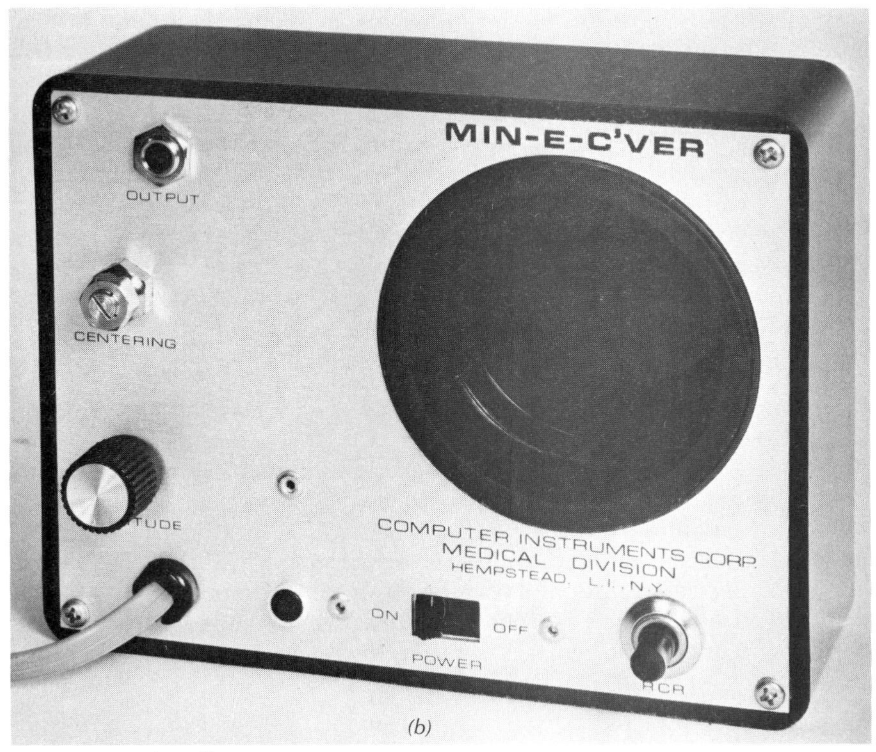

(b)

Fig. 6-26 (continued)

6-29
MEPC

We have just learned how telephone telemetry can be useful to the hospital or doctor that needs to receive outpatient data. Another interesting system allows a physician or hospital to gain access to a regional medical computer. A Mini Electrocardiogram Processing Center (MEPC) will receive telephone ECG data from a hospital or doctor's office. The technician dials the regional computer, which sends a signal indicating it is ready to receive data. The patient's identification and ECG are transmitted. This Telemed computer analyzes four or five groups of three leads each. The computer then signals whether it has received satisfactory data or must reject unacceptable data. The computer can monitor incoming data for noise, missing leads, calibration, and other quality factors. Prior to interpretation by the computer, it converts the incoming data to digital format and queued-on disk storage. The system can process over 100 ECGs per hour.

After interpretation, the reports may be sent to both local and remote printers. Transmission of interpretations to remote locations is fully automatic; any mixture of local, WATS, and dedicated lines may be used.

MEPC systems can be expanded to receive data simultaneously from up to four interfaces. Noise-level monitoring and all other real-time quality controls are applied to each ECG. The number and complexity of line-queuing devices attached to the ECG interfaces are unlimited. The system is capable of controlling ECG direct writers (recorders) automatically: simple keyboard commands determine which ECGs are to be recorded.

TELEMED PROGRAM

The Telemed electrocardiogram analysis program is derived from the largest data base of ECGs and specific ECG abnormalities in existence, thus providing extremely accurate and complete analyses of contour and rhythm. The program's diagnostic criteria, representing the collective opinions of a board of cardiologists, are continuously updated as newer, more clinically relevant information is developed. The ECG analysis, based on the patient's age, body build, clinical history, and current drug therapy, provides interpretive statements which offer the various diagnostic possibilities in their decreasing order of probability, assuring clinical validity and usefulness.

IBM/BONNER PROGRAM

The IBM/Bonner ECG Interpretive Program has been translated from IBM Model 360/370-compatible language to a form which operates on InterData computers. Interpretations produced by the MEPC system are identical with those produced by the corresponding release of the IBM/Bonner program when run on Models 360 or 370. Criteria and logic changes may be made by systems users, aided by IBM documents which explain the principles used in developing the program.

STORAGE

The Telemed electrocardiogram storage system is based upon high-capacity, magnetic-disk storage devices. The disk system is capable of storing over 150,000 ECGs; multiple disk packs allow unlimited storage capacity.

Retrieval is accomplished by simply entering, via a keyboard, the patient's identification. The stored digital record is then instantly recalled and converted to an analog tracing. Full identifying information is printed on the reproduced tracing.

QUESTIONS

1. Describe the theory of the reflection coefficient.
2. According to the propagation velocity of each, separate the following into three of the most-dense materials, then three of the least-dense materials. List in the order of declining density: muscle, liver, kidney, fat, brain, blood.
3. List the following materials in the order of their decreasing ability (at a given frequency) to convert ultrasonic energy into heat: blood, brain, fat, kidney, liver, muscle.
4. An ultrasonic wave encounters a boundary between blood and fat. What kind of angle of incidence is required for the greatest reflectance?
5. When a 1-MHz radiated signal is reflected from a moving reflector, the reflected frequency is 1.1 MHz. What does the Doppler effect tell us about the movement of the reflector?
6. Calculate the Doppler shift (F_c) when velocity = 100 ms, frequency = 800 kHz, and speed of sound = 1088 ft/s.
7. Considering the low reflectance of blood, is the Doppler technique practical when blood is the reflecting medium? Explain your answer.
8. Calculate the Doppler frequency shift with blood-flow velocity equal to 0.01 s and the transmitting frequency equal to 1 MHz. The transducer beam has an angle of 41.3° to the flow of blood.
9. What characteristics and specifications would be desired for an operational telemetry system as compared to an experimental telemetry system?
10. Answer *yes* where you would use telemetry, and *no* where you would not use telemetry, after the following applications. (*a*) Multiple ground-path leakage cannot be eliminated, leaving questionable ground current loops. (*b*) Nearby elevators and the hospital heating system transmit strong transient signals into the power line which cannot be eliminated. (*c*) The patient is extremely restless and many data channels must be recorded with high resolution (definition).
11. Find the average modulated FM carrier power when the carrier amplitude $C = 8$ V.
12. We can break a telemetry carrier into separate pulses. List three ways these pulses can be manipulated to provide data.
13. You designed a three-channel, multiplexed telemetry system based on the frequency-division principle. Subcarrier 1 operated at 800 Hz, subcarrier 2 at 1600 Hz, and subcarrier 3 at 3200 Hz. To obtain more power, transmitter and receiver transistors were operated in their extremely nonlinear regions. To keep the receiver simple, its selectivity was not sharp. As soon as the system went operational, you were fired. Explain why.
14. What is a slew-rate limiter?
15. Calculate how many days the telemetry transmitter battery will last. Transmitter current drain is 675 μA. The battery has a rating of 0.2 A·h.
16. Indicate true or false after the following telemetry safety procedures. (*a*) Do not replace the transmitter battery until the old one has half the voltage output. (*b*) Store the telemetry transmitter with its battery connected. (*c*) Check battery voltage without the transmitter connected. (*d*) Always determine if the voltage output from new transducers or sensors will fully modulate the telemetry transmitter. (*e*) Always store the transmitter in a very warm place.

17. Describe the function of a demodulator or discriminator.
18. With the subcarrier technique, how many demodulators would be required for an eight-channel telemetry receiver? How many subcarriers for the same system?
19. List three problems sometimes found with subcarrier telemetry systems.
20. Answer true or false. (*a*) 10,000 Ω of skin resistance is satisfactory when using skin electrodes in telemetry applications. (*b*) Make certain that electrode wires are pulled very tight so that they are not flexible. (*c*) Metal electrodes should be pressed tightly into the skin to make good contact. (*d*) Any commercial jelly may be used for long-term telemetry applications. (*e*) Always place electrodes near large muscles in ECG telemetry.

chapter 7

Biomedical Computers and Microprocessors

7-1 THE COMPUTER AND HEALTH-CARE DELIVERY

In the past, medical data were organized and coordinated manually. The physician's memory had to be depended on to produce accurate patient-related data. Hospital administrative and financial affairs were managed as they had been for decades. With the sharply accelerating growth in today's health-care delivery system, however, the continuation of the methods used in the past would have surely resulted in unmanageable chaos. Computers now keep patient records, perform administrative functions, and monitor patients on-line. The programmable CRT terminal is integrating the patient-history data base and covering the conventional admissions and accounting functions. Computerized, clinically oriented data systems assist with personnel, medical records, and outpatient registration. Intelligent computer terminals at nursing stations generate new patient data and communicate with terminals in other parts of the hospital or in other hospitals. In the hospital pharmacy, the computer is an aid in dispensing drugs.

Using combined voice, data, and TV links, HEW is promoting a program to deliver health care to remote rural areas and even to space capsules on trips to distant planets. Doctors at a central hospital can receive a complete patient data profile for diagnosis. Then paramedical personnel can be guided toward the correct procedure. Pathology reports, radiology reports, and medication reactions can instantly be processed to expedite fast and flexible changes in medical procedure.

The physician's memory is now supplemented by data storage and retrieval. The organization of patient data is completely up to date at all times and is focused on solving the patient's problems. Eventually every ward and hospital service area will have its own terminal and microprocessor. This will enable every specialist, nurse, technician, and pharmacist to coordinate effectively. Their performance will be based on the most significant and relevant information available.

The data revolution is spreading far beyond the confines of the hospital. Every specialist and practitioner will have a desk-top terminal. These intelligent terminals will independently correlate patient records with medication prescriptions. These terminals will also be linked to central data banks where exhaustive and specialized data will be available.

Last, but not least, outpatients are wearing computer monitors which automatically set alarm limits for ECG, EMG, and EEG activity. Computations compensate for the amount of physical activity and other stress factors.

7-2 COORDINATING PATIENT DATA

Traditionally, medical records are organized with documents sorted according to their origin, such as doctor's notes, laboratory reports, x-rays, and so on. However, physicians cannot trace the course of a medical problem from such source-oriented records. Not only are such source-oriented records awkward to use, but they fail to reveal why various actions were taken, and so they do not preserve the logical connection to medical care. Computerized medical records are divided into four phases which define the structure of medical records. These records are then organized to make health-care delivery most effective.

To maintain a patient's health and correct any disorders, one must develop a data base on that individual. The data base defines a complete list of problems, develops a plan of action for each problem, and keeps titled, numbered progress notes (flowsheets when necessary) on each problem.

Medicine has evolved from the days of the country doctor without changing the basic assumption that doctors can remember how to identify all medical problems and recall from memory the appropriate treatment for each. American medicine has not modified this assumption in the face of an "information explosion," but has chosen, instead, to break itself into pieces called specialties. Experience gained with current terminals suggests that, to support effectively the flow of medical activity of an experienced medical user and thereby replace human memory as a major factor in the quality of health care, a very fast response to service requests is essential. The response time (screen touch to appearance of the next display) is less than $\frac{1}{2}$ s for 70 percent of the selections. An average display currently requires the transfer of 600 characters from the computer to a terminal, so that even if half the $\frac{1}{2}$-s response time was available for data transmission, a data rate of 2400 characters/s (24,000 bits/s, serial asynchronous) would be needed. Present terminals are connected via a parallel data bus which operates at 50,000 characters/s, with an average display transfer time of 12 ms. Coordination of the efforts of various specialists, nurses, pharmacists, and technicians in the care of a patient can be achieved through the common use of a problem-oriented medical record, in which the logic of each action has been preserved. However, this record must be available in various places, often simultaneously. The record must be kept in an electronic form and communicated promptly to the doctor's office, the patient's room, the pharmacy, the operating room, or the business office.

7-3 THE COMPUTER TERMINAL FOR DATA RETRIEVAL

New patients enter the electronic data processing (EDP) system before they physically enter the hospital. Advance-reservation patients are sent admission questionnaires which, when completed, form the nucleus of their hospital data base. This information is basically sociological/demographic. Data assembled on outpatients are essentially similar to those collected for admissions. However, an important difference is that the system must keep track of where in the hospital the patients are treated (in the emergency room, the outpatient clinic, or as referrals from private physicians' offices). It must register them into the system as they come into the hospital. As with admissions, the terminals are used to input basic information on their financial records and begin the medical data base. As far as personnel are concerned, the display functions principally as a retrieval system. Personnel information is entered by employee name, number, or position and can be retrieved for such assignments as payroll computation and vacation time.

7-4 NURSING STATION APPLICATIONS

Nursing stations are used to maintain the basic patient census. Diet orders are entered on the station and used, in turn, to update the patients' records. As part of the patient data base, the new dietary information is of use both to the nurses on the floor and to the hospital's kitchen.

Nursing stations also maintain a current diagnosis, which is displayed on the diet sheets and various other formats where appropriate. Nursing stations enter messages to indicate patients discharged from the unit or about to be discharged, transfers, room condition, and other information related to the maintenance and availability of beds. Some of these messages may be switched to admissions, for example, or the pharmacy, depending upon what kind of action is required. Nursing stations also enter drug-allergy indications and patient weights. This information is used for the development of a drug profile. The terminal in the pharmacy is used to enter all drug orders. In association with the allergy and patient weight information, the entry of all orders permits display, upon request, of a patient's drug profile (all drugs currently ordered for the patient).

7-5 SERVING REMOTE PATIENTS WITH A VISITING MOBILE VAN

Modern hospital facilities can be made available to widely dispersed patients via medical electronic techniques. Through remote health clinics and mobile health units, physician's assistants and nurses can tend a patient's needs under supervision of a doctor at a distant location. Communications are via VHF and microwave. Radio transceivers for audio communications and a microwave relay and transmission station for TV are available to the rural centers. Data can also be transmitted over dial-up phone lines, using acoustic couplers and modems.

NASA mobile health clinics visit on a scheduled basis. In an actual situation, a patient enters the van's reception area and is interviewed by a physician's assistant as to complaint and symptom. At this time the medic determines the need to call up a patient's history or other pertinent information by using the data terminal keyboards available in the van. Subsequent patient examination takes place in the van's examining room, where the medic is in radio contact with the physician. During the examination, the physician can view the patient via TV (as the medic uses the color TV camera above the examining table). Other facilities available in the van include the patient-viewing microscope, which utilizes fiber optics, and a special assembly which permits views of microscopic blood smears or slide cultures to be transmitted to the physician. X-rays taken in the van can also be sent to the physician via TV. Also carried in the van is a pacemaker, a defibrillator, an ECG monitor, and an aspirator, as well as eye, ear, nose, and throat diagnostics, an acoustic phone coupler, and an RF transmitter. Datacom hardware includes the physician's console, which is the focal point of the system. This console includes a storage scope and strip-chart recorder for ECG viewing. Two additional scopes are available for multichannel data reception and redundancy. There is also a television monitor and control panel for image selection, remote control of the TV cameras, and data call-up. Additionally, the console includes a video tape recorder and a stop-motion video disk recorder. Using the console, the doctor at the control center will be able to communicate with the mobile units. In the admitting office, a GE 1200 TermiNet printer is used. At the hub, the data center minicomputer is used for on-line retrieval and medical record processing.

X-rays or pictures of the patient's lesions are transmitted via slow-scan TV, using existing phone lines. These same phone lines also provide capability for voice communication and data transmission. This slow-scan capability provides x-rays or picture transmission in 45 to 90 s. It inherently records the transmission which enables almost unlimited playback capability for extensive, repetitive studying by the distant physician.

NASA's interest in the program is specifically to "determine the most effective way to administer health care to a remotely located population." The crew and passengers on future long-duration earth orbital and interplanetary missions must be provided quality health services to combat illnesses and accidental injuries, and for routine preventive care.

In remote areas on earth, the physician and allied health personnel must administer health care under conditions that are not usually optimum, including limited clinical equipment and a lack of surgical and therapeutic facilities.

7-6 SENDING MEDICAL DATA TO THE COMPUTER WITH A UNIQUE TERMINAL

To send information to the computer from a light-pen terminal, the operator aims the light pen at a word, which registers a bright feedback signal, then presses the activating button and the word is recorded. The item recorded might be a single word, several words, or a whole page of information that could be selected at one stroke of the light pen. The keyboard is used for information that cannot be entered with the light pen. Typically, the data base is generated with the keyboard, but after that, the light pen is used almost completely. Doctors use it to write orders, to look up lab and x-ray results, and to order immediate printouts such as a 7-day summary and comparative format of all lab work. Nurses use the system to do charting and for patient-care planning; the computer produces care plans just prior to every shift. Nurses also participated to a great extent in the system design, particularly with the displays. We have variable displays according to nursing specialty—pediatric nurses have one kind of display and obstetrics nurses have a different kind. Hospital personnel have their own identification minicodes. If the operator is a physician, the computer puts the names of the doctor's patients on the screen, along with their bed numbers and case numbers. The physician would use the light pen to aim at a particular name. After pressing the button on the pen, the screen would change to register the particular patient at the top of the display. It would also present a doctor's first display or "master guide." A nurse, lab technologist, or other user would get a different display. This is how access is controlled. All abbreviations used on the display screen are expressed in medical terminology. If the screen does not supply the statement wanted, anything the doctor has in mind can be typed in. Once a doctor has finished any order, it must be reviewed before the terminal will release it. In a typical case, upon release of the order, the system immediately prints the appropriate documents throughout the hospital, such as gummed labels in the pharmacy, requisitions in the laboratories, ECG, radiology and so on. The system also prints all new orders at the nursing station.

7-7 COMPUTERIZED BATCH SAMPLING

In the hospital laboratory large numbers of samples are being processed by computerized batch systems. A typical example would be the blood-sampling autoanalyzer described in Chap. 3. Data from the au-

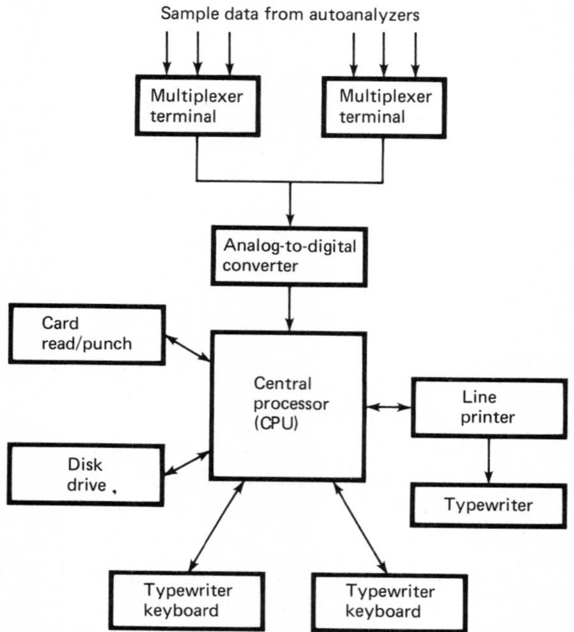

Fig. 7-1 Batch-process computer system stores data taken from blood-sampling autoanalyzer output. Sample data from six autoanalyzers are multiplexed at the input, then converted into digital pulses.

toanalyzer are reduced and transferred to the multiplexer. These terminals then become a limited-capacity storage device, but essentially make the data accessible to the CPU (central processing unit) shown in Fig. 7-1. This typical system could be programmed using a language known as *assembler language*. As the name implies, assembler language has a great deal of flexibility. It can readily be reassembled or modified and updated.

The lab sample would be accompanied by a multiple-copy request form. Each sample would have its own four-digit lab accession number which would identify that sample. The lab accession number is entered in a log-book. Long after the original sample has been centrifuged, split, and analyzed, the complete data are readily available for access or correlation with relevant medical data.

Autoanalyzer data are multiplexed at the input, allowing 12 samples to share two inputs to one analog-to-digital (A/D) converter. This converter further reduces the variable data into binary information that the CPU can understand. The CPU contains its own main-core memory system. It also acts as a receiver from a transmitter to a line printer, card reader, disk drive, and two typewriter keyboards. The variety of input/output (I/O) devices gives the clinician a great deal of flexibility.

7-8 COMPUTER TERMINOLOGY

Before we explore computers and microprocessors in great detail, we need to understand basic terminology. Whether the electronics is in a calculator that fits in the palm of your hand or in a giant IBM 370, the system is digital. This means that the electrical design is based on words of data. Analog information such as a variable voltage is far less important. In the data domain, only a state or space relationship exists. That is, only *yes* or *no* counts. A pulse is either present or absent. There is nothing in between. The whole computer language of words begins with the bit.

Bit: The smallest data unit recognized by the computer. Bit is an abbreviation of BInary digiT. It must be either a 1 or a 0. Binary bits correspond to digits in the decimal system. The decimal number 9811 is 4 digits, and the binary number 1110 is 4 bits.

Character: When 4 bits are put together, a character is formed. 1010 is 4 bits and also a character which represents the number 10.

Byte: When 4 or 8 bits are combined to form a character, this combination is called a byte.

Parallel Data: When pulses are sent in a group at one time, they are being transmitted in a parallel format. This system offers high speed but requires more data channels or data lines. For example, to process seven pulses sent simultaneously, seven separate channels would be needed.

Serial Data: When pulses are sent one at a time, or sequentially, speed is sacrificed, but greater economy is achieved because only one data channel is necessary. In Fig. 7-2, each format is serial. In Fig. 7-2*a*, each bit occurs separately in time so that the bits are serial; in Fig. 7-2*b* each byte occurs separately in time so that each byte is serial; and so on.

Words: Bits and characters combine to make a word. A word may be either data or merely instructions to the computer. Data bits in a stream all look alike. One pulse is distinguished from another by how it is organized into a word, or its format. In Fig. 7-2*a*, 8 bits, each 1 μs long, are combined serially to make a word which is 8 μs long. In Fig. 7-2*b*, 4 bits are sent simultaneously (parallel), making byte 1. Byte 2 is another 4-bit byte which completes the word. In Fig. 7-2*c* all the bits are sent in parallel, but each word is separated in time. In these examples, the computer will process a word composed of 8 bits. How fast each word is processed depends on the rep rate, clock rate, or pulse rate.

Computer Speed: The clock generates pulses that are processed by the memory and input data. The more clock pulses available, the faster the

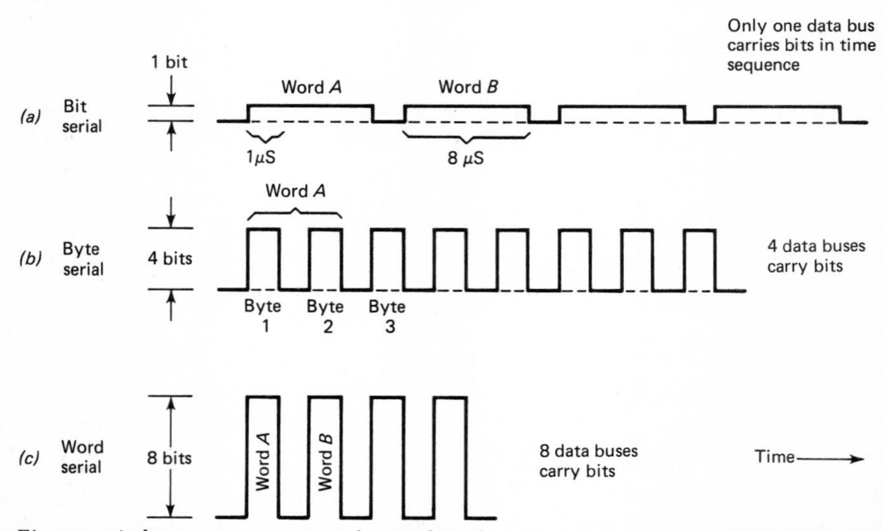

Fig. 7-2 A data stream consists of many bits that can only have two variations. Pulses are distinguished by their format, or how they are organized into words. An 8-bit word might be 8 serial bits (*a*), or 8 parallel bits (*c*), or 4 parallel bits followed by 4 more parallel bits (*b*). These three formats are also called *bit serial, byte serial,* and *word serial.*

potential speed of the computer. The clock also generates a timing pulse. This pulse triggers a new word or word group. The timing pulse keeps the operation on schedule and establishes the computer's pulse rate or speed. If the clock (a very stable oscillator) generates a 1-μs pulse (1-MHz frequency) the computer could potentially handle almost a million pulses per second, depending on the timing pulse.

Parity: A means of detecting errors uses a parity bit. When an odd number of bits precedes the parity bit, the parity bit should be 0. When an even number of bits precedes the parity bit, it should be 1. The reverse, or odd-parity, systems also exist.

Register: Stores the computer instructions while they are being interpreted and executed. Instruction registers may be flip-flops (devices that remain in one or the other state once set).

Decoder: Takes the instructions from the register, interprets the instructions, and controls the circuits required to carry out those instructions.

RAM: The random-access mode addresses the memory directly. Its access time is how long it takes to pick up a piece of data being stored, or the interval between the request and the delivery. In this mode, data can be addressed much faster than in the sequential mode. A tape drive must be addressed sequentially (must wait for the tape to reach the right place), but the tape's storage capacity can be extremely high. As opposed to read-only memories, the RAM has read-write capability.

ROM: Using read-only memory, inquiries are addressed to the memory, then a particular piece of data is retrieved by questioning the stored data at the proper address location. Once the data have been read, they are automatically rewritten so that they are still available. ROM can only be read, not changed or replaced.

PROM: Programmable read-only memory is ROM which can be altered and changed by the circuitry.

TTL: Transistor-transistor logic is an earlier form of logic circuitry that uses transistor switches.

MSI: A system having a medium density of components is medium-scale integration.

LSI: A system having a high density of components is large-scale integration.

Microprogram: A type of program that directly controls the operation of each functional element in a microprocessor.

Microinstruction: A bit pattern that is stored in a microprogram memory and specifies the operation of the individual LSI computing elements and related subunits. Subunits can be main memory or I/O interfaces.

Microinstruction Sequence: A series of microinstructions that the microprogram control unit (MCU) selects from the microprogram to execute a single macroinstruction or control command. Macroinstruction sequences can be shared by several macroinstructions.

Macroinstruction: Conventional computer instruction such as ADD MEMORY or INCREMENT or DELETE. Can also be a device controller command, such as SEEK or READ.

Source Language: Programming language which cannot be directly understood by the processor but is intelligible to the programmer.

Assemble: To translate source language into a written language of instructions understood by the main processing unit (MPU).

7-9 MICROPROCESSORS

Diagnostic patterns and test routines can be generated in a flexible and accurate manner by the microprocessor (MP). These miniature computers can monitor patient data, recognize artifacts and errors, and even identify faulty hardware. Where frequent calibration of biomedical equipment is mandatory to ensure the accuracy of medical measurements, the MP can automatically recalibrate biomedical instruments.

Data developed by the MP extend the effectiveness of human decision making. MPs can interface with large computers, as does the intelligent terminal. Human fatigue often overlooks meaningful symptoms, while the MP scans its input data looking for particular early warning symptoms. Repeated mechanical and electrical adjustments can be done automatically and with great accuracy by using MP control. The MP can read and store transducer output data, calculate the offset, then make the mechanical adjustments.

SPECIFIC MEDICAL APPLICATIONS

The MP has been used to process and monitor arrhythmias and postural disturbance, as well as EMG, EEG, ECG, and ERG (electroretinogram) activity. MPs are used to analyze respiratory gas and to monitor tissue perfusion. The MP may be an adjunct to a major system, or it may be the heart of a complex system. The latter is the case at Massachusetts General Hospital in Boston.

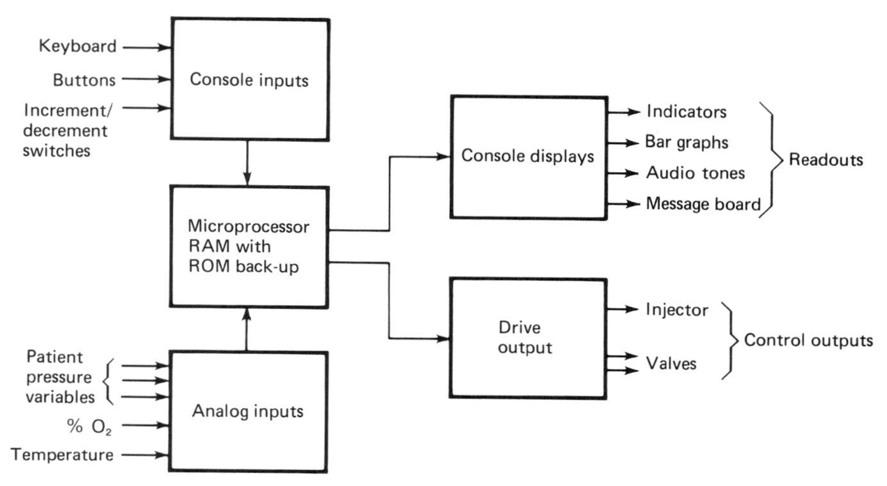

Fig. 7-3 Simplified diagram of an MP-based anesthesia delivery system. The anesthesiologist has a choice of four different readouts. In addition, there are three separate control outputs.

An MP-based anesthesia delivery system at this hospital is illustrated in Fig. 7-3. This system minimizes or eliminates potential safety hazards resulting from human error, especially in such functions as the reading of flowmeters and operating controls. The system will supply oxygen, anesthetic gases, and volatile anesthetic liquids in controlled flows. It will also control patient ventilation. Prior systems had mechanical subsystems for control and display of gas flow and anesthetic concentrations. They could not communicate with other parts of the system. By using an MP-based system, new ideas and technologies can be incorporated as they become available, without creating confusion and clutter in the system.

MICROPROCESSOR PROGRAMMING

The explosion of MP technology in biomedical electronics is based on its high degree of flexibility. This is possible because the MP operates in accordance with *instructions* which are defined in a sequence by the biomedical engineer. Thus the BMET must learn how to *instruct* or program the MP.

The ROM in the MP holds the instructions. They are "fetched" (by addressing the memory) into the MP one at a time to be decoded. Any sequence of instructions that is self-contained and is a complete solution to a particular problem is called a *program*.

Whenever a set of instructions performs a part of the main program, it is a *routine*. A very large routine has subroutines. For example, a program for a complex data processing task may have four separate routines: an input routine, a main routine, an error routine, and an output routine.

Each of these functions is an independent section of the total program and can be written in isolation from the rest of the program. In Fig. 7-4, we can see the terms, program routine, and instruction. We also can see the structure of a program and how each routine is self-contained.

Every MP has a unique set of instructions it is designed to understand and obey. The size of this instruction set is a valuable criterion in comparing one MP with another. In the main processing unit (MPU) each instruction is a combination of 1 and 0. The combination specifies an operation. An MP with an 8-bit byte and an 8-bit instruction code has two possible instruction sets. However, not all possible bit combinations may be used. Instruction sets are usually quoted according to the number of executable instructions that may be assembled into up to 3 bytes of machine code. For example, 72 executable instructions in source language can be assembled to form 197 machine codes, out of a possible 256.

MP word length is very important. A 16-bit-word MP can perform a 16-bit manipulation with one instruction. However, an 8-bit MP would need three instructions to process the same data. Before a program can

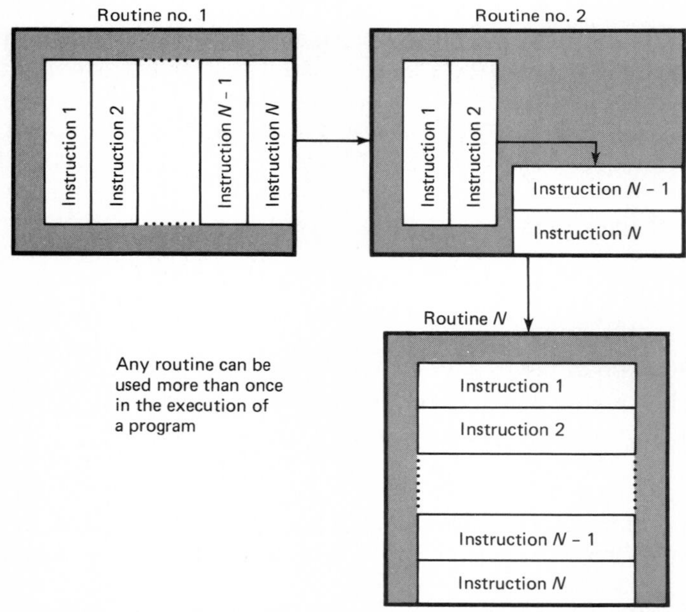

Fig. 7-4 Basic MP program structure. Each program routine contains its own set of instructions. Those labeled as N and N − 1 might be executed into more than a hundred instructions, depending on the number of gates the MP contains.

be written, the problem to be solved must be defined. This definition should include descriptions of the input parameters that must be processed, what processing is required, and the details of the output to be produced. Defining the program is simplified with a decision table.

THE DECISION TABLE. This table is a graphic representation of the relationship between variable conditions to determine the action required under differing circumstances. The decision table is based on a condition, then questions and possible responses are offered. For example, there are three conditions that affect a decision and four possible results depending on certain parameters. The conditions are written into a four-block table. Each condition is thus written, and more conditions necessitate more four-block tables. This format is followed even for the most complex problems.

Block 1 defines the condition. Block 2 gives the condition values (yes or no). Block 3 gives the action which occurs when the condition is met. This could be a recalculation of the subtotal or the beginning of another calculation. Block 4 gives the values for the actions. For example, action A should be taken, not action B.

Some problems may have more than one set of conditions and action values. Figure 7-5 shows the basic decision-table structure for a simple problem. It may be necessary to repeat a sequence of instructions until a count reaches a specific value or an external condition is fulfilled. The sequence can be continued until either of these states has occurred, or until the task is completed. A very complex problem can be broken

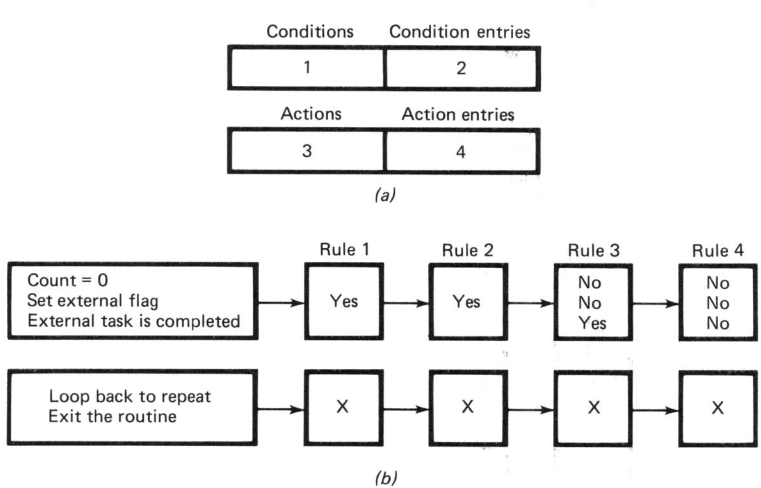

Fig. 7-5 In (*a*) we see the method of presenting the relationship between variable conditions to specify the required action in different circumstances. It is actually a very simple decision-table structure. The decision table is then translated into the various rules for the execution of a subroutine, as seen in (*b*).

into small separate sections. It can then be further defined, even by different people, if the workload has become a problem. If the problem is straightforward, it may be written as one procedure. In that case, the program is prepared without a flowchart. At this point, the programmer chooses which program language to use. However, there would be no choice when there is only one method of translating a program into machine code.

The programmer needs an understanding of what takes place in the CPU (central processing unit) and a knowledge of the data paths between the CPU and each memory element. This way, the advantages of the various instruction formats can be evaluated and the best instruction can be chosen. As defined in this text, an instruction is taken to mean that the source program defines the required action and the data or the address of the data upon which the action should be completed.

The sequence of the program is governed by the contents of the program counter (PC). During the execution of the program, the PC holds the address of the next instruction to be taken from the program's memory space. The instruction and its data are stored in one location of the memory. The PC then becomes PC + 1. After the instruction has been taken, the PC is then ready to address the next instruction in sequence. An instruction may consist of the operation code (op code), which is decoded to determine what operation is to be performed, and the address in the memory to be operated upon. The complete execution of this one instruction is enacted in three separate stages. The sequence of this operation is known as the *operating code.*

OPERATION SEQUENCE. The operating code begins as the CPU puts the contents of the PC on to the address bus. The memory responds by sending the first instruction into the instruction decoder. Part of the op code will be information that tells the CPU that an address is now required. The CPU then increments the PC by 1 and prepares to load the address register.

The CPU (with its new contents from the PC) fetches the most significant part of the address and then increments the PC again. Finally, the least significant part of the address is fetched into the address register. Having addressed the memory with the address of the required data, the data bus sends that data into the CPU. Here they are loaded into the appropriate register as defined by the instruction op code. After the PC is again increased by 1, the instruction can be completed by obeying the op code contained in the instruction decoder.

MICROPROCESSOR TECHNOLOGY

MP technology currently takes many forms. N-channel metal-oxide-semiconductor (MOS) technology has been popular for some time. LSI is being used where speed is important. However, even higher speeds are achieved using integrated-injection-logic (I^2L) technology. The BMET will be faced with more and more MP applications. Decision making will require an understanding of MP technology. A basic knowledge of the various MP technologies thus becomes extremely important.

N-CHANNEL MOS. The N-channel MOS microprocessor is designed to work directly with a minimum number of memory and peripheral support chips. These chips are supplied in coordinated families to allow them to operate off the same power supply as the CPU. A typical group of chips contains the CPU, a RAM for fast scratch-pad logic control, ROM for storing the system's program parameters, and a set of I/O chips. These I/O chips enable the CPU to control a large variety of biomedical applications.

THE MOTOROLA MC6800. This MP family consists of five chips, a single-chip CPU, a 128- by 8-bit static RAM, a 1024- by 8-bit ROM, and an I/O interface circuit. The MC6800 is packaged in a 40-pin dual inline package (DIP) and is shown in Fig. 7-6. It is built with ion-implanted, N-channel, silicon-gate technology. This chip has functions for multi-instruction processing, an arithmetic and logic unit, instruction decode and address registers, all the clock and logic circuits required for timing, a full complement of data-bus input and output matrices, and address bus drivers. The chip shown in Fig. 7-7 provides 72 self-contained basic instructions with decimal and binary arithmetic capability. The variable-length instructions include double-byte operations (such as increment, decrement, store, and compare) and enough registers to provide seven addressing modes. Instruction time is less than 5 μs, and there is direct memory access on the chip. Up to 64 bytes of memory can be addressed in any combination of RAM, ROM, or peripheral registers.

THE INTEL 8080. This MP can achieve an execution time of 2 μs, which is comparable to the speed of a minicomputer. It will trigger on a lower amplitude of signal input than previous generations of MPs, with threshold voltages as low as 0.8 to 1.4 V. Only six interface chips are required to receive 78 instructions. The internal memory holds 104 bits. The 8080 RAM and ROM have an extremely high size-to-speed ratio.

THE PACE MP. The Pace, made by National Semiconductor, allows referencing of three sequences of 256 words located anywhere in the 65,536-word memory as well as another 256 words in fixed positions. Other MPs that use an 8-bit word length are handicapped in applica-

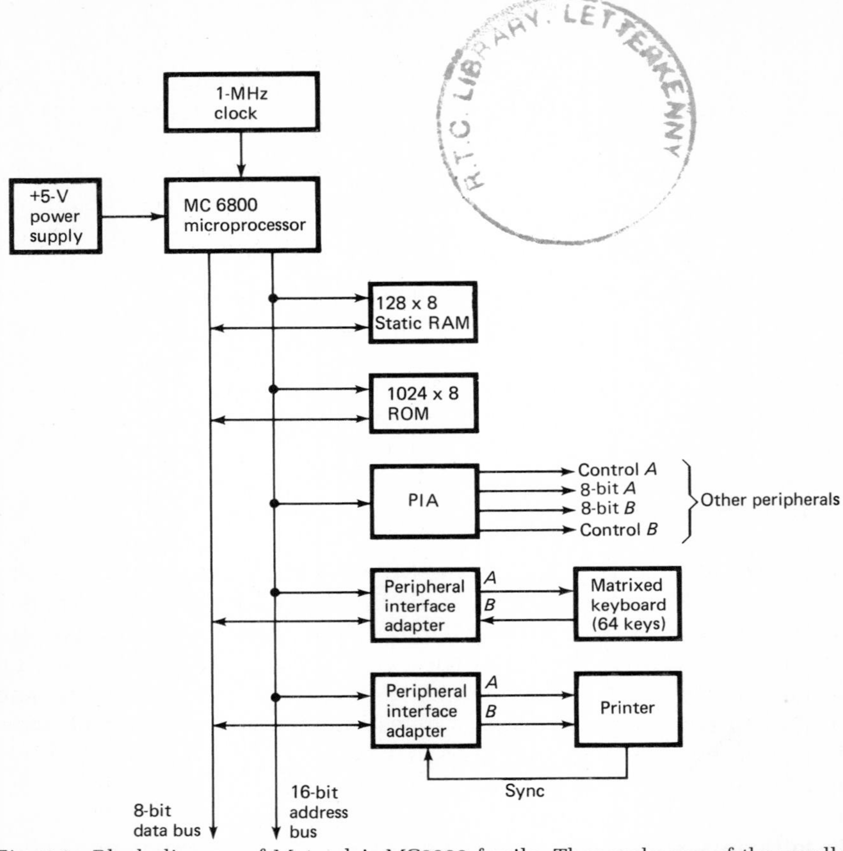

Fig. 7-6 Block diagram of Motorola's MC6800 family. They make use of the parallel data-bus concept. All PIA (peripheral interface adapter) chips are designed to hang on its CPU's eight bidirectional data lines.

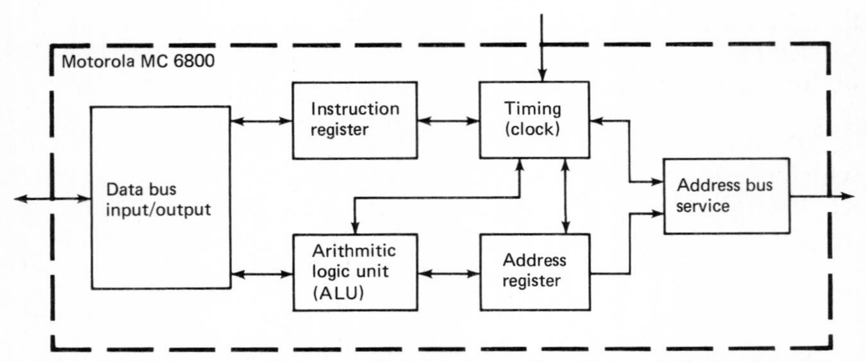

Fig. 7-7 Inside the CPU of the Motorola MC6800 MP chip. This is the heart of the microcomputer system shown in Fig. 7-6. The I/O data bus can connect to communications and telephone circuits through a UART or interface adapter. The UART (Universal Asynchronous Receiver-Transmitter) facilitates sending and receiving data through unrelated equipment.

tions requiring 16-bit words for instructions and memory address. The Pace, shown in Fig. 7-8, offers a choice of either 8- or 16-bit data processing. Since shorter programs are possible with a 16-bit word, less memory is required. Pace output buffers can drive current-sensing amplifiers. For internal data storage, Pace has seven 16-bit registers; four of these are directly available to the programmer for data storage and addressing. Additional storage for over 10 words is accomplished by storing the contents of the PC during subroutine execution. The Pace can add (four-digit word) binary-coded-decimal (BCD) data as well as straight binary, thus eliminating BCD-to-binary conversion. Using a status-flag option, the programmer can execute 8-bit applications on an 8-bit data bus and read-write memory. Also, address instructions can be implemented in 16 bits.

PROGRAMMABLE LSI. LSI technology has become a replacement for discrete logic and custom ICs. Intel's bipolar LSI chip can be faster and more flexible than MOS technology. A 16-bit processor can be assembled on a 6-in-square PC board. The processor in Fig. 7-9 has a speed of 125 ns. When choosing the right MP component, the BMET must consider such factors as gate complexity, power dissipation, and propagation delay. MOS technology alone allows a high functional density and low power dissipation. When MOS is combined with LSI technology, the MP can be placed on a single chip using a conventional control section and fixed instructions. These MPs use standard memories that are

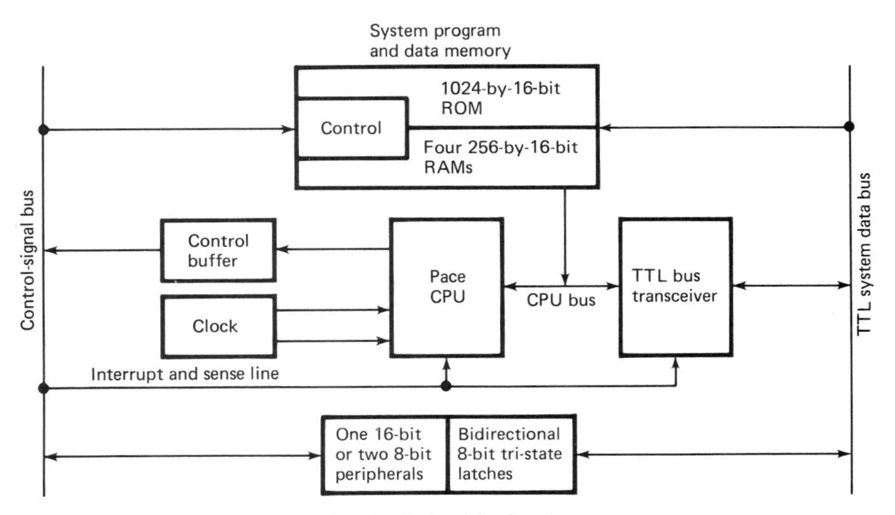

Fig. 7-8 The Pace chip allows a complete microcomputer system to be built with a minimal parts count. This system requires five ICs for the 16-bit CPU, clock, and buffering circuits, plus six ICs for the memories and two ICs for interfacing.

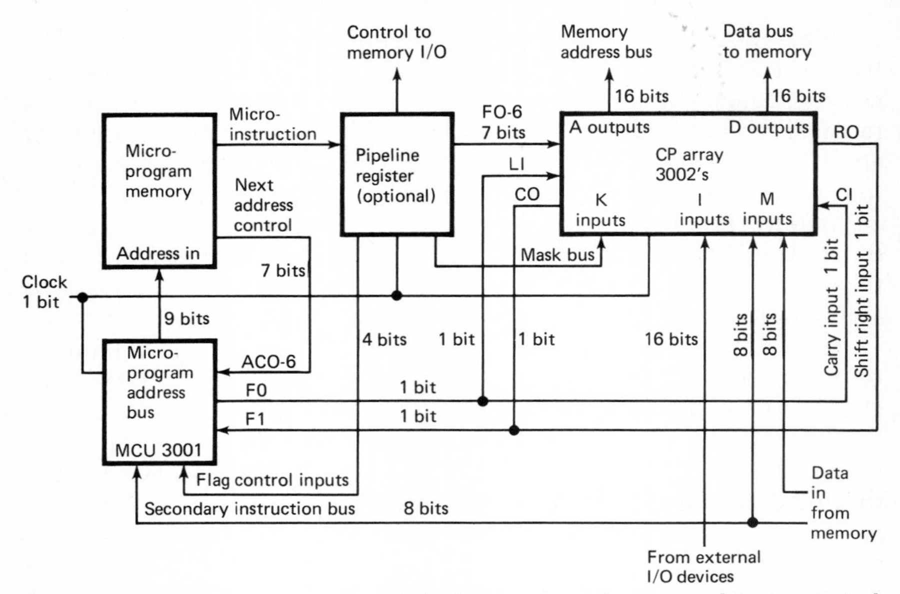

Fig. 7-9 A bipolar microcomputer. Block diagram shows how to implement a typical 16-bit controller processor with bipolar computer elements. An array of eight central-processing elements is governed by a microprogram control unit (MCU) through a separate ROM that carries the microinstructions for the various processing elements. This ROM may be a fast, off-the-shelf unit.

electrically programmable and mask programmable. RAMs hold the microprograms in experimental systems to simplify debugging. PROMS (programmable read-only memories) are used to build and test prototypes. LSI and MOS technology reduces the amount of transistor-transistor-logic (TTL) packages needed to support custom devices. This is accomplished with multiple independent data and address buses that eliminate time multiplexing and external latches. Three-state output buffers with high fan-out (load-carrying capacity) make bus drivers unnecessary. Separate output-enable logic permits bidirectional buses to be formed simply by connecting inputs and outputs together.

INTEGRATED-INJECTION LOGIC (I^2L). This recent technology allows more than five times the speed of N-channel MOS microprocessors and allows the simulation of 4-bit controllers to 16-bit minicomputers. Integrated-injection-logic gates do not require isolation between elements within the gate. In this nonisolated I^2L form, gates shrink to the size of a single transistor, so that together with their low-power capabilities, digital I^2L structures may contain thousands of gates on a single high-performing bipolar chip. I^2L changes direct-coupled transistor logic into a single complementary transistor equivalent. In Fig. 7-10, the resistor in the transistor gate is replaced by an active current source. The emitter-grounded output transistor pair is replaced by a single multicollector transistor, and a simple PNP transistor is added to serve as the current-injector source. Six transistors in the older three-input gate now become a single I^2L transistor pair. Q_1 is an inverter, and Q_2 is a current source and an active load. The base of the multicollector NPN transistor is made common with the emitter of the multicollector NPN. Consequently, the entire I^2L gate takes up the same space as a single multiemitter transistor.

Isolated I^2L allows standard bipolar and MOS design techniques to be combined with I^2L gates. Along with I^2L digital functions, a single low-cost monolithic chip can hold light-emitting-diode (LED) drivers, memory decoders, current regulators, op amps, comparators, oscillators, and TTL logic. Electronic watches use this technique. Isolated I^2L can be combined with TTL and emitter-coupled-logic (ECL) memory to provide fast, low-cost bipolar memory designs. The I^2L gates would form the internal array of the memory, while the TTL transistors would form the peripheral interface elements. I^2L arrays combined with RAMS (Texas Instruments 74S209) provide low-cost 100-ns memories. Using the single-transistor switch design of Fig. 7-10, nonisolated I^2L capitalizes on the high carrier mobility inherent in bulk silicon structures. No isolation or ground metalization is needed because (Fig. 7-10) the output of one gate serves as the input of the next. These gates operate at nanosecond speeds and microwatt power dissipation. The I^2L gate has the lowest speed $\times$ power product of any MP technology. Since its theoretical limit is 0.001 picojoule (pJ), 100-ns propagation delays at 100-nW consumption per gate has been achieved.

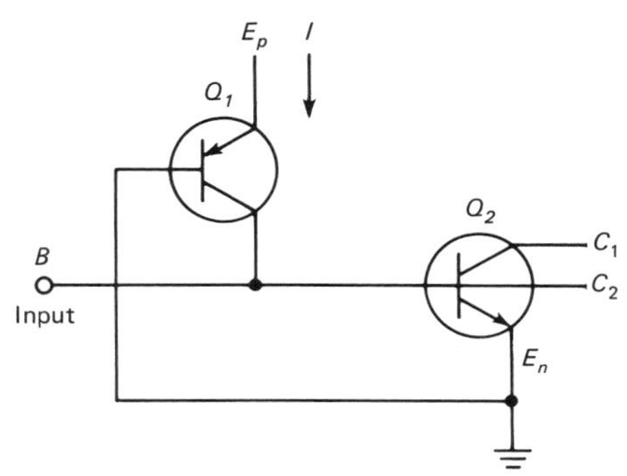

Fig. 7-10 The equivalent transistor circuit of digital I^2L would consist of a vertical NPN transistor Q_1, with multiple collectors C_1 and C_2, operating as an inverter. The lateral PNP transistor Q_2 operates as a current source and a load.

I²L POWER SUPPLIES. I²L gates resemble silicon switching diodes when they are observed on a curve tracer. Their power requirements are thus extremely low. Any power supply may be used that provides the desired current at 850 mV or more, such as a dry cell battery. Rectified power supplies should have good regulation and an extremely low noise level.

THE TI SPB 0400 MP. This 4-bit processor, shown in Fig. 7-11, is expandable in 4-bit multiples. It has larger multichip systems and parallel access to all control, data, address, and I/O functions. It is this parallel access, with the 110- to 500-ns speeds, that gives this device its short-cycle-time capability. The factory-programmable logic array (PLA) offers 512 one-clock operations. This compares to a fixed-instruction capability of less than 80 operations. Any set of instructions is available in a 1-μs-clock cycle. For example, any one of 459 nonredundant operations can be selected, including tasks like transferring data from the processor's register to the external memory or to a register. The PLA decodes the 9-bit operation-select word input lines and generates a 20-bit internal control word. This control word is stored in the operations register and contains the appropriate logic operation —functional block, bus enable, and bus select—for execution of the decoded instruction. The registers are used for temporary storage of source data. A separate register is a PC, is presettable, and may be externally controlled for incrementation by 1 or 2 on the next clock transition. Fetch and command are simplified as the contents of the PC are directly available at the address-out bus (AOB). Regardless of the conditions established by a present instruction, a PC priority input overrides and routes the PC data on the AOB input terminal.

MICROPROCESSOR SELECTION

To appreciate the advantages of various MPs, the BMET must have a basic knowledge of the field alterations that are possible with microprocessors. Unlike larger processors, the MP is fabricated as one IC or a small number of ICs. A PROM allows the existing system to be changed in a few hours. The speed, addressing modes, interrupt capabilities, and number of internal registers of the popular MPs are listed in Table 7-1. As more addressing modes and more internal registers are present, less memory capacity is required. Usually, memory cost dominates other considerations. If the MP can handle interrupts, it can perform more than one task at a time and can do single tasks faster because it can overlap processing and I/O operations. The pointer-address mode allows a machine with a short word length to address a large memory array. These large arrays may require more bits in an address represen-

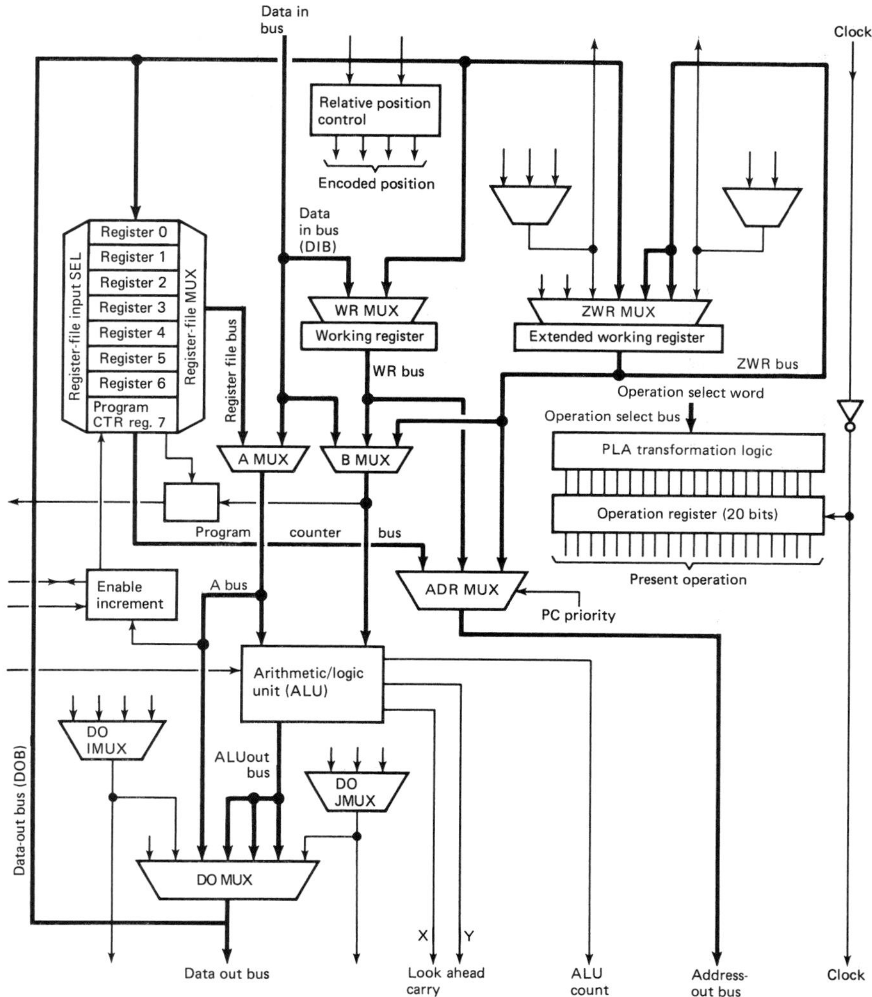

Fig. 7-11 The Texas Instruments I²L microprocessor lends itself to many biomedical applications. This SPB 0400 chip contains a 16-function arithmetic logic unit (ALU) and the factory programmable logic array (PLA), which provides 512 standard one-clock operations. This 40-pin, 4-bit microprogrammable binary processor element has over 1450 gates and has all the functions for 4-bit parallel processing (except for sequencing controls). Using TTL technology, it would take over 40 circuits to accomplish the same thing.

tation than can be contained in one instruction word. Thus the address is kept in a separate register. This register is preloaded by an instruction in the program. Subsequent instructions then refer to locations in the memory which are addressed by the pointer register. In its indirect-address mode, the processor executes an instruction on data found, and at the address specified by the part of the instruction word

Table 7-1 **Microprocessor Characteristics**

	Intel MCS-4	**Rockwell PPS**	**Intel MCS-8**	**Intel 8080**	**Signetics PIP**	**National GPC/P**	**AMI 7300**
Word size (bits)	4	4	8	8	8	4–16	8
Instruction time (microseconds)	10.8–21.6	5–10	7.5–22.5 12–44 (Note 1)	2–6	<5–<10	3.3–9.6	4–32 (Note 2)
Memory size — Pgm	4096 bytes	16,384 bytes					4096 words (Note 4)
Memory size			16,384 bytes	65,536 bytes	8192 bytes	65,536 bytes	
Memory size — Data	1280 nibbles (Note 3)	8192 nibbles (Note 3)					65,536 bytes
No. of instructions	45	54	48	48+	64	Microprogram	Microprogram
Interrupt capability	Reset to 0 only	None	1-level vector to 8 locations	Multilevel vector to 8 locations	1-level stack to store machine state	1-level stack to store machine state (Note 5)	3-level
Address modes	Pointer Indirect Immediate Register	Pointer Immediate	Pointer Immediate Register	Pointer Immediate Register	Direct Indirect Relative Immediate Register Indexed	Direct Indirect Relative Immediate Register Indexed	Direct Indirect Relative Immediate Register Indexed

Registers	16 × 4 bits pc + 3 stack	2 × 4 bits pc + 2 stack 1 pointer	5 × 8 bits pc + 7 stack 1 pointer	5 × 8 bits pc + Unlimited stack 1 pointer (Note 6)	4 × 8 bits pc + 7 stack	4 × 16 bits pc + 16 stack (Note 7)	16 × 8 bits pc + 32 × 8 stack (Note 7)
RAM & ROM	Special or standard (Note 8)	Special	Standard	Standard	Standard	Standard	Standard and special microprogran
TTL chips	Clock only	None	20–40	Clock & buffers	4–6	15–20	Clock & buffers

NOTES:
1. 8008-1 instruction times are 0.6 × (8008 instruction times).
2. Executes microinstructions from 512 × 22 microprogramed ROM at 4 μs/microinstruction.
3. 1 nibble = 4 bits = $\frac{1}{2}$ byte.
4. Microprogram.
5. Conditional jump MUX external to chips allows 2-level interrupt very simply.
6. Pc stack is stored in main memory and is accessible to programer.
7. Stack is general-purpose to store pc, registers, and flags.
8. 4008 & 4009 chips allow easy interface to standard RAM & ROM.

SOURCE: Laurence Altman, ed., *Microprocessors*, Electronics Book Series, McGraw-Hill Book Company, New York, 1975.

to be operated upon (the operand code). If the MP can be microprogrammed, its control sequences are stored in ROMs in the same way as object programs, which determine the machine's function. The program is written in assembler language, then converted to binary or machine language. Assembly language is executed on the same machine that is to run the machine program.

When selecting the central processing unit (CPU), a decision must be made how to process the data. The processor can have either a fixed word length or chip paralleling capability. A 16-bit CPU chip might be programmed into 4-bit words for BCD display or control in calculators or cash registers. An 8-bit word would most likely be used for CRT terminals or data concentrators. A 12-bit word would be used for handling the output of analog-to-digital (A/D) converters. A 16-bit word would be used for general-purpose processing, as might even 24- to 32-bit words for high-accuracy or high-throughput applications.

The only way to compare instruction sets is to compare their execution time and the number of bits of storage they use. The medical application will determine the necessary processor interface structure. A simple low-cost bus (parallel or serial) with separate input, output, and address lines may be used, or a high-speed, bidirectional bus with addresses and data multiplexed over the same lines can be used. Processor I/O circuitry should directly interface with the 5-V bipolar logic required to drive I/O lines; otherwise buffers will be needed. Read/write memories (RAMs) are best used for variable data storage and for program storage during the development of a new program.

GENERAL-PURPOSE MPs. MP selection can sometimes be simplified by considering systems with a high degree of flexibility. Such a system is shown in Fig. 7-12; it is an 8-bit system. It consists of a CPU, RAMs, ROMs, a clock generator, a direct memory-access controller, and an assortment of general-purpose I/O devices. All of them are accessible on the same bidirectional data-instruction bus. This bus provides 8-bit parallel communication within the computer at 500 kHz. Over 90 instructions can be executed in 4 μs each, which covers a ROM access for instruction fetch and a RAM access for data fetch as well as the processing of the data. Special I/O devices such as a telephone modem or a keyboard-display controller with independent input and output buffers are available.

National Semiconductor's IMP-16 provides computing power from a simple 4-bit keyboard address capability right up through full 16-bit minicomputer capability. Processing is done by four 4-bit arithmetic logic units (ALUs) controlled by microprogrammable ROMS (Fig. 7-13).

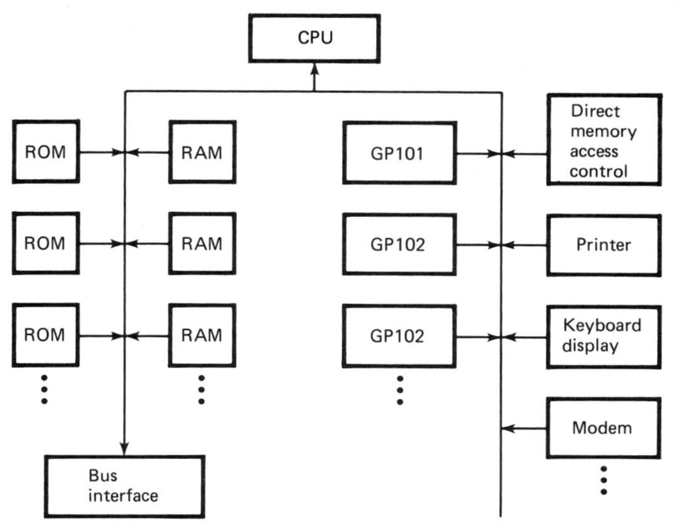

Fig. 7-12 This 8-bit microprocessor chip set, made by Rockwell, contains more than 90 instructions with 4-μs execution times. All the components shown work directly off the CPU.

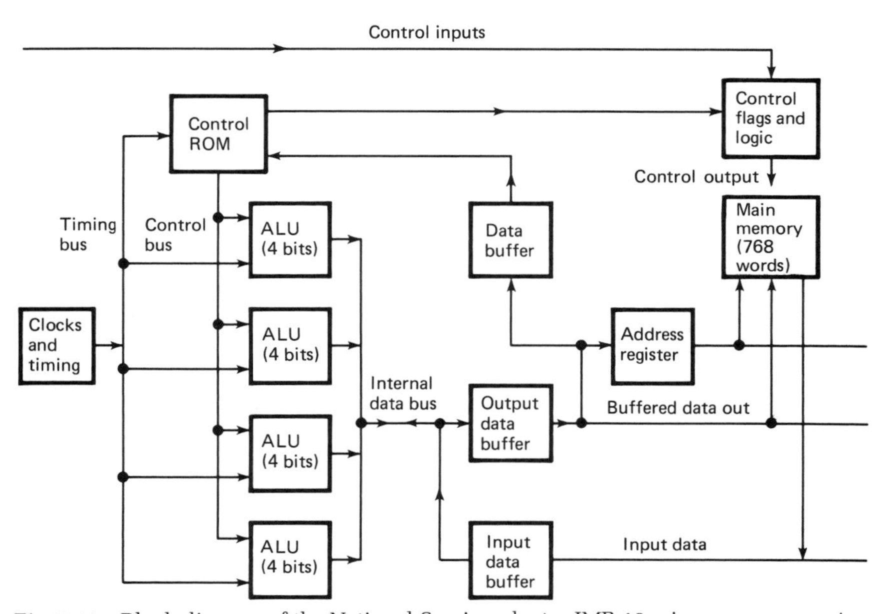

Fig. 7-13 Block diagram of the National Semiconductor IMP-16 microprocessor system shows the system of four 4-bit ALU slices with control registers, ALU logic, and I/O data lines. Altogether 43 instructions are available.

With this arrangement, data exchange takes place over a 16-bit-wide data bus. However, all I/O and control operations occur over a set of 16 addressable registers or flags. The five-chip board has 256 words of random access memory and 512 words of read-only on-card memory. Also on the card are interfaces such as an address bus, data I/O buses, additional control flags, system timing lines, and an interrupt input.

AVAILABLE ASSISTANCE. Armed with this very basic knowledge of processors, the BMET can now seek additional assistance from equipment vendors. Users' manuals, programming manuals, and biomedical application notes are available from MP manufacturers and distributors. Many electronics distributors now stock the various MPs described in this chapter. They also have an MP application specialist who can interpret your biomedical application into the proper hardware. Thus a working MP system can be developed with the medical data requirements being the sole guide.

QUESTIONS

1. What part of the computer generates pulses to be processed by the CPU and to synchronize the various data-bus lines?
2. Describe the function of the computer's timing pulse.
3. If we are interested in economy, not speed, and we use only one data line (channel), what data format would we use?
4. Which bit would be checked to determine if noise has obscured a pulse?
5. In the random-access mode, what is the execution time or address time?
6. A disk is an example of __________ addressing, with a __________ storage capacity.
7. A computer language that is not understood by the processor but is intelligible to the programmer is called __________ language.
8. What is a routine?
9. To process 16-bit data with a single instruction, what type of MP should be ordered?
10. In writing an MP program, give three items to be considered.
11. What is a graphic representation of the relationship between variables that determines the action to be taken under different circumstances?
12. Why should the programmer know what goes on in the central processing unit and also know the data paths between the CPU and each memory element?
13. What is a function of the program counter?
14. An instruction enacted in three stages determines which operation should be performed and the correct address to be operated upon. What is this sequence called?
15. Correct the following operating sequence. (*a*) The memory responds by sending the first instruction to the decoder. (*b*) The CPU puts the contents of the program counter on the address bus. (*c*) The data bus sends data to the CPU, where it is loaded into the appropriate register.

16. If you wanted a shorter program along with less memory, would you order a 4-, 8-, or 16-bit MP?
17. To eliminate external latches and time-multiplexing circuits in an MP, what should be included in the MP circuitry?
18. Give at least two advantages of I^2L technology.
19. If an MP using MOS circuits were replaced by one using LSI, what would be gained?
20. List at least three general, technical considerations the BMET should review when investigating a new MP purchase.

chapter 8

Common Biomedical Circuits

INTRODUCTION

Presently there are some 2000 corporations manufacturing medical electronic instrumentation. It would hardly be possible to explain each circuit in every instrument which has been manufactured.

Yet in every instrument made, there is a power supply, amplifiers, oscillators, and other basic circuits. Armed with a knowledge of the most common biomedical circuits, the BMET will be able to approach a strange piece of equipment with confidence. The instrument's basic circuit concepts will become clear with some amount of study. If the instrument is extremely complex, a basic circuit may be repeated several times. However, the basic elements are nevertheless present. In many cases, the circuits given in this chapter have been oversimplified. Components have been omitted to facilitate an understanding of the basic circuit concept.

Power supplies and their regulators are described. Techniques for voltage multiplication up to 400,000 V for use in nuclear medicine are covered. The principles of common-mode rejection and differential amplifiers are discussed. Chopper circuits used in low-level applications are included. Analog-to-digital (A/D) converters are being used more and more as technology advances. Basic thermometer and pacemaker circuits give the reader a glimpse into these frequently encountered biomedical devices.

A radio pill circuit is given which could actually be constructed by an enterprising BMET. Basic remote control circuits are included, as more applications are being found for these devices. Since the BMET will undoubtedly encounter dated equipment using vacuum-tube circuits, basic tube circuits have been included.

Under safety circuits, a floating power supply is described which is powered by ultrasonic energy. Several different safety circuits will be found in this one isolated power source.

8-1
THE POWER SUPPLY

Unless the medical instrument is battery-powered, it must have some type of power-supply circuitry. Such circuits change the 60-Hz power source into usable voltages for vacuum tubes, photomultipliers, CRTs, transistors, ICs, LEDs, etc. Essentially, most power supplies can be identified by the center tap on the power transformer secondary. In Fig. 8-1, a series regulator can be switched to any one of three popular power-supply circuits. With the switch in position *A*, the vacuum-tube full-wave circuit is working. When the top of the transformer secondary is +, the top rectifier conducts. Then 180° later, when the bottom of the secondary is +, the bottom rectifier conducts. At the cathodes, alternating half-cycles are combined. The result is full-wave output. With the switch in position *B*, the same sequence of events occurs. Only this time, the tubes have been replaced by solid-state diodes. If the transformer secondary did not have a center tap and there was only one diode, rectification would only occur on a half-cycle. Regulation and ripple would not equal a full-wave rectifier system. However, if the transformer secondary does not have a center tap and four rectifiers are seen, then we have a bridge rectifier. This is seen in switch position *C*, Fig. 8-1*a*. When the switch is in either position *A* or *B*, the output voltage is half the full transformer secondary voltage. However, in the bridge circuit, the output voltage is the full transformer secondary voltage. For moderate and heavy current applications, there is considerable transformer cost economy when using the bridge circuit.

In the series regulator (Fig. 8-1*b*), all the power must pass through Q_1, which becomes a series gate. Q_2 amplifies current on the way to the "main gate," so that this gate will be extremely sensitive to the output of dc amplifier Q_3. Transistor Q_3 senses the difference between the current in Q_5 and Q_6. The power-supply output is continuously sampled by R_1. When the voltage at the base of Q_6 is equal to the voltage generated by the zener reference on the base of Q_5, then the differential amplifiers Q_5 and Q_6 are said to be balanced. However, when there is a difference voltage, it is amplified by Q_3, changing the current in Q_2 and consequently in the gate Q_1. Thus a feedback loop between R_1 and Q_1 regulates and stabilizes the power supply. This regulation may be as precise as 0.001 percent against a wide range of line or load variations. For instruments used in nerve-conduction studies, the variation of several microseconds in a nerve's response time could mean the difference between a healthy and a diseased patient. A fault in the power-supply series regulator could cause a time-base error, leading to an incorrect diagnosis.

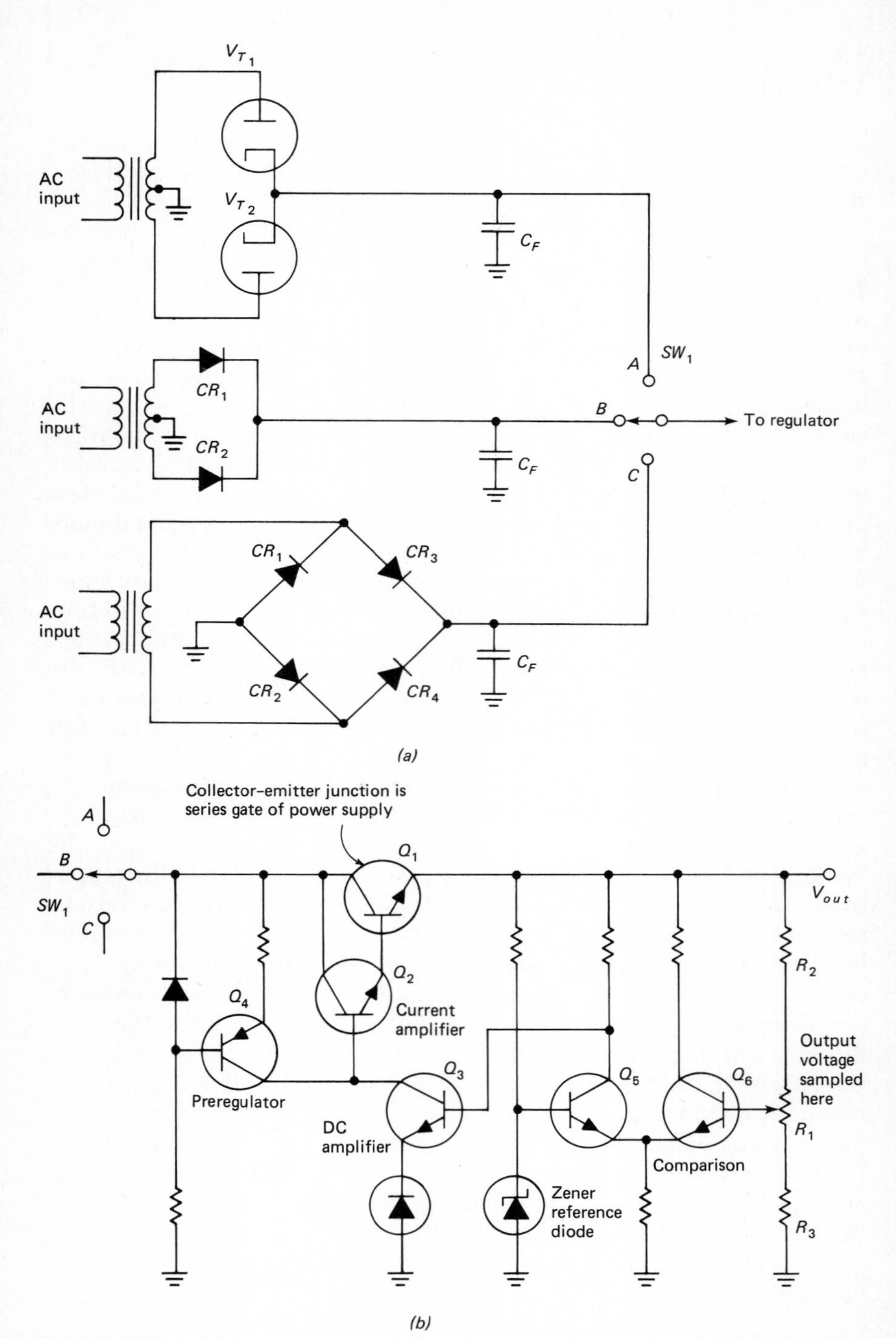

Fig. 8-1 Switch SW_1 enables the series regulator to be switched to the most common power-supply circuits. Switch position *A* goes to a vacuum-tube full-wave rectifier. Switch position *B* is a solid-state full-wave rectifier. Position *C* is a bridge rectifier.

8-2 VOLTAGE MULTIPLICATION

The power supplies in Fig. 8-1 could be made with special transformers to give us power with a voltage up to 5000 V. Above these voltages, however, transformer cost would become prohibitive and the circuit would be subject to voltage breakdown. If we need voltages for CRT tubes, photomultipliers, scintillation counters, or precise electrostatic fields, new circuits must be devised. Ordinary TV sets use an oscillator and flyback-transformer arrangement to generate high voltages for the CRT tube. A color TV may generate up to 35,000 V this way. However, these voltages are not stable under varying load conditions.

In medical instruments, the stability of the power source must be beyond question. We must then generate high voltages that are extremely stable. One technique is to design a flyback-transformer-type oscillator to provide a relatively low voltage (5000 V) with a regulator (similar to Fig. 8-1) to ensure stability. The regulator senses the output voltage and feeds this information to a feedback loop. This loop controls the oscillator bias so that the oscillator output is precisely regulated.

Diode multipliers are added to the 5-kV output. These circuits increase voltage and isolate the power supply from the load. The voltage doubler is seen in Fig. 8-2*b*, the voltage tripler in Fig. 8-2*c*, and the quadrupler in Fig. 8-2*d*. All these circuits have capacitors (*C*) connected in such a way that they charge in phase with the input voltage, thus adding their charged voltage (equal to the input voltage) to the input voltage itself. Each capacitor-diode section consequently doubles its input voltage. The sextupler (Fig. 8-2*e*) works on the same principle. Sextupler sections can be stacked or combined. For example, 36 capacitor-diode (*C*-CR) sections would change 5 kV into 400 kV. In high-precision supplies of this type, the output voltage (in addition to the oscillator output voltage) is again sensed and fed back to regulate the oscillator bias. This technique provides voltages that are stable to within a fraction of 1 percent of the output voltage. For medical applications where the diagnosis depends on the reliability of the power-supply voltage, this stability is imperative.

8-3 DIFFERENTIAL AMPLIFIERS

Biomedical amplifiers often handle physiological data in the low-microvolts region. EEG amplifiers are required to detect signals as low as a microvolt. Aside from the stringent noise requirements for such high levels of amplification, 60-Hz interference is a formidable

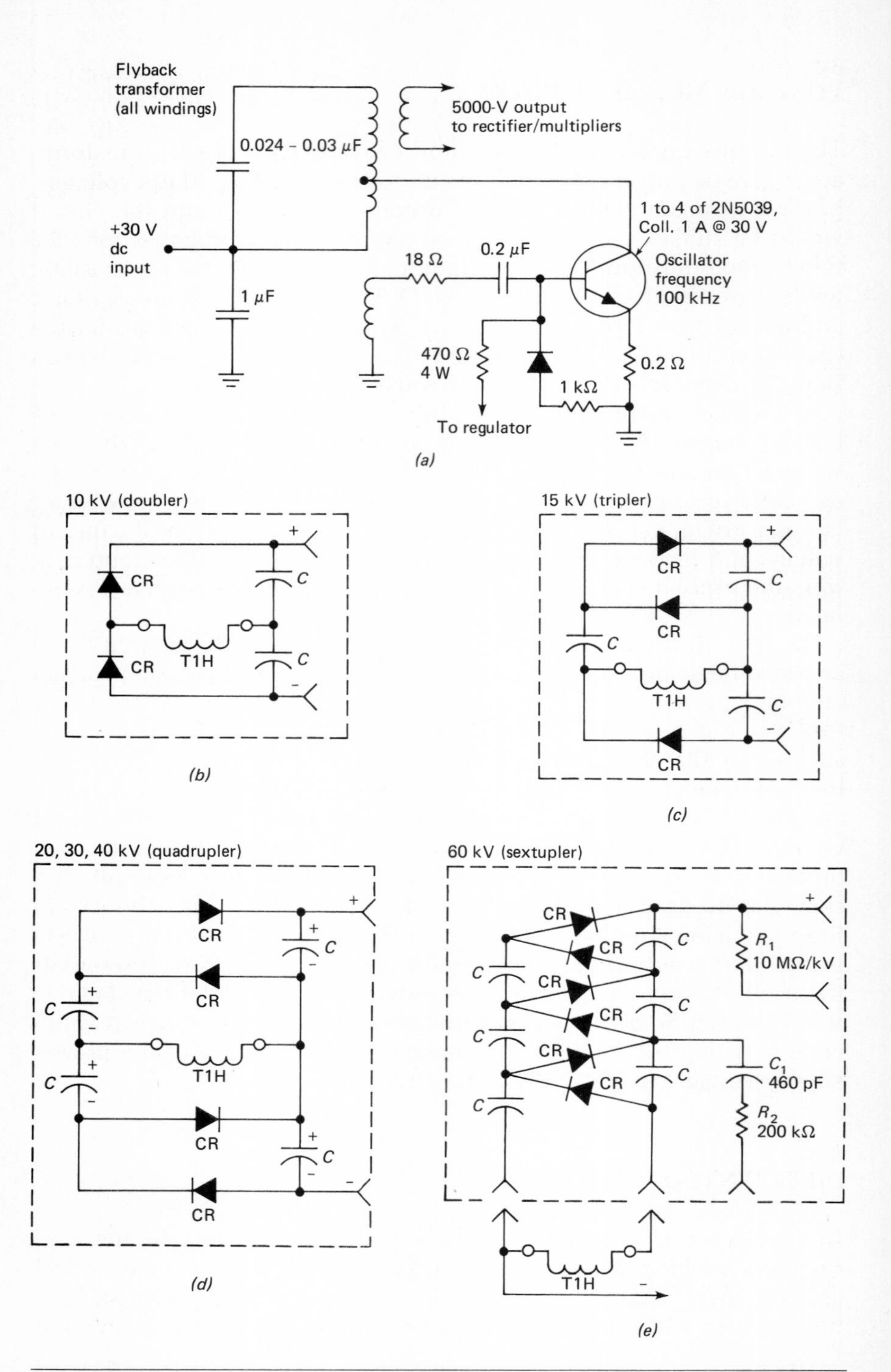
Flyback
transformer
(all windings)
5000-V output
to rectifier/multipliers
0.024 – 0.03 μF
1 to 4 of 2N5039,
Coll. 1 A @ 30 V
+30 V
dc
input
18 Ω
0.2 μF
Oscillator
frequency
100 kHz
1 μF
470 Ω
4 W
0.2 Ω
1 kΩ
To regulator
(a)
10 kV (doubler)
CR
C
T1H
(b)
15 kV (tripler)
(c)
20, 30, 40 kV (quadrupler)
(d)
60 kV (sextupler)
R_1
10 MΩ/kV
C_1
460 pF
R_2
200 kΩ
(e)

problem. AC interference might easily have a magnitude 500 times that of the desired medical data. If there is one single circuit primarily responsible for medical instrument progress, it would be the differential amplifier. This circuit responds to the differential input, or the medical data, and discriminates against interference, or the common input.

COMMON-MODE REJECTION

A linear active device might have two input signals, V_1 and V_2, and one output signal, V_0. All inputs and the output are measured with respect to ground. In the ideal differential amplifier, the output V_0 would be stated as

$$V_0 = \text{gain of the differential amplifier } (V_1 - V_2)$$

Accordingly, a signal which is common to both inputs (V_1 and V_2) will not affect the output V_0. The figure of merit of a differential amplifier is its common-mode rejection ratio (CMRR). In the linear device, the output was a linear combination of the two input voltages; thus

$$V_0 = \text{amplification of } V_1 \text{ against ground} + \text{amplification of } V_2 \text{ against ground}$$

also

$$\text{Differential gain} = \tfrac{1}{2} \text{ amplification of } V_1 \text{ against ground} - \text{amplification of } V_2 \text{ against ground}$$

Before we can calculate the CMRR, it is necessary to know the differential gain. This can be measured by applying a 1-V signal across the differential input terminals V_1 and V_2. The common-mode input is now 0 V. Under this condition, the measured output voltage V_0 gives the gain for the differential signal. Now it is possible to determine the quality of the differential amplifier or the CMRR as

$$\text{CMRR} = \frac{\text{amplification of the differential voltage}}{\text{amplification of the common-mode voltage}}$$

To illustrate this, if the CMRR is 1000, then a common-mode voltage V_c of 1 mV and a differential voltage V_d of 1 μV will both produce the

---

Fig. 8-2 (page 250) Oscillator and flyback-transformer circuit in (*a*) can produce 5000 V of highly regulated power. Diode (CR) and capacitor (C) combinations become multipliers which are added to the oscillator power-source output. These additional sections (Fig. 8-2*b* to *e*) can be stacked to produce almost a million volts of highly regulated power.

same output voltage. Another way of saying this is that the common-mode signal (interference) is discriminated against by a ratio of 1000 to 1.

EMITTER-COUPLED DIFFERENTIAL AMPLIFIERS

The circuit in Fig. 8-3*a* would make an excellent differential amplifier if the emitter resistance R_e were very large. In fact, the common-mode gain would be zero if R_e were large enough. Thus the CMRR would be infinite, for R_e would be infinite and the circuit would be perfectly symmetrical. Unfortunately, there are limitations in raising R_e due to the voltage drop across R_e. The emitter supply V_{ee} must become larger as R_e is increased to maintain the quiescent current at its proper value. If the operating current of the two transistors decreases sufficiently, there will be a higher emitter input resistance and thus a lower beta or gain. Both these effects will decrease the CMRR. Therefore R_e must be kept low. This means that the circuit of Fig. 8-3*a* will never be able to yield too high a CMRR.

THE CONSTANT-CURRENT SOURCE

The differential-amplifier emitter resistance R_e in Fig. 8-3*a* can be replaced with a constant-current source, as shown in Fig. 8-3*b*. R_1, R_2,

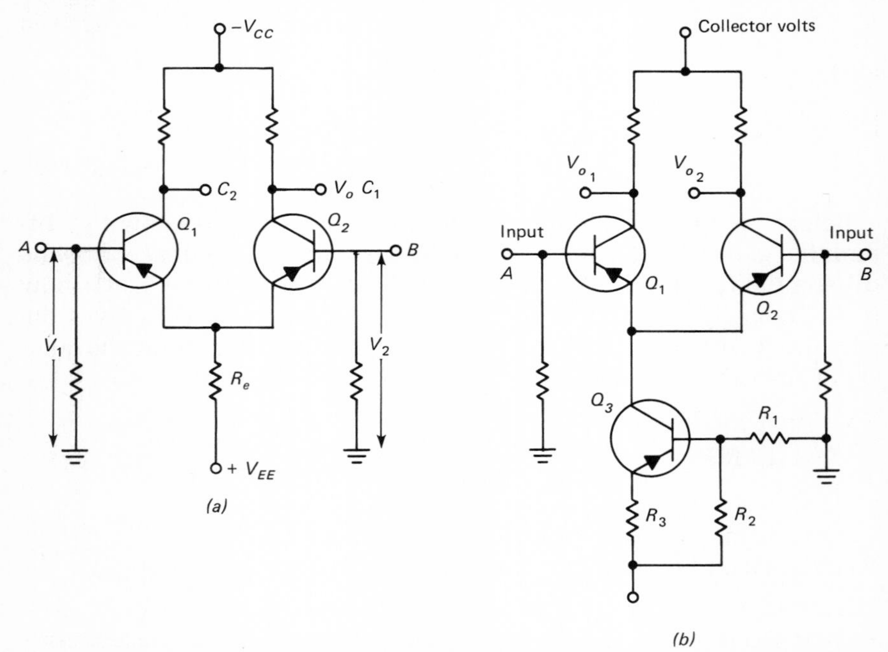

Fig. 8-3 (*a*) The basic differential amplifier configuration. The input is across *A* and *B*; the output is taken across C_1 and C_2. (*b*) A differential amplifier with a constant-current source. Q_3 operates in its constant-current mode.

and R_3 can be adjusted to give the same quiescent conditions for Q_1 and Q_2 as the circuit in Fig. 8-3*a*. The new circuit has a very high effective emitter resistance. R_e is now the effective resistance looking into the collector of Q_3. R_e will be several times 100,000 Ω, even if R_3 is as small as 1 kΩ. Q_3 is a constant-current source, subject to the conditions that the base current and the base-emitter voltage of Q_3 are neglible. The emitter current is independent of the signal input voltage, and Q_3 supplies the two amplifiers with a constant current. If Q_1 and Q_2 were identical and Q_3 were an ideal constant-current source, the common-mode gain would be zero.

The problem with transistor differential amplifiers is that drift due to variations of hf_e, V_{be}, and I_{cbo} with temperature always exists. A shift in any of these quantities changes the output voltage and cannot be distinguished from a change in input-signal voltage. Using IC equivalents of Q_1 and Q_2, greater stability can be achieved. Differential amplifiers can be cascaded to increase both gain and CMRR. In Fig. 8-3*b* the outputs V_{o_1} and V_{o_2} are equal but 180° out of phase. In measuring biomedical signals, the input impedance of the differential amplifier should be as high as possible. The higher the input impedance, the lower the magnitude of current that can flow across the input terminals and through the patient. A higher input impedance also increases sensitivity to low-level signals. Therefore, it is sensible to replace transistors with FET devices, as shown in Fig. 8-4. In this actual biomedical circuit, the 2N3904 (bottom left) stabilizes the base of the constant-current source (2N3904, bottom center). It also is part of the base-stabilization circuit for another constant current source, the 2N3906 (top center). The stabilization built into this circuit gives it a wide dynamic range. The differential pair of FETS (2N5519) have an extremely high Z and low noise level. This circuit can detect biomedical signals in the low-microvolts region.

8-4 CHOPPER CIRCUITS

The input circuit in Fig. 8-4 can be coupled to an ac amplifier whose frequency response is as low as 10 Hz. However, if this high sensitivity must be used to amplify dc signals, then stability becomes a severe problem. Transistors are temperature and current sensitive. Their parameters change with age. To obtain a high gain with a dc amplifier, it is necessary to contend with many variable parameters inherent in solid-state devices. It would be extremely difficult to know if our measurement reflected true medical data or merely unstable component variables.

The chopper solves these problems by permitting an ac amplifier to

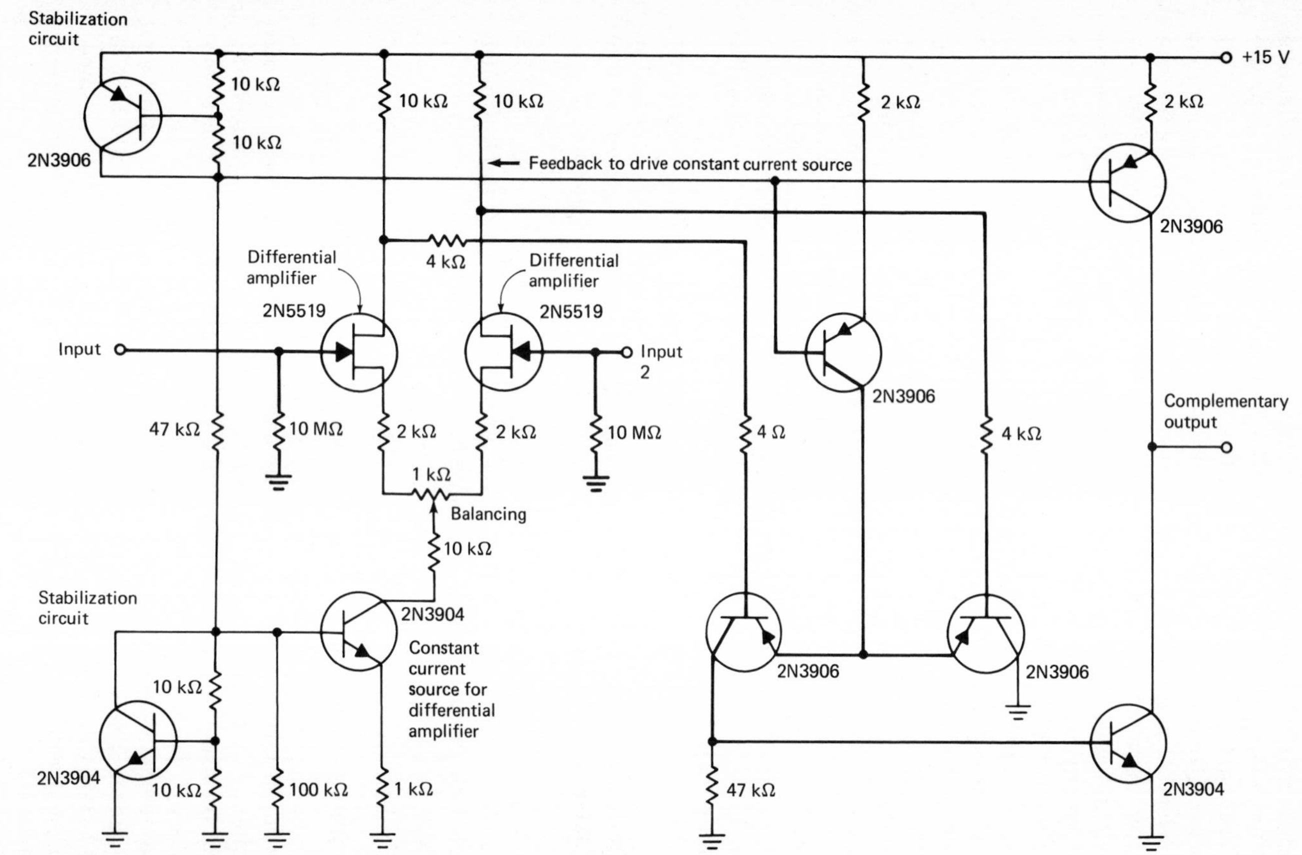

Fig. 8-4 An actual high-gain biomedical differential amplifier. The N-channel FET devices have a low noise figure and an extremely high input Z.

look at (or sample) the dc signal we wish to observe. The ac amplifier is not plagued by the heat and instability problems of a dc amplifier, yet it can read the dc data. In Fig. 8-5*a*, the left-hand pair of MOSFETS forms an astable multivibrator whose period of oscillation is determined by values of *R* and *C*. The multivibrator output drives a simple shunt MOSFET chopper switch. When this switch is ON, the circuit looks at the dc input. The MOSFET at the right provides signal gain and transforms the high chopper impedance into a low impedance for ac output.

If our medical application requires an extremely stable input device that will drift less than 0.35 μV/°C, then we might use the op-amp

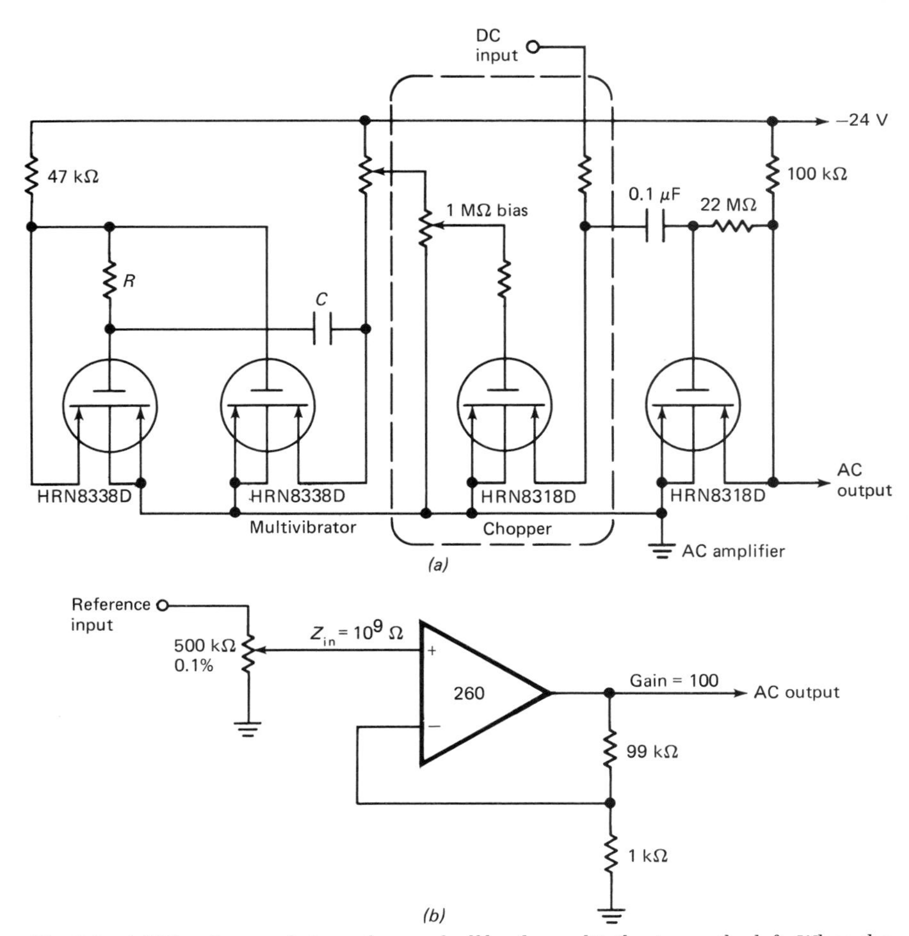

Fig. 8-5 (*a*) The chopper is turned on and off by the multivibrator on the left. When the chopper is on it samples the dc input. The ac output then becomes an analog of the dc input. (*b*) A noninverting chopper amplifier is in a mode of operation which gives high accuracy with high-impedance signals. Maximum current drift of the op amp is 10 pA/°C. The CMRR is 300,000. Choppers are common in multichannel medical oscilloscopes.

arrangement in Fig. 8-5*b*. It has an input noise level of approximately 0.5 μV. The multivibrator and dc sampling switch technique is used here as it is in Fig. 8-5*a*. However, in this case, the entire circuit is built into a single IC made by Analog Devices.

8-5 A/D CONVERSION

In every medical data application, we begin with variable or analog data. The only exception to this rule would be using a transducer with a pulsed output. These pulses could be fed directly into digital counting circuits. However, in all other situations, our medical data are analog. There are many reasons why it may be necessary to convert these analog data into digital information. We might want to feed a computer which only understands a digital language. We might wish to critically analyze the data-frequency spectrum via a digital technique, or we might wish to feed digital readout devices. An increasing number of instruments provide a digital output for external equipment or peripheral storage devices. In all the applications outlined, an analog-to-digital (A/D) converter will be called upon for A/D conversion.

The block diagram in Fig. 8-6 is a typical A/D conversion circuit. A low-level analog signal (0 to 10 V) enters the converter at bottom left. It is fed to the converter itself, which provides sequential pulses to both counters. These pulses relate to the amplitude (analog) of the medical data. The input also feeds the voltage comparator, which provides reference pulses to both 4-bit counters to sync their operation. The clock supplies a stable time base for both counters. In this particular A/D conversion technique, the converting is accomplished close to the signal source. An advantage of this technique is that the data cannot be affected by unstable circuits preceding the converter. A possible disadvantage is that a minimum signal amplitude is required to trigger the system; also interference and artifacts as well as actual medical data may show up in the output. A Precision Monolithics CMP-OIC comparator samples the input providing up or down counts to the counters.

In some medical instruments, the A/D converter will be found farther along in the circuit where a stronger signal is found. However, no matter where in the circuit the converter is located, the basic principle remains the same as in the block diagram in Fig. 8-6. When checking A/D converters, refer to the instrument maintenance manual or the IC manufacturers' specifications to determine the critical parameters. Critical parameters include noise level, drift rate, resolution, linearity, and power consumption. If any of these parameters have departed sharply from the correct value, then the IC is probably defective.

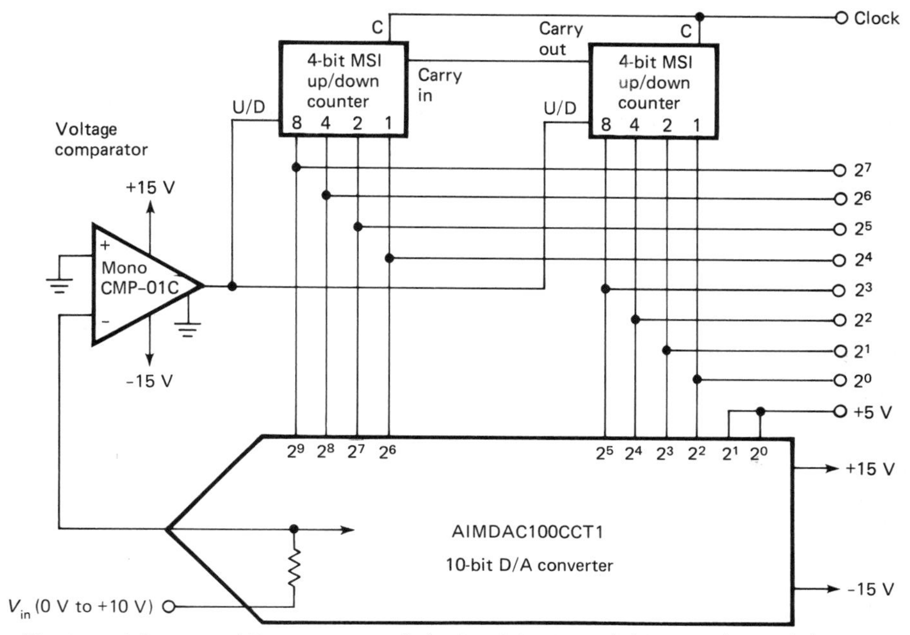

Fig. 8-6 A low-cost A/D converter made by Precision Monolithics. Analog signals enter at bottom left. Converted digital bits are taken off at the output lines on the right. This output may drive a digital display or a memory device. It might also be transmitted over communications circuits, then later reconverted back into the original analog data. Remember, all physiological data are originally analog.

8-6 THERMOMETER CIRCUITS

Hundreds of different types of electronic thermometers are in use today. While it is impossible to describe every circuit, the basic principle is the same. A typical hospital thermometer circuit is described in Fig. 8-7. The reference diode establishes a reference temperature. The silicon diode (probe diode) senses the temperature of the patient. If the temperature sensed is lower than the reference, the output will go positive, and vice versa. The accuracy is determined primarily by the specifications of the reference diode. The circuit drives a panel meter or can drive an A/D converter for digital readout.

Let us explore the circuit of Fig. 8-7 in somewhat greater detail. The output of the IC will vary in accordance with its differential input, or the difference between inputs A and B. The reference diode along with the connected IN5288 form a stable voltage source. Resistor R_1 senses the fixed junction voltage which then appears at input A. The resistance of a silicon junction will decrease with increased temperature. Thus a temperature increase will decrease the voltage across the

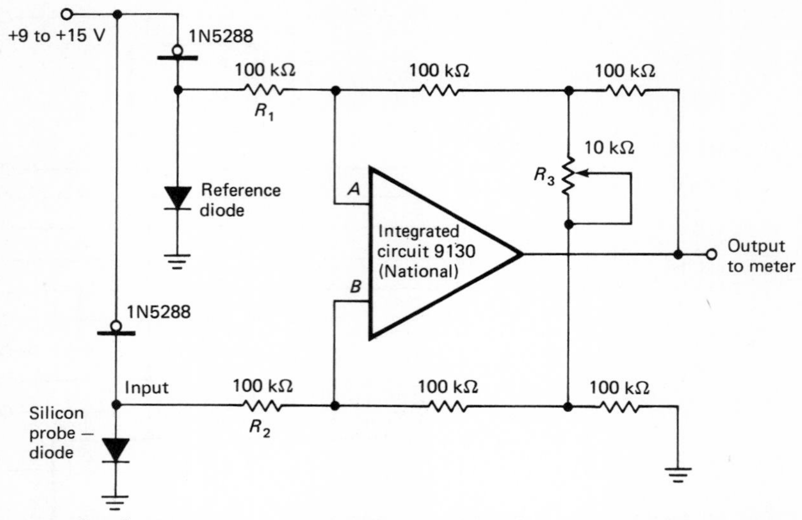

Fig. 8-7 This thermometer circuit compares a stable reference diode to the temperature sensor (probe diode). The output meter displays the temperature difference in terms of absolute temperature.

divider consisting of the silicon probe and its connected IN5288. Resistor R_2 senses this voltage, which becomes input B. Potentiometer R_3 adjusts the offset voltage at input B so that the probe indicates ambient temperature when the sensing probe is not connected to a patient. A single 9-V battery powers the thermometer.

8-7 PACEMAKER CIRCUITS

As in the case of electronic thermometers, there are a great variety of pacemaker circuits in use. The two circuits shown in Fig. 8-8 are simplified versions of circuits that are basic to all heart pacers. Understanding the theory of these circuits will give the BMET the ability to recognize and comprehend all pacemakers.

In Fig. 8-8*a* a TV type of blocking oscillator Q_1 generates a fixed pacing pulse at a rate determined before implantation and connection to the heart. The oscillator generates very low-powered pulses for triggering Q_2, which then delivers a 1-ms pulse to the heart through C_2. A pulse amplitude much lower than the manufacturers' specification might indicate a weak battery, shorted turns in the blocking transformer, or a collector-base short in Q_2. A pulse whose timing is way off might reveal that C_1 or R_1 has changed value.

In Fig. 8-8*b*, the pacemaker generates 70 pulses per minute at 10 mA. The pulse duration is 1 ms. A conventional multivibrator would have,

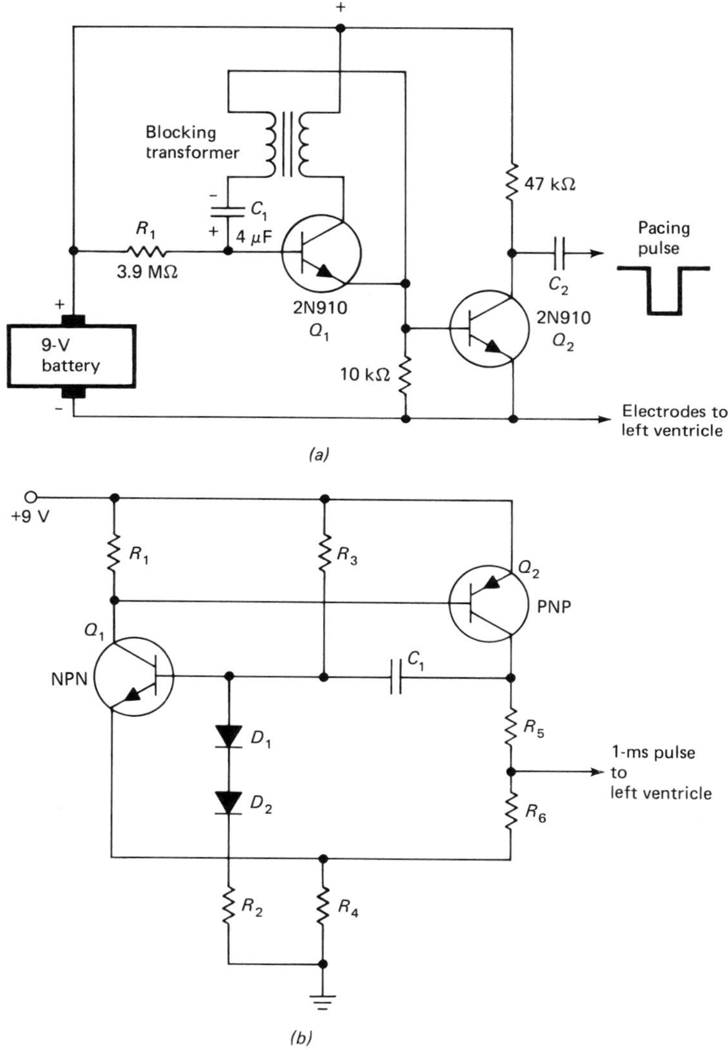

Fig. 8-8 (*a*) A typical pacemaker circuit. Q_1 serves as a blocking oscillator, with the blocking transformer providing feedback. Q_2 is a pulse amplifier. (*b*) This pacemaker circuit generates a 1-ms pulse at 70 pulses per minute. The absence of a transformer permits ultraminiaturization. C_1 and R_3 determine the pulse rate.

at best, a mark-space (on-off) ratio of 1000 to 1, which is not sufficient for a pacemaker. In this circuit, the unsymmetrical configuration has only one timing capacitor and permits a mark-space ratio of up to 10,000 to 1. This extremely low duty cycle (on time) permits low current drain. C_1 charges, turning on Q_1. This increases the voltage across R_1, turning on Q_2. When Q_2 turns on, a positive pulse appears across resistors R_4, R_5, and R_6. This pulse is carried by the timing capacitor C_1 back to the base of Q_1, causing regeneration, and both transistors go into saturation (switch on). The pulse width or the period during which the transistors conduct is determined by the potential across D_1, D_2, R_2, and the rate of C_1 and R_3. This modified multivibrator pacemaker circuit does not have the stability of the blocking-transformer circuit in Fig. 8-8*a*. It is nevertheless used in thin-film circuits (ultraminiaturized) where the size of the blocking transformer in Fig. 8-8*a* would be a disadvantage.

8-8 TELEMETRY CIRCUITS

Telemetry from the body's surface was discussed in Chap. 6. The Endoradiosonde sends signals from inside the body. This device, often called a radio pill, is used to measure digestive tract pH, local temperature, blood flow, intestinal mobility, intracranial pressure, internal bleeding, etc. The ingested pill is a single-channel, modified Hartley oscillator which is frequency-modulated. The radio pill in Fig. 8-9 has two variable capacitors or varactors (C_1 and C_2). They are part of the transmitter's resonant circuit and alter the carrier frequency according to the modulating medical signal. Components are protected by a hermetically sealed capsule which can be used for a long-term implant. The transmitter is operated from a mercury cell and can be switched on and off by means of a magnetic switch. A good FM receiver can be used for reception. The operating range depends on the receiver's sensitivity. A high-quality FM receiver will allow reception from 4 to 20 ft away from

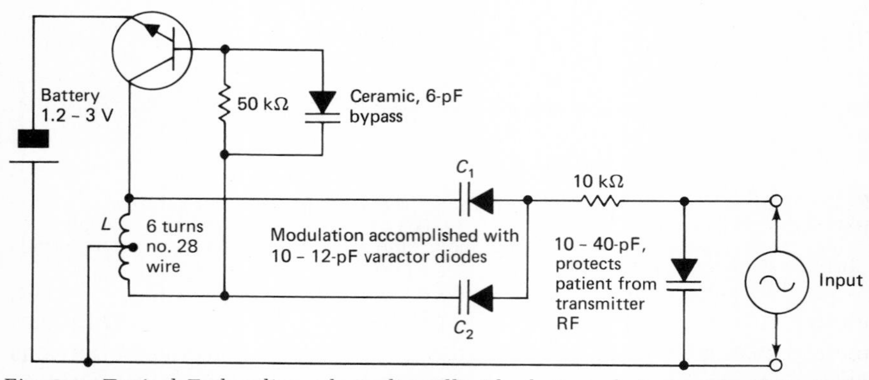

Fig. 8-9 Typical Endoradiosonde (radio pill). The battery drain is only 420 μA. Its operating frequency can be 108 MHz at the top of the commercial FM band. The noise level, with 1-kHz bandwidth, is 1 μV RMS. Its size is 20 by 12 by 5 mm. Modulation sensitivity is 15 kHz/mV. Bandwidth is 20 to 10,000 Hz, and input impedance is 1 MΩ in parallel with 30 pF.

the patient. Although the radio pill is commercially available, BMETs may wish to build their own to their own special requirements. For example, an audio-amplifying stage preceding the oscillator will give the pill greater modulation sensitivity.

In Fig. 8-10 we find other basic telemetry circuits. The discriminator in Fig. 8-10*a* changes the incoming frequency variations into a dc potential. Thus the FM carrier is demodulated. The voltage from the transformer will be positive if the modulated frequency is higher than the carrier, and negative if the modulated frequency is lower than the carrier. As the output is taken off above and below ground, the output potential adds or subtracts (algebraically) the individual voltages on both sides of the transformer secondary. The output is then the analog equivalent of the frequency deviation at the input. It has been returned to the form in which it originally entered the transmitter.

In Fig. 8-10*b*, the voltage E_s is generated by a piezoelectric transducer. C_c represents the cable capacitance, and C_s is the cable's series capacitance. The inverting amplifier isolates and amplifies the transducer signal to produce a large voltage swing. This voltage alters the frequency of a voltage-controlled oscillator (VCO). As its name implies, a VCO is an oscillator whose frequency is varied by a variable voltage. Another VCO is shown in Fig. 8-10*c*. Here the modulation input is not sensitive to a common-mode signal such as interference. However, the physiological data (differential signal) change the varactor capacitance to produce frequency modulation. Going a step further, in Fig. 8-10*d*, the previous *LC* oscillator is now crystal-controlled. The quartz crystal guarantees that the oscillator's carrier frequency will be extremely stable. The receiver's discriminator center frequency can now be adjusted with a high degree of precision. In addition, the receiver's IF (intermediate frequency) can have a narrow bandwidth to decrease noise and eliminate interfering carriers. This crystal-controlled VCO requires more modulating voltage than the previous *LC* version. To compensate for this, the gain of the modulation amplifier will have to be higher.

8-9
REMOTE CONTROL CIRCUITS

Many biomedical applications require the remote control of servos, motors, instruments, recorders, and other circuits. A typical remote control system is shown in Fig. 8-11. Like the radio pill, these systems are available commercially or can be homemade. These circuits were originally designed for the citizens band, and some commercial remote control circuits do operate on 27 MHz. If these circuits are to be changed to a higher frequency where there is less congestion, crystal Y_1

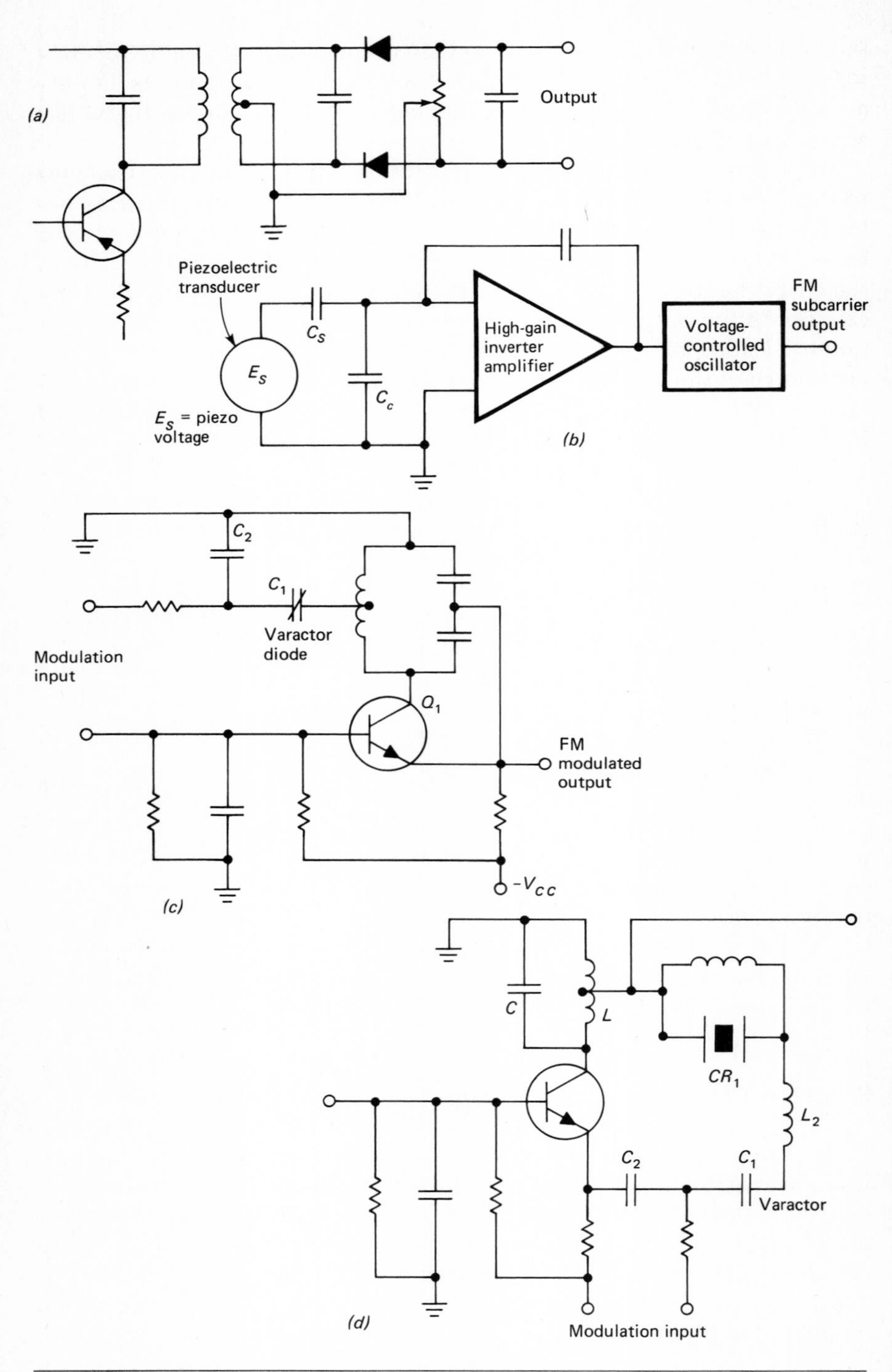

(a)
Output
Piezoelectric transducer
C_S
E_S
C_c
E_S = piezo voltage
High-gain inverter amplifier
Voltage-controlled oscillator
FM subcarrier output
(b)
C_2
C_1
Varactor diode
Modulation input
Q_1
FM modulated output
$-V_{CC}$
(c)
C
L
CR_1
L_2
C_2
C_1
Varactor
Modulation input
(d)

can be changed. Also, turns can be taken off L_1 (both receiver and transmitter) and L_2 in the transmitter.

The transmitter is a crystal-controlled oscillator (Q_3) and RF amplifier (Q_4) modulated by a tone oscillator (Q_1, Q_2). The receiver is a superregenerative detector, quench filter, audio amplifier, and control relay (K_1). If the transmitter control signal is strong enough, Q_4 may be omitted. This system will work over 100 yd. Transmitter power can be increased to 5 W, or even higher at the higher frequencies. The superregenerative receiver shown here could be replaced by a sensitive superheterodyne receiver. With these modifications, this system could control devices and circuits over a 5-mi range. Patient data could be remotely sampled at periodic intervals using a remotely controlled transmitter at the patient site. In another application, this system could inquire as to the function and calibration of medical instruments at a remote location.

8-10 VACUUM-TUBE CIRCUITS

Although recent biomedical instruments consist of solid-state circuits, the BMET will nevertheless encounter some vacuum-tube equipment. Figure 8-12 describes the vacuum-tube circuits most often found in biomedical instrumentation. Although nonessential components have been omitted for simplification, the basic circuit will be easily recognized in the medical instrument.

The differential amplifier in Fig. 8-12*a* is theoretically the same as its solid-state counterpart in Fig. 8-3. As in the solid-state version, this circuit may be cascaded to increase CMRR and gain. The essential difference between the circuits is that a high-voltage power supply is necessary in this case.

Oscillators are often found in medical instruments. They are used to generate a sync clock signal, to establish a time base, as a calibration marker, as a sine-wave or square-wave source, etc. The oscillators in Fig. 8-12*b*,*c*, and *d* all generate a sinusoidal waveform. The Hartley oscillator is the simplest of the three. Its drawback is that a tap must be provided on the tank coil (L_1), and that cathode current flows through

---

Fig. 8-10 (page 262) Typical telemetry circuits. (*a*) All demodulators and FM or phase detectors use some form of this Foster-Sealey discriminator to demodulate the FM carrier, so that the original data can be reproduced. (*b*) The high impedance of a piezoelectric transducer becomes an asset in a telemetry modulator, as shown here. The transducer drives a charge-controlled oscillator. (*c*) This inexpensive telemetry transmitter achieves a fair amount of common-mode rejection, as its output is proportional to the difference between its two inputs. (*d*) This simple telemetry oscillator has high stability, as it is crystal-controlled. The modulating voltage changes the varactor *C*, thus frequency-modulating the oscillator.

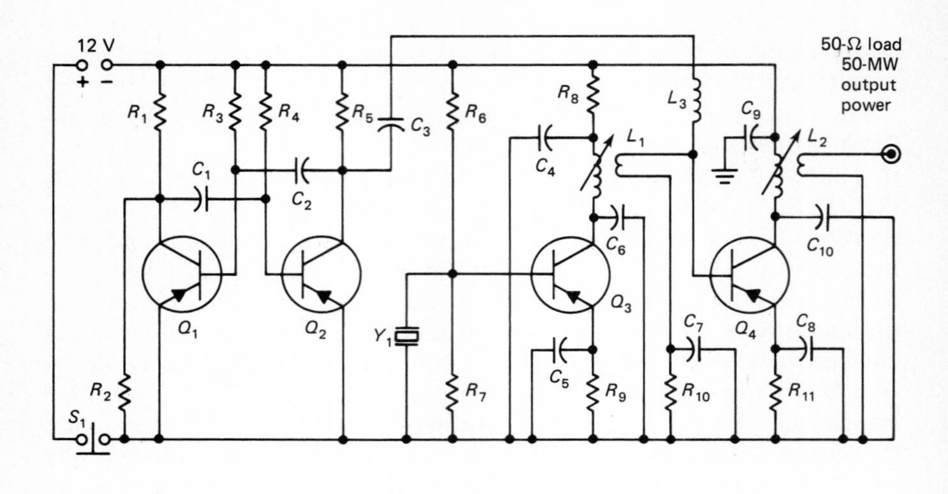

Parts List

Resistors	*Kilohms*	*Watt*
R_1	6.8	½
R_2	20	½
R_3, R_4	100	½
R_5	6.8	½
R_6	47	½
R_7	4.7	½
R_8, R_9	150 Ω	½
R_{10}	1	½
R_{11}	47 Ω	½

Capacitors	
C_1, C_2	0.01-μF disk
C_3	0.1-μF disk
C_4, C_7, C_8, C_9	0.05-μF disk
C_5	56-pF disk
C_6, C_{10}	33-pF disk

Transistors	
Q_1, Q_2	2N1274
Q_3, Q_4	TI 395

Inductors

L_1, L_2	Adjustable RF coil (J. W. Miller 4403 or equivalent). Add 2 turns of No. 24 enameled wire on cold end.
L_3	RF coil, 15 μH (Delevan 1537-40 or equivalent).

Miscellaneous

S_1	Push-button switch (normally open)
Y_1	27.255-μHz crystal

(*a*)

Fig. 8-11 (*a*) Remote control transmitter is capable of controlling medical instruments, patient devices, motors, lights, etc. If the 50-mW power output were increased, a range of 2 miles would be possible. (*b*) Remote control receiver drives relay K_1, which then controls electric and electronic circuits or devices.

the bottom part of this coil. The heat generated causes L_1 to expand, limiting the oscillator's stability. The Colpitts oscillator (Fig. 8-12*c*) provides a solution to this problem: The tap on L_1 has been eliminated. However, even in the Colpitts circuit, L_1, C_1, and C_2 dissipate energy, thus making stability less than perfect. Colpitts and Hartley oscillators are tuned by the values of L and C in their tank circuit.

When stability is extremely critical and the ability to vary the oscillator frequency is not important, a crystal oscillator is used. In Fig. 8-12*d* the *LC* feedback path has been replaced by a quartz crystal. To change the frequency, several other crystals will have to be switched into the circuit.

When troubleshooting any oscillator, the important thing to remember is that an *in-phase* feedback path must exist. The Pierce oscil-

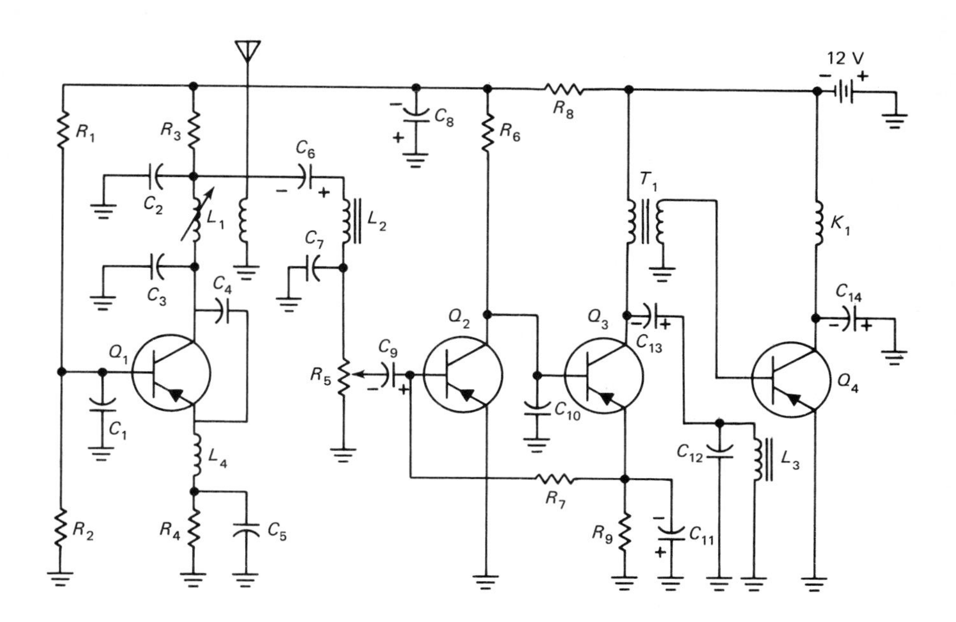

Parts List

Resistors	*Kilohms*	*Watt*
R_1	22	½
R_2	2.2	½
R_3, R_4	1	½
R_5	10	Potentiometer
R_6	2.7	½
R_7	10	½
R_8	270 Ω	½
R_9	150 Ω	½
Transistors		
Q_1	2N2188	
Q_2, Q_3, Q_4	2N1274	
Capacitors		
C_1	0.001-μF disk	
C_2, C_7, C_{10}	0.05-μF disk	
C_3	15-μF disk	
C_4	18-pF disk	
C_5, C_{12}	0.002-μF disk	
C_6, C_9, C_{13}	5-μF electrolytic	
C_8, C_{14}	100-μF electrolytic	
C_{11}	40-μF electrolytic	

Transformer	
T_1	10-2 kΩ (Thordorson TR7 or equivalent).
Inductors	
L_1	Adjustable RF coil (J. W. Miller 4403 or equivalent). Add 2 turns of No. 24 enameled wire on cold end.
L_2	30-mH choke (Bud CH 1228 or equivalent).
L_3	8.5 H (Stancor C1279 or equivalent).
L_4	RF coil, 15 μH (Delevan 1537-40 or equivalent).
Miscellaneous	
K_1	Typical: Sigma 11F-2300-G/SIL or equivalent).

Fig. 8-11 (Continued) *(b)*

lator circuit can be built to serve as a valuable piece of test equipment. When a crystal oscillator does not function (or has a weak output), plug its crystal into the test oscillator. Checking the oscillator's output on an oscilloscope will determine the existence (or the amount) of crystal activity.

In an FM receiver, a ratio detector acts as a demodulator. In other

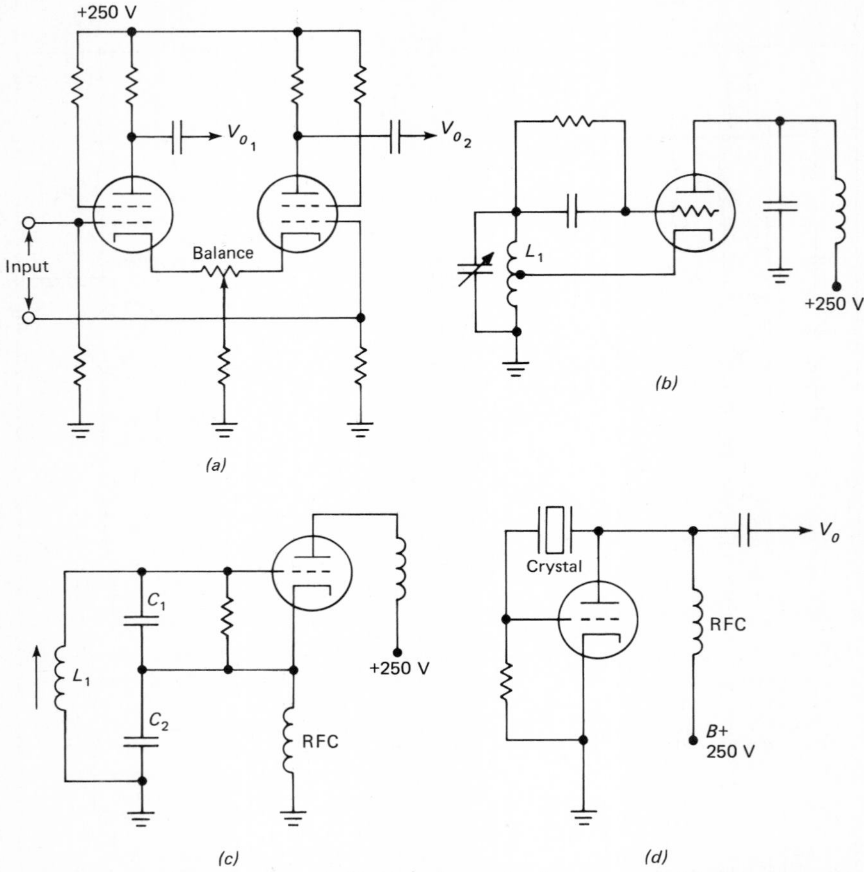

Fig. 8-12 Vacuum-tube circuits found in biomedical equipment. (*a*) The differential amplifier; (*b*) Hartley oscillator; (*c*) Colpitts series-fed oscillator; (*d*) Pierce oscillator, crystal-controlled; (*e*) the ratio detector or demodulator; (*f*) phase or reactance modulator.

medical circuits, a ratio detector translates a minute phase difference into an analog output. Electroencephalography techniques increasingly are concerned with subtle phase differences. The ratio detector in Fig. 8-12*e* recovers an audio signal from the FM carrier. It does not respond to amplitude variations in the input signal. Voltages E_2 and E_3 are each 90° out of phase with E_1 and the same amount of phase as the reference voltage across L. The voltages which are rectified by the diode tubes are additive, with their sum appearing across C_1. C_1 is an RF bypass, grounding one end of L so that only the subcarrier or modulation can drive the deemphasis network.

The ratio detector produces an output voltage which corresponds to the phase variations at its input, or an FM demodulator. Its counterpart

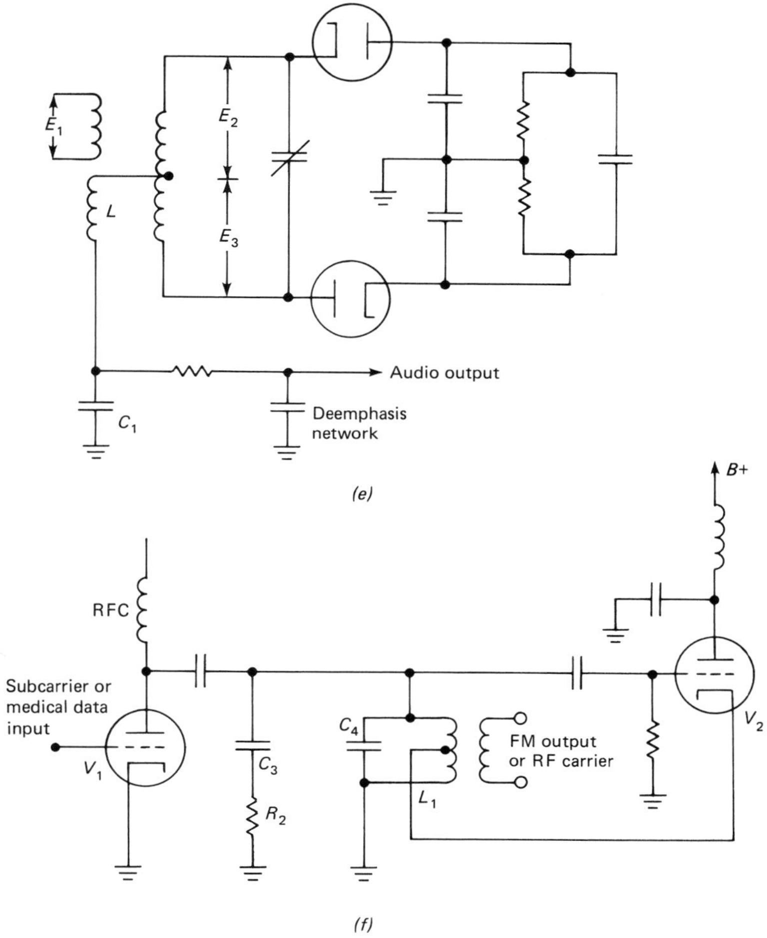

Fig. 8-12 (Continued)

is the reactance modulator (Fig. 8-12*f*), which takes a dc or subcarrier input and varies the phase of a high-frequency oscillator according to this input. The subcarrier or dc analog input is usually the biomedical data; the oscillator output becomes the carrier. The instantaneous plate voltage of reactance tube V_1 is applied across a load consisting of C_3 which is also across the Hartley oscillator tank circuit C_4 and L_1. Medical data on the grid of V_1 change the reactance of C_3 as the resistance of the plate-cathode current of V_1 varies with the input data. The reactance of the oscillator tank (C_4, L_1) will vary above and below the zero-subcarrier signal value. Thus the oscillator (V_2) frequency will vary above and below its center frequency. The amount of frequency or phase deviation (and its rate) depends on the amplitude and frequency of the modulating signal.

Thus far, oscillators have been discussed which produce a sine wave. Pacemakers, sweep generators, and calibration markers are examples of sources that do not produce sine waves. For example, the sawtooth generator in Fig. 8-13*a* produces a sawtooth waveform when

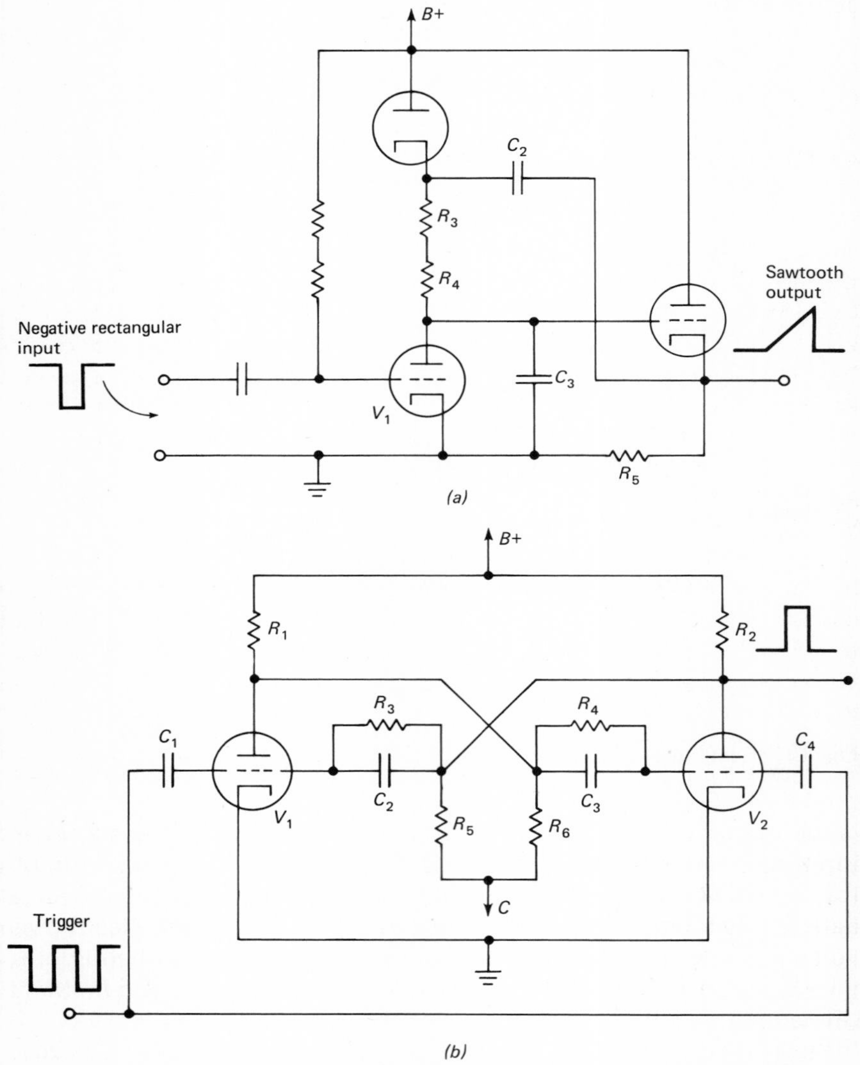

Fig. 8-13 (*a*) This circuit accepts a negative rectangular input pulse and converts it into a ramp or sawtooth. This ramp might provide the time base for a medical oscilloscope or chart recorder. (*b*) This triggered multivibrator is bistable. One output pulse is produced for every two input pulses. The output might stimulate a muscle or nerve.

fed a negative rectangular input pulse. Without an input pulse, both triodes conduct and C_2 is charged. When a negative input pulse reaches the grid of V_1, it cuts that tube off. Timing capacitor C_3 charges through R_3 and R_4. This rising voltage is applied to the grid of the next triode, which is a cathode follower. The diode cathode becomes more positive because the charge on C_3 is added to the charge on C_2. The voltage drop across R_3 and R_4 is constant as C_3 charges and its voltage increases linearly, causing a sawtooth waveshape across R_5. When the diode cathode is more positive than its plate, it ceases conducting. Thus the charging circuit is disconnected from the supply voltage. As the diode cathode is less positive than its plate, the diode conducts until another negative impulse is fed to the first triode grid, or V_1.

In many medical applications, it is necessary to decrease the pulse rate yet retain the same pulse shape. The divide-by-two multivibrator shown in Fig. 8-13*b* produces one output pulse for every two input pulses. When both tubes are turned off, a negative trigger pulse applied to V_1 drives the tube further into cutoff. The plate voltage rise raises the grid voltage of V_2. This tube conducts, causing a drop in its plate potential. This is sensed at the grid of V_1. The next pulse restores the circuit to its original position. By reducing the bias, this bistable multivibrator may be made astable or free-running.

8-11 SAFETY CIRCUITS

In Chap. 2, Patient Safety, we learned how electrodes come in direct contact with the heart when cardiac catheterization is employed and that fibrillation of heart muscles under these conditions can be induced with currents as low as 10 μA. Thus the amplifier connected to the cardiac catheter must be totally isolated from ground. Yet all the other amplifiers and monitors must be completely grounded.

To achieve this complete isolation, an optical transmitter receiver might be used. The patient data activate an optical transmitter that sends light variations to the receiving transducer. Although the patient has been optically isolated from most of the system, preamplification is needed to activate the optical transmitter. The preamplifier might be battery-powered. This might solve the problem of patient isolation but leave us with the problem of battery replacement. The isolation transformer, another solution, leaves the problem of insufficient electrical insulation to prevent patient injury under all conditions.

Superisolation with high reliability is being accomplished by using a floating ultrasonic-powered isolation amplifier. These circuits afford high isolation, high breakdown voltage, low-capacitance leakage, and good power-transfer efficiency. Acoustic energy is transmitted by an

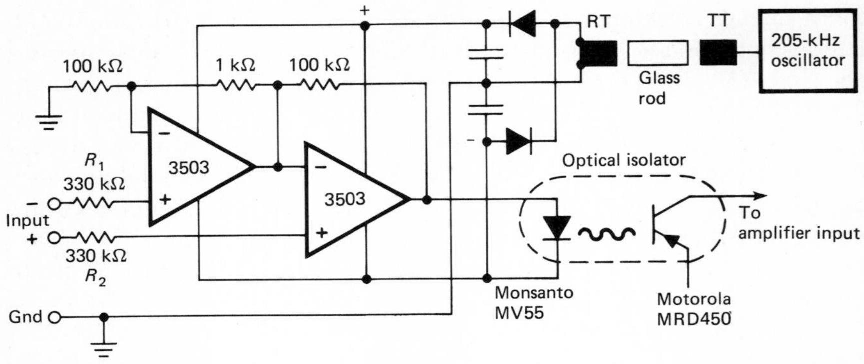

Fig. 8-14 Typical floating power source which assures complete patient isolation without relying on battery power. Transducer RT receives acoustic energy through the glass rod. This energy is rectified and provides power for two Burr-Brown ICs and the optical transmitter. This is a Monsanto light-emitting diode. In critical cardiac applications isolation transformers do not provide sufficient safety. However, the battery which powers an optically isolated amplifier might fail just when it is needed most. This circuit overcomes all these problems.

electrically isolated transducer, TT in Fig. 8-14. Another transducer (RT) then converts the transmitted acoustic energy into electric energy. The transducers may be Brush-Clevite PZT5 or PZT4. Acoustic energy can be made to travel efficiently through a glass rod. Each transducer is 10 mm in diameter and has a 205-kHz resonance mode. The 10-mm glass rod (20 mm long) becomes the acoustic propagation medium. With 7.5 V RMS in the transmitting transducer (TT), 60 mV of power can be transferred to the receiving transducer (RT). The received energy goes to two diodes, producing a positive and negative voltage with respect to ground. This is similar to the dual power supplies often used to power ICs. The rectified direct current powers the preamplifier. An additional precaution is that isolated preamplifier signal output is further isolated from subsequent electronics by an optical isolator. The preamp IC is an FET op amp with an input current of less than 10^{-12} A. The CMRR is 100 dB. Amplification of 100 times occurs, with the resistors R_1 and R_2 limiting current in the input circuit to 2 μA. The preamplifier bandwidth is 5 kHz. When the optical isolator operates in its linear region, signal distortion is less than 1 percent. Although there are isolated preamplifiers that have somewhat different circuits, the basic concept is similar to that of Fig. 8-14.

8-12 LEARNING THROUGH DOING

The circuits described in this chapter are simplified versions of the most typical circuits the BMET will find in the biomedical instrument field. The BMET must understand these circuits in order to effectively troubleshoot components and systems according to the procedures outlined in the remainder of this text.

The bioengineering student may have no electronic background or may already have studied basic electronics. In either case, building simple biomedical circuits will help the student to understand these factors:

1. The use of measuring instruments and a knowledge of construction practices
2. The theory behind the basic circuit
3. How a functioning circuit should perform
4. How a malfunctioning component affects circuit performance

To achieve these learning objectives, a biomedical circuit kit can be extremely helpful. One such kit allows the student to construct the basic biomedical building blocks. It includes 10 working circuits along with their power supply. These circuits are an optical coupler, an ultrasonic isolated power supply, an ultrasonic transceiver, a differential amplifier, an ECG monitor, a phonocardiography telemetry system, an electronic thermometer, an EMG muscle monitor, and an alpha-wave trainer. This kit is available from Neurotronics Corp., Peekskill, NY 10566. It also includes a lab manual which presents a series of questions to determine whether the student fully comprehends the theory involved in each circuit project.

QUESTIONS

1. In Fig. 8-1, the full-wave rectifier is shown. If the full transformer secondary voltage was 24.2 V, what would be the approximate unloaded supply output voltage? Base your answer on the text material.
2. In Fig. 8-1, a bridge rectifier is shown. The full transformer secondary voltage is 82.4 V. What is the approximate unloaded supply output voltage? Base your answer on the text material.
3. A series regulator circuit senses the ________ voltage, then compares it to a(n) ________ voltage.
4. If we wanted to build a precision medical power supply of 400,000 V, would we design a 400,000-V oscillator? Explain your answer.
5. A differential amplifier has a differential gain of 2400 and a common-mode gain of 5. What is the common-mode rejection ratio (CMRR)?
6. Assume a CMRR of 10,000. The common-mode interference is 10 mV. A physiological signal that will give twice the output of the interference will be usable. What is the minimum usable physiological signal? Explain.
7. If we design a differential amplifier, should its common-emitter resistor be as large or as small as is practical? Why?
8. Explain the function of the constant-current source in the differential amplifier.

9. What does cascading do to a differential amplifier?
10. Differential-amplifier output amplitudes are ________ and their phase relationship is ________.
11. True or false: To measure biomedical signals, the input impedance should be as low as possible because a low impedance does not pick up stray interference.
12. A chopper amplifier is needed (*a*) to chop the input signal so that it does not overload the amplifier, or (*b*) to allow a stable ac amplifier to measure dc signals, or (*c*) to allow a stable dc amplifier to measure ac signals.
13. Which is *always* true? (*a*) The instrument output is always analog. (*b*) High-level stages of biomedical circuits are always analog. (*c*) The first stage of a biomedical amplifier is always analog, except when using a digital transducer.
14. If you have doubts about whether an IC is actually an A/D converter, you should (*a*) saw it in half and look at its circuitry; (*b*) analyze the surrounding circuit; or (*c*) refer to the IC manufacturer's catalog to determine its specifications.
15. You are given an electronic thermometer to repair. The meter reads higher when a subject's temperature is being sensed, but the reading is always 10° too low. (*a*) The sensing diode is probably defective. (*b*) The output meter is probably defective. (*c*) Voltage across the reference diode should be checked. An incorrect voltage here will probably indicate a defective reference diode.
16. In Fig. 8-8*a*, why is the oscillator's pulse rate largely controlled by C_1 and R_1?
17. In the same circuit as in Question 16, the pacemaker should generate 60 pulses per minute and C_1 measures 1 μF. What is the value of R_1?
18. In Question 17, if R_1 measured 500,000 Ω, how many pulses per minute would the pacemaker generate?
19. In the radio-pill circuit in Fig. 8-9, explain how a biological signal changes the oscillator frequency or modulates the oscillator.
20. The varactors in Fig. 8-10*c* and *d* are wired into their respective oscillators in a different way than with the radio pill. Explain how each oscillator is tuned by its varactors.
21. If we wish to detect the variations in phase of an input signal, which of the following circuits would we use? (*a*) An AM detector; (*b*) a discriminator; (*c*) a pulse detector.

chapter

9

Troubleshooting Biomedical Components

INTRODUCTION

The problems inherent in interference, instability, and the various readout techniques have been explored earlier. Through those chapters we have also discovered that a variety of solid-state devices and ICs are used in biomedical systems. An entire extremely sophisticated, complex system often fails to operate because one single component is defective, just as "the entire battle was lost for lack of a single nail!" Thus it is imperative that the BMET gain a basic understanding of troubleshooting as it relates to a single faulty component. In addition to describing general troubleshooting techniques, we will focus on the use of the curve tracer. This tool will do everything the more elementary techniques will do. In addition, it will do what no other technique will do. It will permit us to detect a component failure before it actually occurs. In medical electronics, preventive troubleshooting is not of fringe value, it is vital. The patient's life may very well depend on how competent the BMET is in the art of preventive troubleshooting.

The testing of transistors, diodes, SCRs, triacs, etc., will be discussed. Moving beyond discrete devices, the theory and troubleshooting of TTL (transistor-transistor logic) devices will be covered. Last, but far from least, the peculiarities and problems of CMOS (complementary metal-oxide semiconductors) will receive a great deal of attention. As CMOS technology becomes more and more widespread, the BMET will be expected to be fully competent in the troubleshooting of these fascinating ICs.

9-1 TOOLS

The most important tools needed for troubleshooting solid-state devices are an oscilloscope, a solid-state multimeter, a curve tracer, a dipper, and a sine/square-wave generator. The multimeter should be the FET input type to facilitate leakage and capacitor testing. It should have a 0- to 100-Ω resistance scale for low-resistance solid-state measurements and coil-winding measurements. The oscilloscope should have a triggered sweep, dc vertical amplifier response, and provision for external horizontal input. Its high-frequency vertical amplifier response is not as important as its stability for biomedical applications. The sine/square-wave generator must have output down to at least 20 Hz.

If possible, two regulated power supplies should be available, one to cover the 0- to 50-V range at 5 A for solid-state equipment and the other to cover the 50- to 400-V range at 250 mA for tube circuits. These power supplies should have fail-safe overload protection which shuts the instrument down when current exceeds a preset level. You may replace a costly instrument component only to find that the new replacement "blows out" as soon as the instrument is turned on again. If the power-supply overload protection is set to cut off near the instrument's correct load, this unfortunate experience can be avoided.

In instances where components are no longer recognizable, or circuit changes have been made, a substitution box will be a valuable tool and a time saver. This box contains known values of resistors and capacitors. Several of these known values are switched into a circuit until the one is found which yields the most correct results.

9-2 TROUBLESHOOTING STARTS AT THE POWER SUPPLY

When equipment does not function, a low, high, or absent power-supply voltage will give us many clues. If the power-supply voltage is abnormal, measure the resistance of its load with the instrument turned off. Examining the instrument's circuits should give you an approximate idea of its correct current drain. The manufacturer's manual, which gives the correct power-supply voltages, may also specify the correct current drain. If the load resistance is approximately correct but the power-supply voltage is abnormal, then look for a defective component in the power supply. If the power-supply voltages are normal, then that part of the circuit can be eliminated as a source of the problem. A low voltage in the load may indicate a shorted component; a high voltage indicates an open component. Either way, once we know all circuits are receiving their proper voltages, we can make use of the signal-substitution method.

9-3 SIGNAL SUBSTITUTION

Using a sine/square-wave generator as a substitute for the missing signal, connect its square-wave output to the last stage before the readout. Set the generator frequency (repetition rate) to 20 Hz or pulses per second. If the medical instrument has a CRT display, observe the square-wave generator output on the instrument display. If the instrument has another type of display, then connect an oscilloscope across its output. Now look for some indication of the square-wave generator output. No indication tells us that the last stage of the instrument or the readout (if it is used for viewing) is defective. If there is some indication of the test-generator output, then connect the generator to the input of the previous stage and repeat the previous procedure. Keep moving the generator signal back toward the data input until the defective stage is located. Once this is accomplished, passive components (resistors, capacitors, chokes, coils) can be checked with the instrument turned off. Using a curve tracer, active components such as transistors may be tested with the instrument on.

9-4 THE TRANSISTOR

Transistors will amplify because a small change in base current causes a proportionately larger change in collector current. The ratio of change is the *current gain*. A current gain of 100 means that a base-current change of 1 part will produce 100 parts of collector-current change. DC or static current gain is H_{FE}, and dynamic or current gain is H_{fe} (lowercase subscript for ac gain). Another way of expressing transistor gain is the greek letter beta, (β). The ac current-gain measurement is more useful than dc beta as it duplicates actual operating conditions. Transistor performance is predicted from these tests.

OPERATING POINT

Beta depends on the collector current of a transistor, as we will see when we test with the curve tracer. Thus the bias or operating point of a transistor is critical if a specified gain is to be achieved. The basic transistor bias circuit is shown in Fig. 9-1. Its simplicity might lead one to believe that this circuit is not a common source of trouble. This is not so. Resistors often increase in value. When R_1 increases, Q_1 base current and collector current decrease. The result is nonlinearity, distortion, negative clipping, amplification loss, or oscillator problems. On the other hand, when R_2 increases, Q_1 base current and collector current will increase. This will create nonlinearity, positive clipping, distortion, and increased power dissipation in Q_1. This will also establish the preconditions for the eventual breakdown of Q_1.

BREAKDOWN

The most common transistor breakdown is between the collector and the emitter. In small-signal transistors, the resistance between these

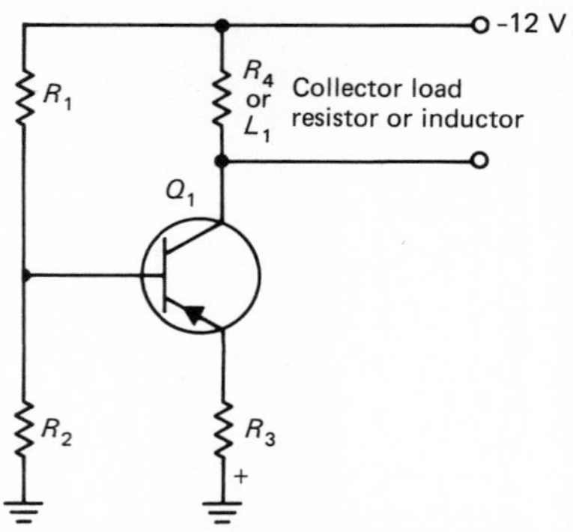

Fig. 9-1 Basic transistor circuit. R_3 is the emitter-bias resistor. R_1 and R_2 form the divider circuit that furnishes bias to the base of Q_1.

elements in one direction (reverse-biased or negative collector for PNP and positive collector for NPN) should be between 100 and 20,000 Ω. For power transistors this resistance can be between 5 and 400 Ω. A dead short in both directions between collector and emitter indicates a breakdown. Collector-to-base breakdown is also common. In small-signal transistors, the collector-to-base resistance, when reverse-biased, should be 1 to 100 kΩ. In power transistors, this resistance can be as low as 300 Ω. These resistances are found in *out-of-circuit* tests with the base and collector disconnected from the circuit. A quick *in-circuit* test procedure is to measure voltage between the base and the emitter. This voltage, with power applied, should be approximately 0.8 V. A noticeable variation in either direction usually indicates a problem. Zero volts indicates that the transistor is operating at cutoff. The collector voltage will equal the source voltage. A higher than normal emitter-base voltage might reveal a leaky transistor or an increase in R_2 (Fig. 9-1). When a collector-to-emitter breakdown occurs, the full source voltage will appear across the emitter-stabilizing resistor in Fig. 9-1. This resistor will then act as a fuse and burn out.

LEAKAGE

I_{ceo} or current flow in the reverse direction between collector and emitter (with the base open) should not exceed 50 μA for germanium transistors or 0.001 μA for silicon transistors. This leakage applies to small-signal transistors. I_{CEO} for power transistors should not exceed 300 μA (germanium) or 0.5 μA (silicon). More critical than collector-emitter leakage is the collector-base leakage I_{cbo}, or simply I_{co}. The I_{co} for small-signal transistors should not exceed 1 μA (germanium) or 0.001 μA (silicon). Power transistor I_{co} should not exceed 10 μA (germanium) or 0.01 μA (silicon).

Leakage testing falls into the category of preventive maintenance. BMETs must learn to develop some of the qualities of a prophet. They may be expected to detect component failure before it occurs. As surgical procedures become more dependent on electronics, the consequence of equipment failure at a critical time becomes increasingly more serious. Unexpected failure in life-support equipment could become a matter of life or death.

An increase in leakage values is a clue to future component failure. In FET-type devices, increased "on" resistance is another valuable clue. Low transconductance in JFETs and depletion-mode MOSFETS is yet another signal. A falloff in breakdown voltage, indicated by nondestructive tests, is also a key indicator, as is negative resistance of a tunnel diode.

9-5 CURVE TRACERS

Figure 9-2 shows the B&K semiconductor curve tracer, Model 501A. This instrument will indicate solid-state breakdowns both in and out of circuit. It will also reveal excessive leakage and other key parameters, such as current gain, output admittance, saturation voltage, cutoff current, temperature effects, and saturation resistance. The Model 501A has two sockets into which small-signal transistors or FETs may be inserted. The collector, base, and emitter of the transistor (drain, gate, and source of the FET) are inserted into the correspondingly labeled pins of the curve-tracer socket. For transistors with a grounded case, the fourth pin can either be inserted into the socket along with the emitter lead or externally jumpered to either of the emitter jacks. Test leads are provided for semiconductors with rigid leads. All jacks, probe tips, and plugs are color-coded for easy identification.

IN-CIRCUIT TESTING

An extremely valuable feature of the curve tracer is its ability to test components while they are in the circuit. In-circuit testing is tricky, as other components may have a large effect on the results obtained. Familiarity with the curves observed on an oscilloscope allows the BMET to discount the effect of other components in the circuit. The B&K 501A is supplied with a probe with three tips. These tips permit contact with the collector, base, and emitter of the transistor (or drain, gate, and source of a FET). By manipulating the probe, all three connections can be made using only one hand. Troubleshooting is thus accelerated.

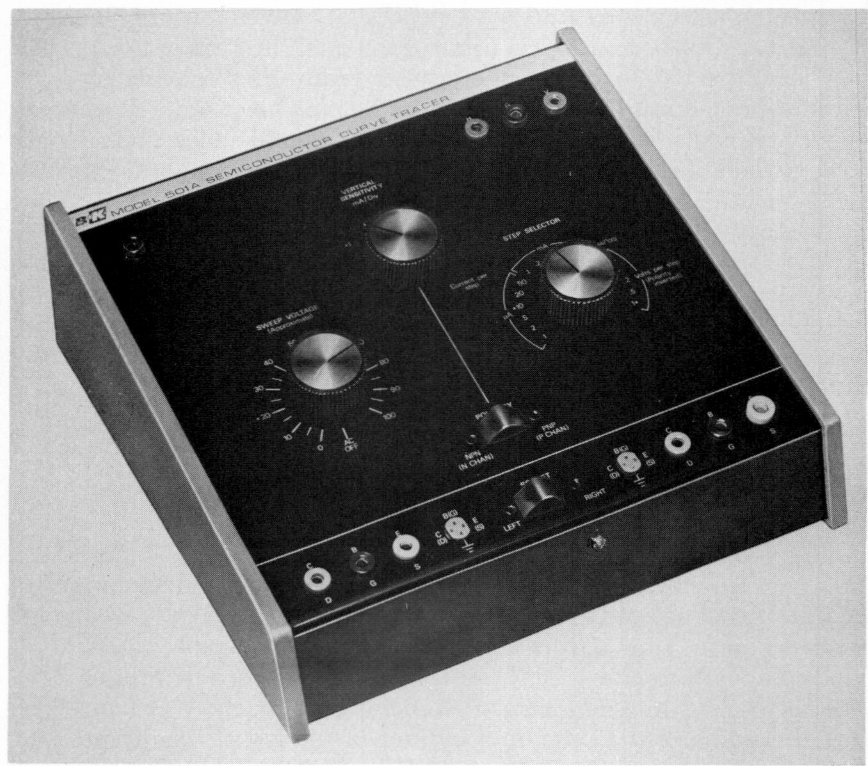

Fig. 9-2 The B & K semiconductor curve tracer. This instrument will reveal a breakdown, leakage, gain, admittance, and conditions of saturation or cutoff. In-circuit or out-of-circuit testing is possible. Transistors, FETs, zener diodes, unijunctions, SCRs, triacs, tunnel diodes, diacs, and ICs may be tested with this instrument.

THEORY OF OPERATION

The curve tracer is essentially a signal generator that generates precision test signals for application to the device under test. The results are displayed on an oscilloscope. Figure 9-3 shows the basic block diagram of a curve tracer. A variable-amplitude 120-Hz sweep voltage is applied to the transistor collector. The transistor base receives a constant current in steps from 1 μA up to 2 mA per step. In testing a FET, constant-voltage steps are fed into the FET gate. Current or voltage steps are positive in the NPN position and negative in the PNP position. An N-channel FET would receive negative voltage steps, and a P-channel FET would receive positive voltage steps.

The sweep voltage applied to the collector is also applied to the horizontal input of the oscilloscope. Thus the same sweep voltage provides

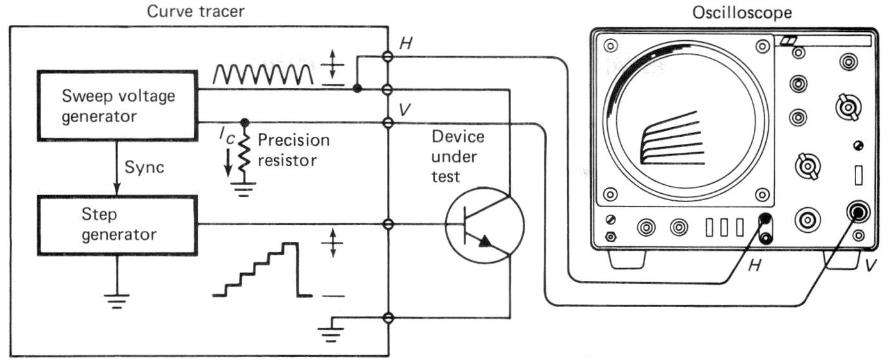

Fig. 9-3 Curve tracer block diagram. The sweep voltage is applied to the transistor collector, while its base receives a constant current from the step generator. A family of curves showing collector current vs. collector voltage is obtained.

the horizontal sweep for the scope. The precision resistor in the sweep generator develops a voltage proportional to the resultant collector current. This voltage is applied to the oscilloscope vertical input. Thus vertical deflection on the oscilloscope represents collector current. Actually, different resistors can be chosen to display a wide range of collector current.

The steps of the step generator are synchronized with the pulses from the sweep generator. The base current is held at one value while a single sweep is executed. The base current then steps up to the next higher value and the sweep generator begins another cycle. Thus a family of six curves is obtained. Each curve or base-current step shows the collector current for that particular step. The display is a dynamic collector current I_c versus collector voltage V_c graph.

THE OSCILLOSCOPE

The oscilloscope used in this test makes use of the sweep-generator voltage, so it must have provision for external horizontal input. It should also have dc-coupled vertical circuits, since capacitor coupling produces phase shift and loss of low-frequency response. Vertical bandwidth should be at least 10 kHz. The vertical divisions of the scope should accurately represent the sweep current supplied to the semiconductor under test. The curve tracer has a built-in calibration source, which is another valuable circuit in this inexpensive instrument. The calibrator can be used to calibrate other instruments as well. The scope vertical gain is calibrated for 1 V full scale (0.1 V/graticule). The scope horizontal-gain control is calibrated so that full scale represents full collector sweep voltage. Each graticule is then 10 percent of maximum sweep voltage.

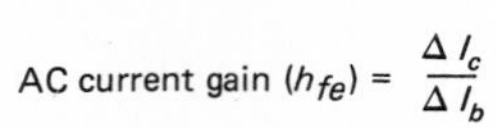
AC current gain (h_{fe}) = $\frac{\Delta I_c}{\Delta I_b}$

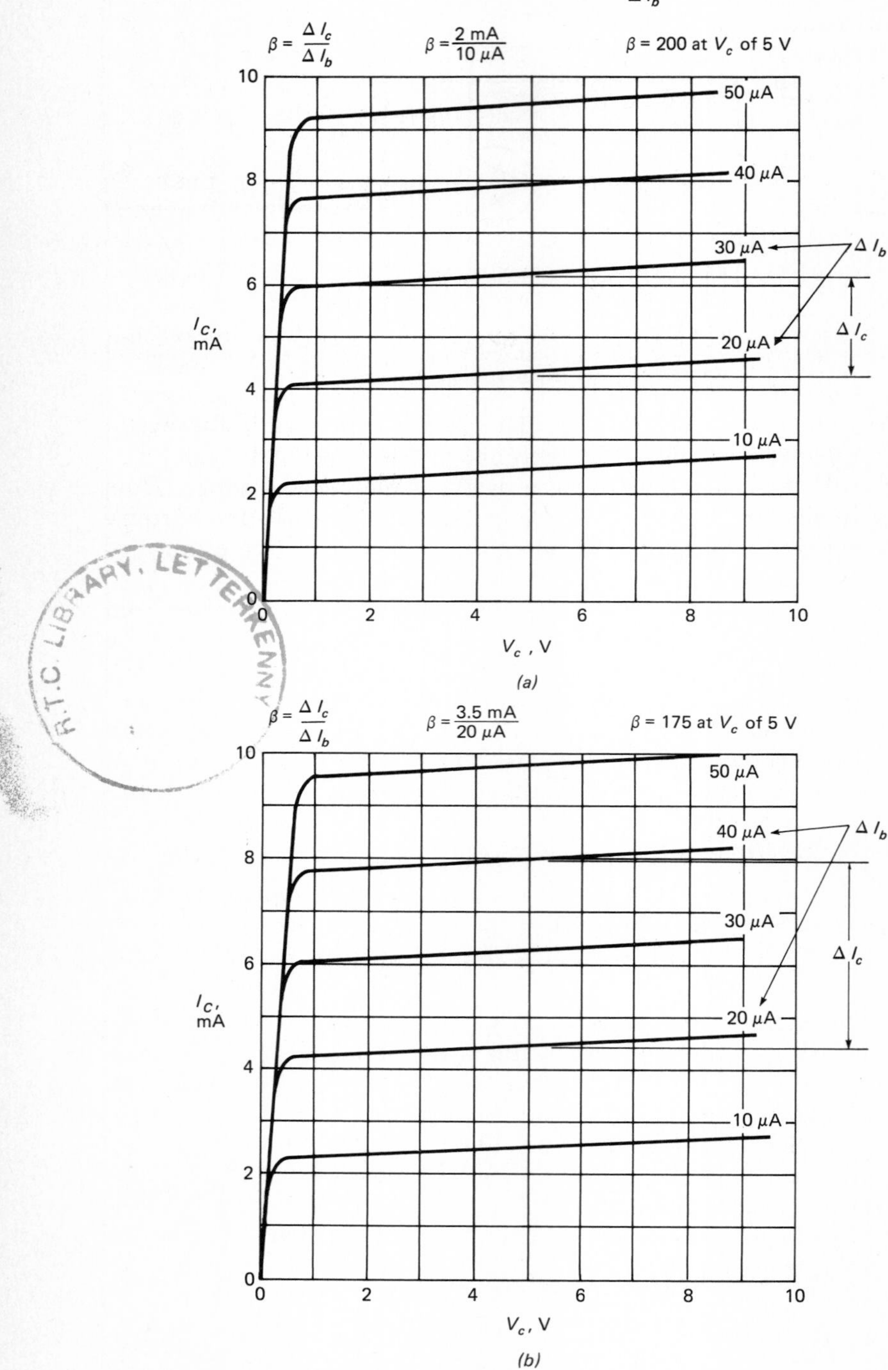
$\beta = \frac{\Delta I_c}{\Delta I_b}$
$\beta = \frac{2 \text{ mA}}{10\ \mu\text{A}}$
β = 200 at V_c of 5 V
50 μA
40 μA
30 μA
20 μA
10 μA
ΔI_b
ΔI_c
I_C, mA
V_c, V
0
2
4
6
8
10
(a)
$\beta = \frac{\Delta I_c}{\Delta I_b}$
$\beta = \frac{3.5 \text{ mA}}{20\ \mu\text{A}}$
β = 175 at V_c of 5 V
50 μA
40 μA
30 μA
20 μA
10 μA
ΔI_b
ΔI_c
I_C, mA
V_c, V
0
2
4
6
8
10
(b)

TYPICAL CURVES

The family of curves of an NPN transistor is in the positive direction. That is, zero volts is at the left and zero current at the bottom of the display. Each curve sweeps to the right and then upward with increasing collector voltage and current. The collector sweep voltage has a positive polarity.

The family of curves of a PNP transistor, by contrast, is in the negative direction. Zero volts is at the right and zero current at the top of the display. Each curve sweeps to the left and downward as collector current and voltage increase. The collector sweep voltage has a negative polarity.

Typical ac beta curves in Fig. 9-4 show that gain is not constant and depends upon the point of measurement. The distance between the curves is seldom equal. This means that ΔI_c is not the same at various regions of base current and, to a lesser extent, at various collector voltages. Base-current values that produce curves closer together are seen in the lower region. Gain is highest in the normal operating region and drops off both above and below this region. It can now be seen how a change in either R_1 or R_2 in Fig. 9-1 will change transistor gain as well as linearity.

LINEARITY

Measuring linearity or distortion is an extension of the gain or beta test. As gain will vary with collector current, the transistor is nonlinear and will introduce distortion. Only a few transistors show a uniform gain over a wide range of collector current. These devices show low distortion and a wide range of linearity. The curves of such transistors would be equally spaced in the vertical direction.

Not all circuits require good linearity and distortion-free characteristics. Before replacing a nonlinear transistor, determine the function of that particular stage. Switching transistors, some class C amplifiers, and frequency multipliers actually depend on nonlinearity for their operation, although class A and B amplifiers (medical data amplifiers) require a high degree of linearity over the entire dynamic range of the biomedical data. Linearity becomes more critical in later stages because larger signals require a larger linear region.

BREAKDOWN VOLTAGE

As the curve-tracer sweep voltage (producing horizontal scope lines) increases, a collector breakdown point will be reached. At the break-

Fig. 9-4 (page 280) Typical ac beta curves indicate that transistor gain changes with base current and also with collector voltage.

down voltage, collector current becomes independent of base current and rises sharply to the current-limiting point of the curve tracer. This feature prevents the transistor under test from being destroyed. This is called *nondestructive* testing. Figure 9-5 shows a typical family of curves with the sweep voltage set high to cause collector breakdown. In both examples, breakdown occurs at 40 V. Note that the base current has little effect when the collector current goes into breakdown. When new semiconductor devices roll off the production line, manufacturers use nondestructive tests to divide devices of the same family into various types, according to quality. A curve-tracer display showing a breakdown voltage lower than is specified for that type device indicates the device has deteriorated.

OUTPUT-ADMITTANCE TEST

The dynamic output admittance of a transistor is the measurement of the change in collector current ΔI_c resulting from a specific change in collector voltage ΔV_c at a constant base current. Admittance is measured in siemens. The *h* parameter for output admittance in the common-emitter configuration is stated as

$$h_{oe} = \left.\frac{\Delta I_c}{\Delta V_c}\right|_{I_B=\text{const}}$$

A change in collector voltage normally causes a change in collector current. For some transistors, this effect is quite apparent because the curves have a noticeable slope. These transistors have a high output admittance. Other transistors display a nearly horizontal curve with a small change in collector current. These devices have a low output admittance.

Output admittance is measured from the same family of curves shown for gain measurements. A constant base current is used. The base current should be typical for the normal operating range of the transistor under test.

THE LEAKAGE TEST

I_{ceo} is the collector-to-emitter current flowing when the transistor base is open. If the transistor is leaky, increasing collector voltage will cause the collector current to increase independently of the base current. Refer back to Sec. 9-4 on transistor leakage to determine allowable leakage for various transistor types. For specific tests, it would be wise to refer to the device manufacturers' specification for I_{ceo}. These specifications will also give a collector voltage and temperature figure at which leakage tests were taken. Leakage is measured by observing the zero-base-current line (ignore the remaining curves). A slope in this line in-

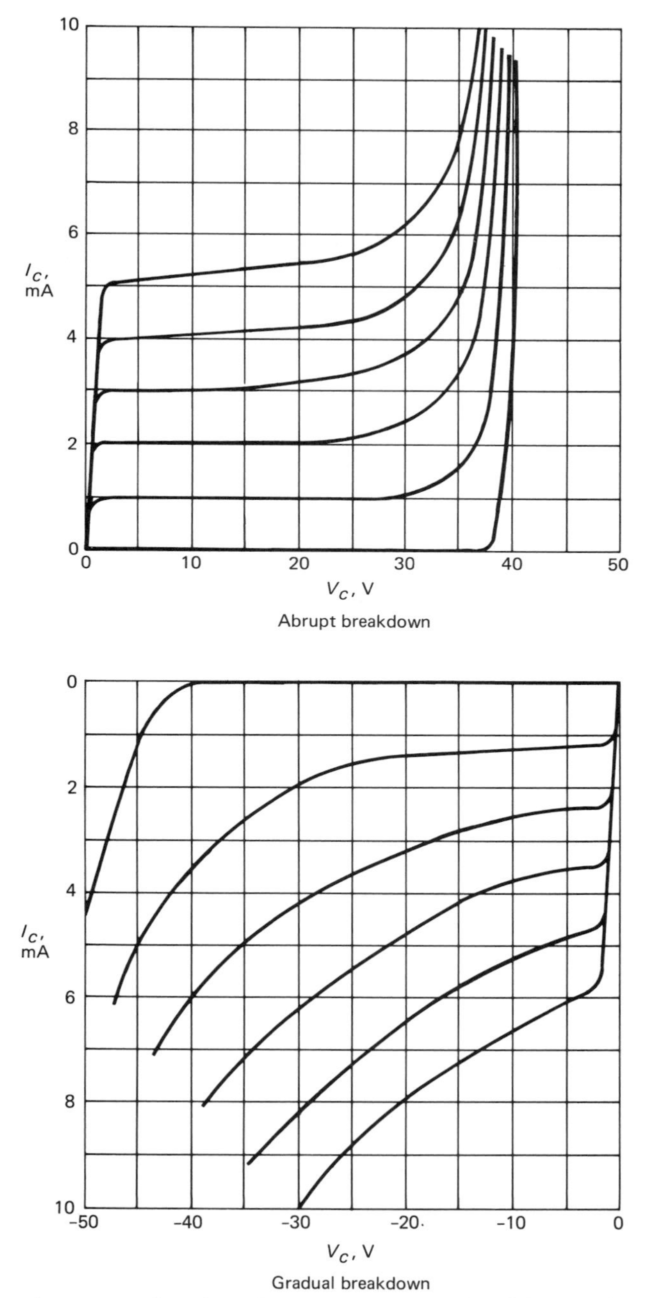

Fig. 9-5 In these examples of nondestructive testing, a breakdown voltage lower than that specified by the manufacturer indicates that the device will probably fail in the near future.

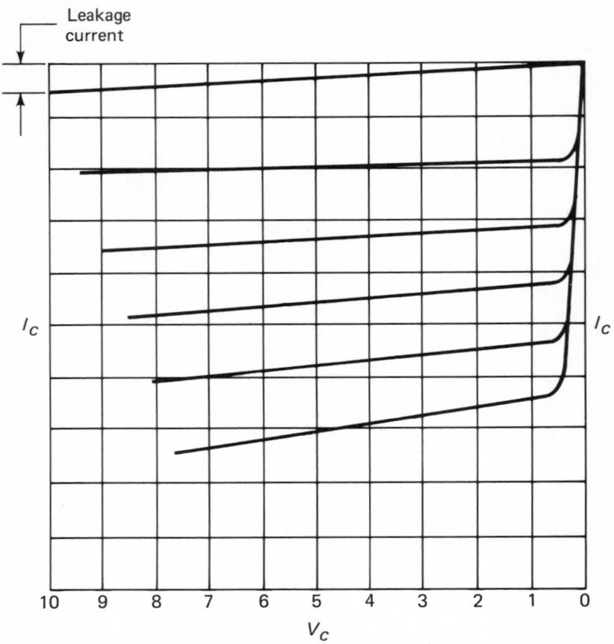

Fig. 9-6 Leakage current from collector to emitter. Study only the top line or zero-base-current line. If this line slopes downward, as it does in this figure, then leakage exists.

dicates a leakage current. In Fig. 9-6 the zero-base-current line (the top curve) shows a downward slope. In other words, collector current is increasing (downward slope) even though no base current has been applied.

9-6
TESTING A FET

FET curves show drain current vs. drain voltage at various gate voltages. In Fig. 9-7, the FET breakdown voltage may be observed and measured by the same method used for transistors. For the FET, the step generator delivers constant volts instead of constant current. The polarity of the step voltage is reversed. The zero-base-current step of a transistor produces no collector current unless the device is leaky. However, the zero-volt step at the FET gate yields the highest drain current. When the gate voltage is sufficiently high, drain current is "pinched off." The pinchoff point is measured with the curve tracer. The forward transconductance of an FET has a voltage-input characteristic which cannot be compared to transistor beta.

Some MOSFETs can be damaged by voltage transients from static

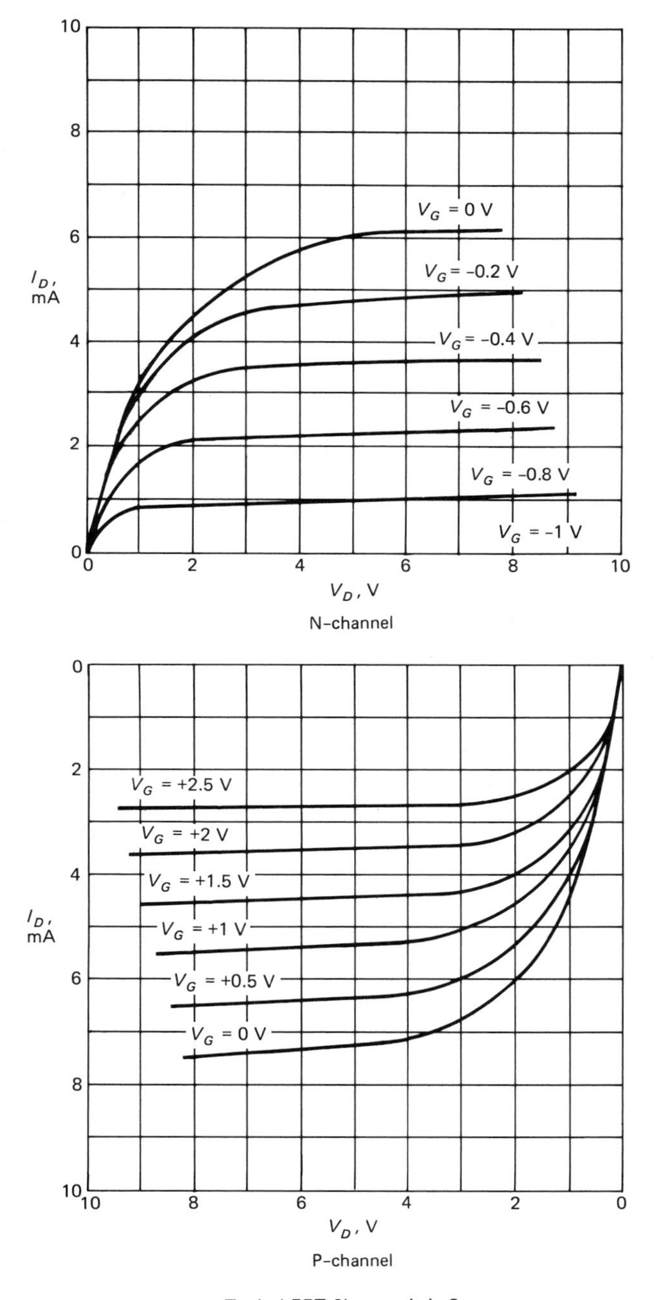

Typical FET Characteristic Curves

Fig. 9-7 Curves show drain current (I_d) against various values of gate voltage (V_g) for the field-effect transistor. When the FET gate is at zero volts, its drain current is highest.

charges. Safeguard against such damage and discharge any static charge by touching ground with one hand before and while handling the MOSFET with the other hand. Most FETs normally operate in the depletion mode with a reverse bias. The constant-voltage steps of a reverse-bias polarity as generated by this curve tracer drive the FET into the depletion mode, with the curves showing lower resultant drain current with each successive step. For testing dual-gate MOSFETs, one gate should be grounded or biased while the other gate is being tested; do not leave the gate open-circuited.

TRANSCONDUCTANCE (GAIN) MEASUREMENT

The most useful and common measurement to be made for an FET is the gain measurement. The dynamic gain, or gate-to-drain forward transconductance (g_m) in the common-source configuration, is the ratio of change in drain current to the change in gate voltage at a given drain voltage.

$$g_m = \left.\frac{\Delta I_d}{\Delta V_g}\right|_{V_d = \text{const}}$$

Transconductance is measured in siemens (S). As an example, if increasing the gate voltage from 1 to 1.5 V (V_g = 0.5 V) causes the drain current to decrease from 6 to 4 mA (I_d = 2 mA) at a drain voltage of 6 V, the forward transconductance of the FET is 4000 microsiemens (μS). Another example is shown in Fig. 9-8.

To calculate g_m, note the difference in drain current between two curves (ΔI_d) at the same drain voltage from the family of curves. Calculate g_m by dividing V_g into ΔI_d.

As with NPN and PNP transistors, the gain of a FET is not constant over its entire voltage and current range. The gain is normally calculated in its typical operating range. Distortion and linearity may be determined by the same method as described for transistors; if the spacing between curves is equal, the FET is linear.

PINCHOFF VOLTAGE (V_p) MEASUREMENT

An important characteristic for depletion-mode FETs is the amount of gate voltage required to turn off drain current. This value is called the *pinchoff voltage characteristic* and may be measured from the family of curves.

Figure 9-9*a* shows the STEP SELECTOR set at 0.5 V per step, and the entire family of curves is displayed. Drain current continues to flow at its highest step of 2.5 V. Figure 9-9*b* shows that when the STEP SELECTOR is increased to 1 V per step, the entire family of curves is not

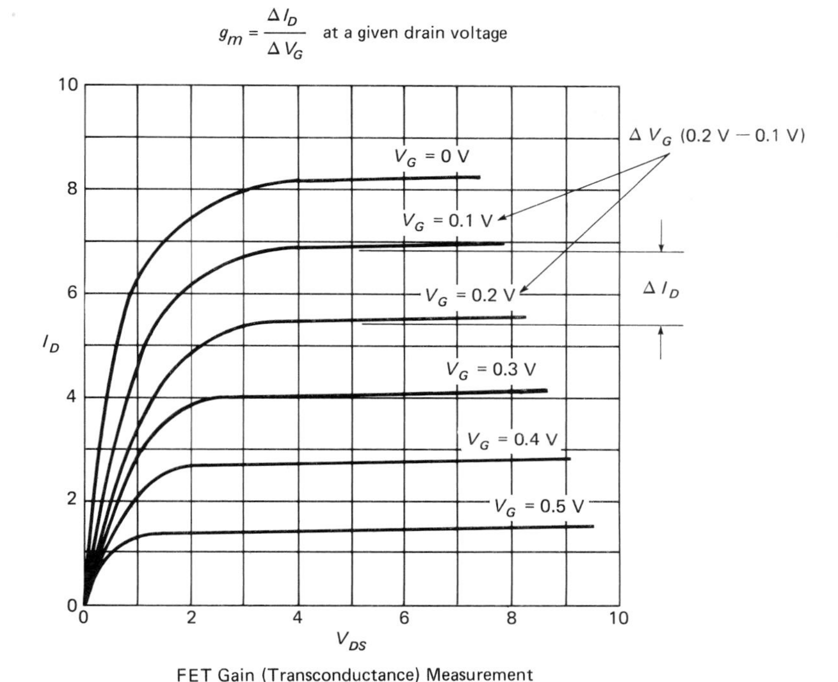

Fig. 9-8 Curve shows the most valuable FET measurement: gate-to-drain common transconductance, or gain. Gain is the ratio of change (△) between drain current I_d and gate voltage V_g.

displayed. In fact, the −3-, −4-, and −5-V curves are superimposed upon each other at zero drain current. All gate-voltage values greater than −3 V prevent drain current. We can conclude that pinchoff occurs between −2.5 and −3 V. A more precise measurement could be made, if necessary, by connecting an external dc bias supply to the gate of the FET, adjusting the bias supply, and observing the exact value of pinchoff voltage on the oscilloscope.

9-7 TESTING SIGNAL AND RECTIFIER DIODES

Signal and rectifier diodes conduct easily in one direction and are nonconductive in the opposite direction. These properties may be tested and observed with the curve tracer and oscilloscope. For testing diodes, the pulsating dc sweep voltage is applied across the diode. The diode current and voltage are plotted on the oscilloscope screen. The step-current–step-voltage signal that was used for testing transistors and FETs is not used in diode testing.

The diode to be tested is plugged into the collector and emitter pins

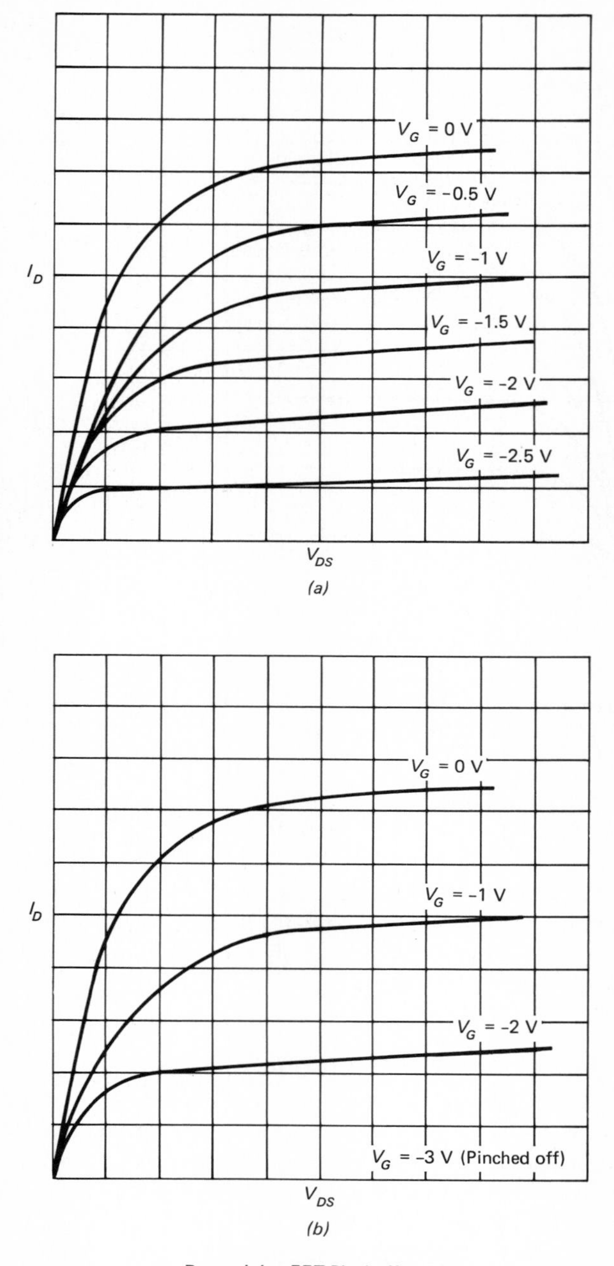

Determining FET Pinchoff Voltage

Fig. 9-9 These curves show how much voltage is needed to turn off FET drain current I_d. At the pinchoff voltage V_g, no I_d flows.

of the transistor socket or directly into the collector and emitter jacks of the curve tracer. Since the polarity of the sweep voltage can easily be reversed, the diode may be inserted into the socket without observing polarity. Of course, diodes inserted at one polarity will produce an oscilloscope display which deflects to the right and upward from its starting point, while the opposite polarity produces a display which deflects downward and to the left from its starting point. A consistent display can be obtained by always connecting the cathode of the diode to the emitter jack. With this polarity connection, the POLARITY switch should be in the NPN position for forward bias of the diode. The display will be the positive-reading type, as shown in Fig. 9-10.

For measuring the forward-diode properties, the oscilloscope horizontal sensitivity should be calibrated to some low-voltage value. A sensitivity of 0.5 V per division or less is necessary to obtain any degree of accuracy in the voltage reading.

When testing diodes, only one curve is displayed, not a family of curves as displayed for transistors and FETs. The forward-bias measurements that can be made are forward-voltage drop and diode resistance. As shown in Fig. 9-10, no current flows until the applied voltage exceeds the junction barrier. This forward-voltage drop is about 0.3 V for germanium diodes and 0.6 V for silicon diodes. Above this point, current increases rapidly with an increase in forward voltage. The current increases more rapidly and the "elbow" has a sharper bend for silicon diodes than for germanium diodes. The dynamic resistance of the diode equals the change in forward voltage (V_F) divided by the change in forward current (I_F). Germanium diodes, with less slope to their curves, have higher dynamic resistance than silicon diodes.

$$R_d = \left.\frac{\Delta V_F}{\Delta I_F}\right|_{\text{at } Q \text{ point}}$$

The reverse-bias condition of a diode may be displayed to check leakage (Fig. 9-10). When the POLARITY switch is set to the position opposite that used for the forward-bias tests, there should be only a horizontal line displayed. The oscilloscope centering must be readjusted because the polarity reversal causes the trace to move offscreen. Leakage current is easier to check with a much higher voltage than that used for forward-bias testing. The oscilloscope may be recalibrated for 10 V per division, which allows display of the test up to 100 V. Any measurable current which is displayed as a slope to the oscilloscope trace can be attributed to leakage current. If peak inverse breakdown of the diode occurs below 100 V, it will be displayed as shown in Fig. 9-10.

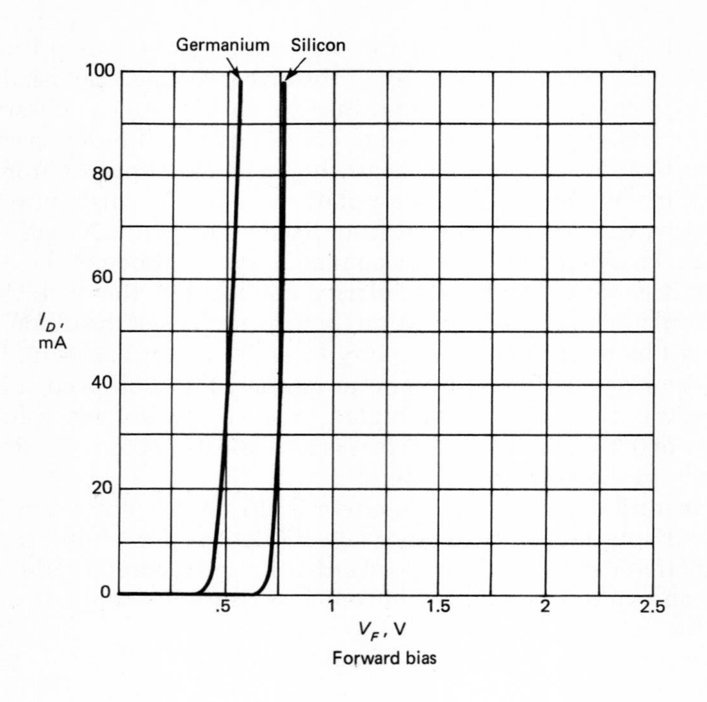

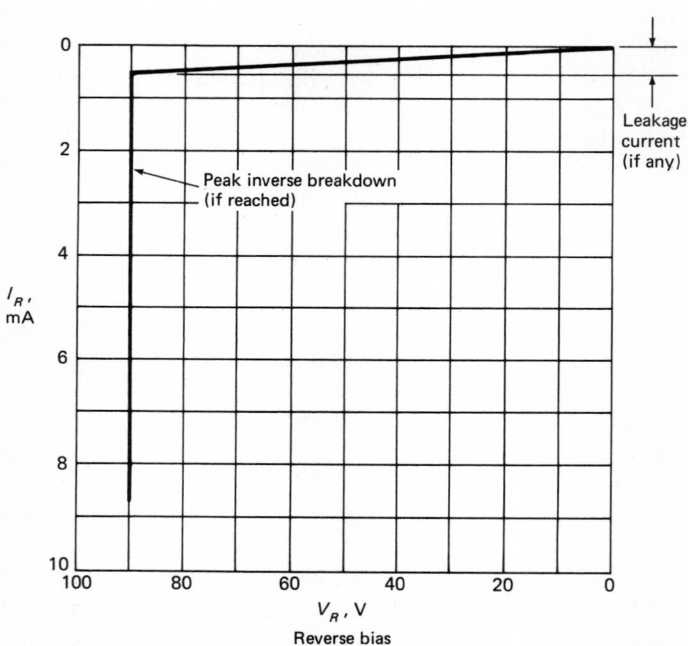

Typical Diode Curves

9-8
TESTING ZENER DIODES

The procedure for testing zener diodes is almost the same as that for testing signal and rectifier diodes. In fact, the forward characteristics of the diodes are essentially identical and the test procedures would be the same, except that forward-voltage measurements are seldom used for zener diodes. Zener diodes are designed to be used in the reverse-voltage breakdown mode. In this region, a large change in reverse current occurs while the zener voltage remains nearly constant. Because of this characteristic, they are most often used as voltage regulators.

The zener voltage value (reverse-voltage breakdown value) may be measured with the curve tracer and oscilloscope. This is the parameter that is most often checked for a zener diode. To obtain the most accurate voltage reading possible, calibrate the full-scale oscilloscope horizontal sensitivity to a convenient value slightly above the zener voltage. For example, for a 6-V diode, calibrate full scale at 10 V; for a 15-V diode, calibrate full scale at 20 V; etc.

Be sure the POLARITY switch is set to display the reverse-voltage condition. Increase the SWEEP VOLTAGE to display the zener region, as shown in Fig. 9-11. No reverse current should flow until the reverse-breakdown-voltage value is reached. At that point, there should be a very sharp "elbow" and a very vertical current trace. If the elbow is rounded or the vertical current trace has a measurable voltage slope, the zener diode is probably defective. Read the zener-voltage value from the display as accurately as possible. There may be variation of zener voltage from one diode to another of the same type number.

9-9
TESTING UNIJUNCTION TRANSISTORS

A unijunction transistor (UJT), as the name implies, is a single-junction device with three terminals. Conduction from base 1 to base 2 is purely resistive until an emitter current is applied. A small trigger current applied to the emitter causes a negative-resistance condition. The value of the trigger voltage is dependent on the voltage between base 1 and base 2. An examination of a UJT's operation can be displayed on the oscilloscope by using the curve tracer (Fig. 9-12*a*).

The curves displayed will appear quite close together, and careful

Fig. 9-10 (page 290) These curves show the important diode parameters: voltage drop in the forward direction and diode resistance. It can be seen that silicon diodes have a higher voltage drop than germanium. With reverse bias, the leakage and breakdown voltages are seen.

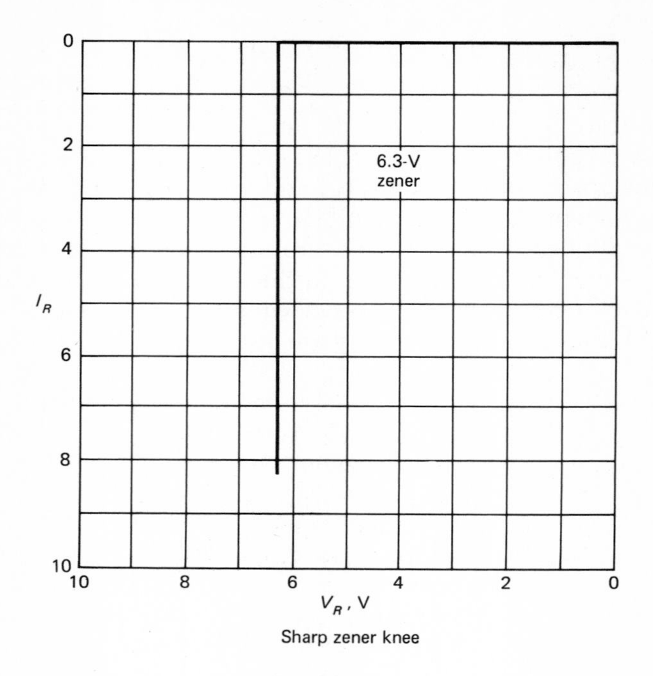

Sharp zener knee

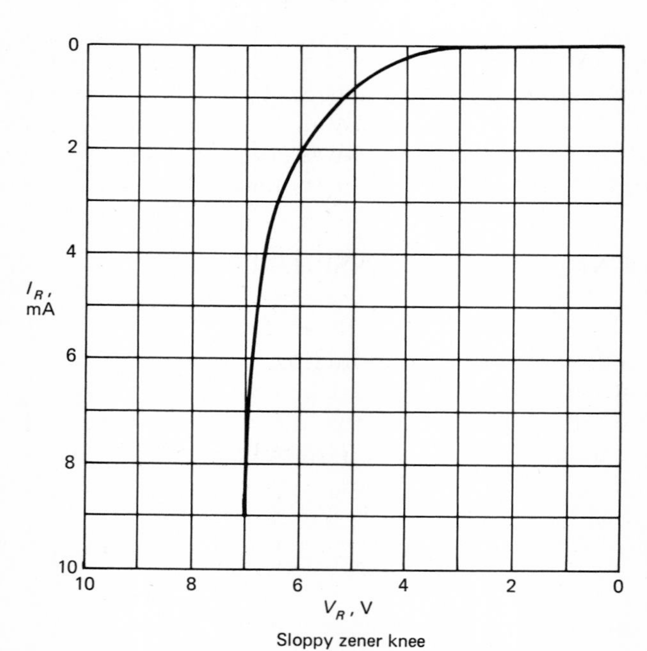

Sloppy zener knee

Typical Zener-Diode Curves

Fig. 9-11 Zener-diode curves show reverse-voltage breakdown. When this region is reached, the large current increase can be seen.

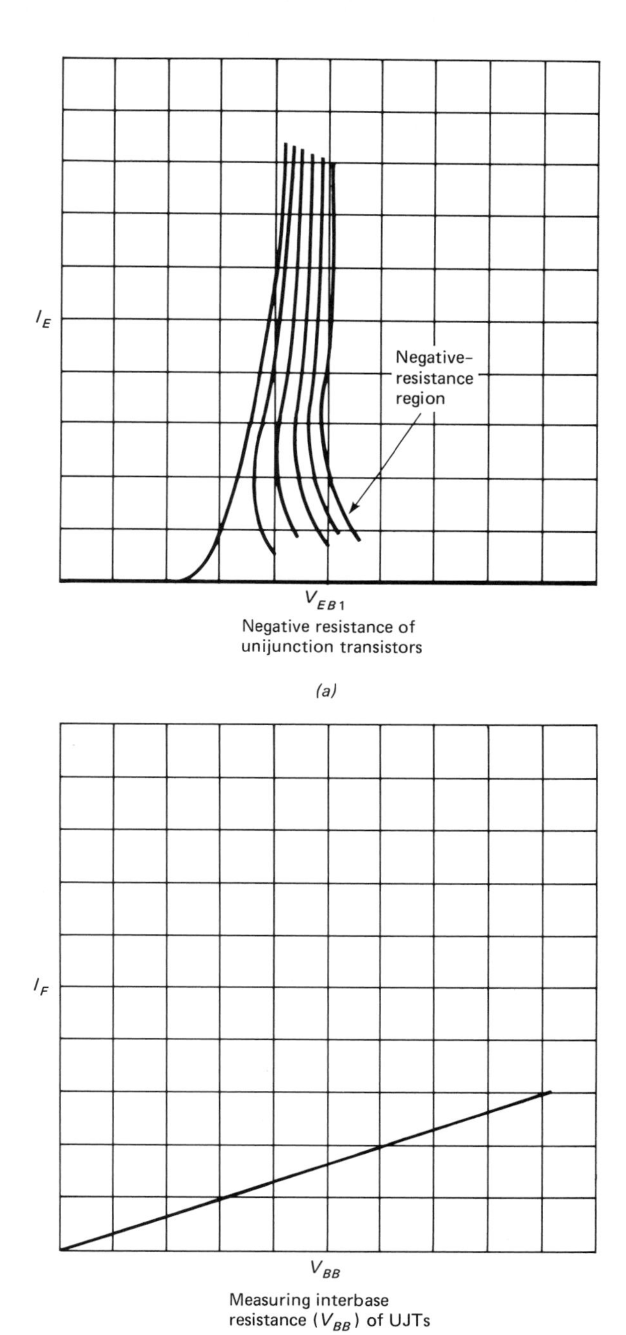

Fig. 9-12 (a) These curves show negative-resistance characteristics of the unijunction transistor. The emitter current I_E is the trigger that causes a negative resistance between base 1 and 2. (b) Interbase voltage V_{BB} affects the amount of forward current I_F that will flow.

observation may be required to distinguish the individual curves. It may be helpful to "spread out" the display by increasing horizontal sensitivity of the oscilloscope. With this test configuration, the step current of the curve tracer is applied from base 1 to base 2, and the sweep voltage applied to the emitter is the UJT trigger voltage. As the sweep voltage is slowly increased from the trigger threshold producing the first current spike, note that the other curves are added one by one. Thus, for each base-current step, the emitter trigger voltage can be measured.

Interbase resistance (R_{BB}) can be displayed (Fig. 9-12*b*) by connecting base 1 and base 2 to the collector and emitter jacks of the curve tracer and leaving the emitter lead of the UJT open-circuited. This displays a linear trace of forward current I_F versus interbase voltage V_{BB}.

$$R_{BB} = \frac{V_{BB}}{I_F}$$

9-10 TESTING SILICON CONTROLLED RECTIFIERS (SCRs)

SCRs (also called *thyristors*) are four-layer PNPN semiconductors with three terminals: cathode, anode, and gate. During conduction, the SCR has the characteristics of two series diodes. However, the device is normally nonconductive until a trigger current is applied to its gate. Once triggered into conduction, the SCR cannot be turned off until the anode-cathode current drops below a holding-current value necessary to sustain conduction. This holding current is usually a small percentage of the permissible peak current.

The following characteristics of an SCR can be displayed and measured with the semiconductor curve tracer:

- Forward blocking voltage
- Reverse blocking voltage
- Leakage current
- Holding current
- Forward-voltage drop for various forward currents
- Gate-trigger voltage for various forward voltages

FORWARD BLOCKING VOLTAGE

Forward blocking voltage (Fig. 9-13) is the maximum anode-cathode voltage in the forward direction that the device will withstand before

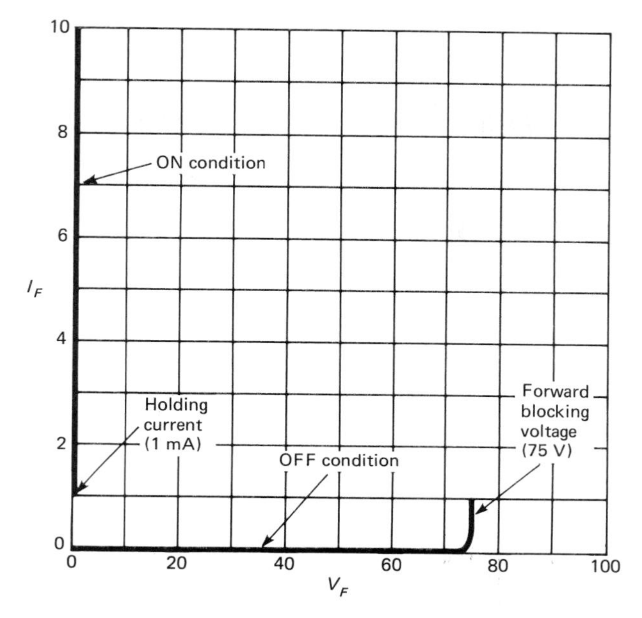

Fig. 9-13 The maximum anode-cathode voltage V_F that the SCR can withstand before conduction is shown. This is the forward blocking voltage. Also displayed is the holding current or the minimum anode current required to maintain conduction after the SCR has fired.

conduction, at zero gate current. The curve tracer will measure forward blocking voltage up to 100 V.

To measure forward blocking voltage, short the gate and cathode to satisfy the zero-gate-current requirement. Increase the *sweep voltage* until the SCR "fires"; that is, the anode current suddenly increases and the anode voltage drops to near zero. Read the highest anode-voltage point in the display. This is the maximum forward blocking voltage. Any anode current at anode voltage below the "firing" point is forward leakage current and can be read directly from the display.

REVERSE BLOCKING VOLTAGE

Reverse blocking voltage is the maximum reverse anode-cathode voltage at zero gate current that the device can withstand before voltage breakdown. It is similar to the peak inverse voltage of a diode. Reverse blocking voltage is normally higher than forward blocking voltage. The Model 501A can measure reverse blocking voltage up to 100 V. The voltage at which voltage breakdown, which is a sudden increase in anode current, occurs is the reverse-blocking-voltage value. Any anode current at voltages below breakdown is reverse leakage and can be read directly from the display.

HOLDING CURRENT

Holding current is the minimum anode current required to sustain conduction once the SCR has been fired. Using the same procedure as for the forward-blocking-voltage test, note the lowest current displayed for the "on" condition. This is the holding current.

FORWARD-VOLTAGE DROP

The forward-voltage drop during the "on" condition at various forward-current levels may be measured by increasing the horizontal sensitivity of the oscilloscope and displaying a low-voltage portion of the forward voltage. Read the forward-voltage drop directly from the display.

GATE-TRIGGER VOLTAGE

The "turn-on" point of an SCR is dependent on the forward voltage and gate voltage. As gate voltage is increased, less forward voltage is required to switch on the SCR. Conversely, as forward voltage is in-

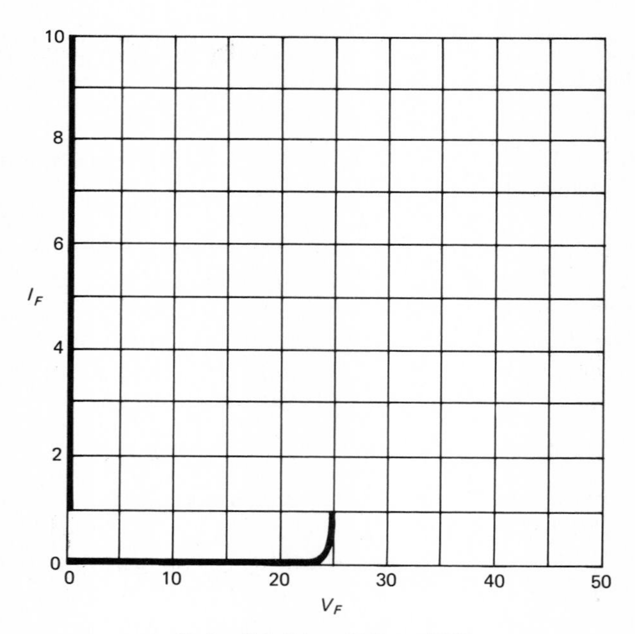

Fig. 9-14 Testing the trigger voltage of an SCR. Its "turn-on" point depends primarily on its gate voltage. However, less gate voltage is needed when the forward voltage V_F is increased.

creased, less gate voltage is required to switch on the SCR. Gate-trigger-voltage values (Fig. 9-14) can be measured by connecting a dc bias supply to the gate terminal of the SCR. Two types of measurements can be made:

1. Set the sweep voltage to a specified forward anode-cathode voltage and increase the dc bias supply until the SCR switches on. Measure the value of gate voltage at which switching occurred.
2. Set the dc bias supply to a specified gate voltage and increase the sweep voltage until the SCR switches on. Read the peak value of sweep voltage which was required.

9-11 TESTING TRIACS

Triacs are four-layer PNPN semiconductors with the same characteristics in both directions, and may be used for ac applications. A triac is the equivalent of two SCRs connected in parallel but oriented in opposite directions (see Fig. 9-15). The device has three terminals: main terminal 1, main terminal 2, and gate. Triacs may be tested exactly as SCRs except that forward tests should be repeated for both directions, and there will be no reverse-blocking-voltage measurement.

9-12 TESTING TUNNEL DIODES

Tunnel diodes are small PN junction semiconductors with a negative-resistance or "tunnel" region. The tunnel region makes it possible to use the diode as an amplifier, oscillator, or pulse generator. The diode conducts very easily in one direction (at much lower voltage

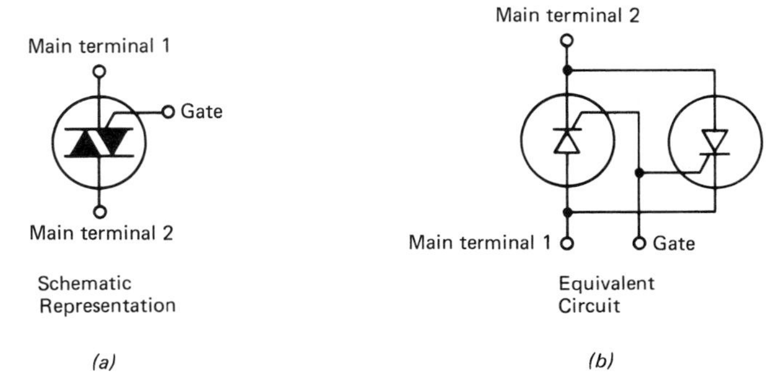

Fig. 9-15 (*a*) The triac schematic. The two SCRs have opposite polarities. (*b*) The equivalent triac circuit; both terminals are in parallel. Also there is a separate connection from two parallel gates.

than conventional signal diodes), but the tunnel region is in the direction of higher resistance. Tunnel diodes are normally operated at very low voltage and current levels.

The characteristics of tunnel diodes may be measured with the curve tracer. Connect the diode between the emitter and collector pins of one of the sockets. A display similar to that shown in Fig. 9-16 should be presented on the oscilloscope.

Several characteristics of the tunnel diode can be measured directly from the display. *Note:* A trace will normally *not* be displayed in the negative-resistance region.

- I_p: peak current, start of tunnel region
- I_v: valley current, end of tunnel region
- V_p: peak voltage, start of tunnel region
- V_v: valley voltage, end of tunnel region

The average negative resistance can be calculated from these measurements:

$$\text{Average negative resistance} = \frac{V_v - V_p}{I_p - I_v}$$

9-13 DIACS AND ICS

A diac is a two-terminal, three-layer semiconductor that exhibits the breakdown characteristic of two zener diodes placed back to back (bidirectional breakdown). It is nonconductive until the applied voltage exceeds its breakdown value, then current avalanches and the voltage drops across the terminals decrease to near zero. Once conduction has started, it continues until the current drops below a holding-current value necessary to sustain operation. Leakage current, breakdown voltage, and holding current can be measured with the curve tracer (the display will be similar to that of an SCR). Since it is bidirectional, a tunnel diode should be tested in both polarities.

9-14 INTEGRATED CIRCUITS

ICs are often multiple transistors or semiconductor devices packaged together. The curve tracer may be used to test such ICs. If the semiconductor devices can be identified and isolated to specific IC terminals, they can be individually tested with the curve tracer. Always be aware that other circuit elements in the IC may cause variation in the test pattern display. These can be seen as additional loops in the curves.

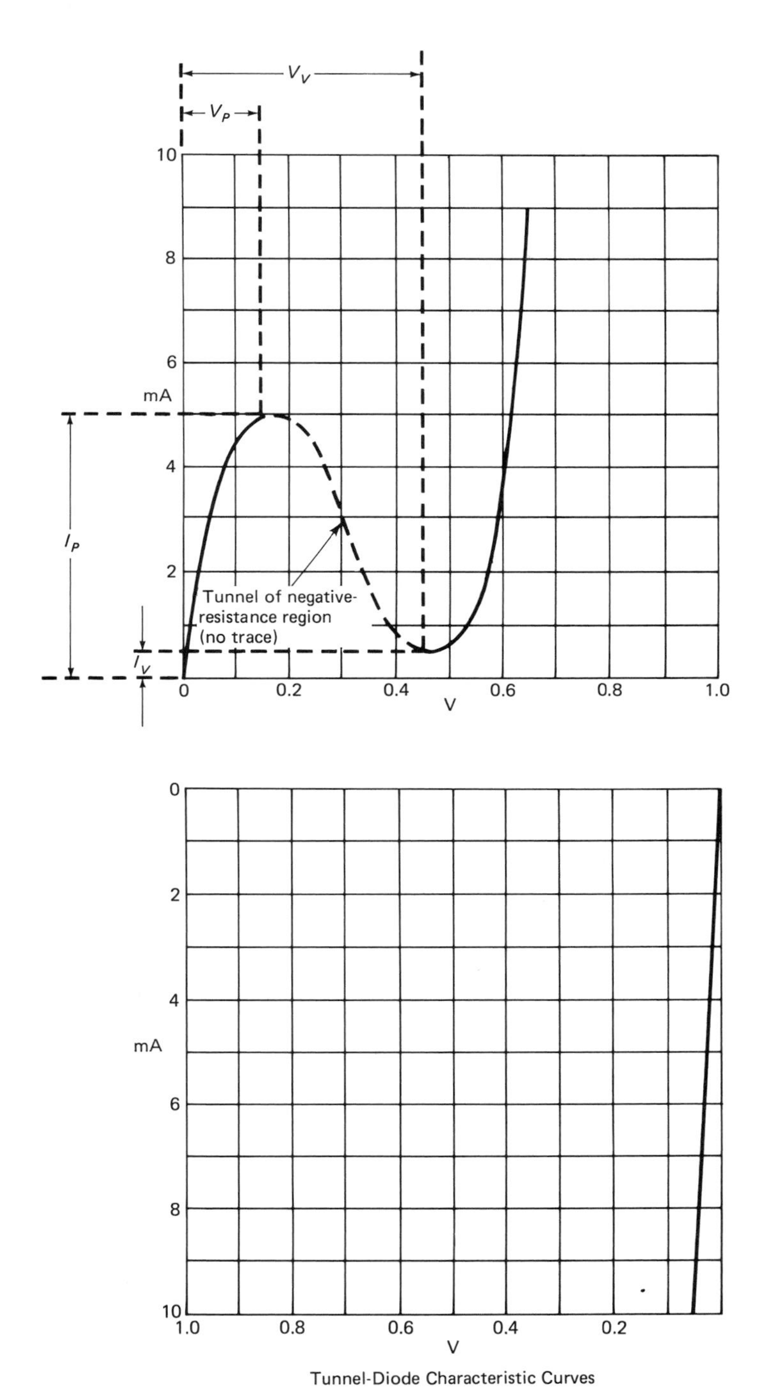

Tunnel-Diode Characteristic Curves

Fig. 9-16 The tunnel-diode peak current I_p is observed. The trace is disrupted in the negative-resistance region. Valley voltage and current and peak voltage can be seen in these figures.

As medical instruments perform more and more logic functions, data processing ICs will be encountered increasingly. Thus it is imperative that the BMET be familiar with the theory and troubleshooting techniques involved in both TTL (transistor-transistor logic) and CMOS (complementary metal-oxide semiconductor) devices.

TRANSISTOR-TRANSISTOR LOGIC

A chapter on troubleshooting solid-state devices would not be complete if ICs were not included. Early in the history of logic functions, diodes and discrete transistors were used. DTL (diode-transistor logic) was soon replaced by RTL (resistor-transistor logic), as the transistor could do everything the diode could and much more. As logic functions increased, it became aparent that RTL consumed too much power. As IC technology advanced, the IC became the solution to the inadequacies of RTL. IC technology permitted TTL to achieve a hundred times the function that earlier discrete components could perform.

TTL GATES. Gates are the basic TTL element. The AND gate will only produce a 1 or high-output pulse when each one of its inputs goes high. The OR gate produces a 1 or high output when any of its inputs is high. The inverter converts a 1 (high) to a 0 or low and conversely changes a 0 or low to a 1 or high. When the AND gate is combined with an inverter, it functions as an AND gate with an inverted output. This is a NAND gate. When the OR gate is combined with an inverter, it functions as an OR gate with an inverted output. This is the NOR gate. Any gate may have from two to eight inputs, and two or more gates are often found in the same IC or dual in-line package. Logic symbols for the various gates are shown in Fig. 9-17.

FLIP-FLOPS. The flip-flop is essentially a memory device. It may be a simple latching circuit or a more complex multivibrator. The latching circuits in Fig. 9-18 are made up from NAND, NOR, and inverter gates. (Letters designating outputs are always toward the end of the alphabet,

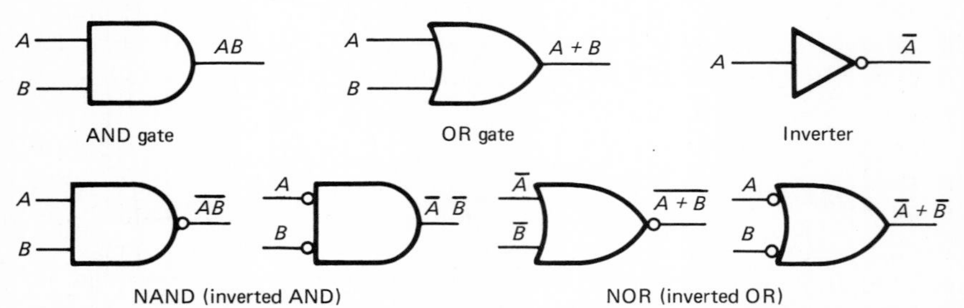

Fig. 9-17 Logic symbols for the various gates. An IC can consist of only these gates or may contain these gates in combination with other circuit functions.

The asynchronous RS latches below operate without a clock pulse

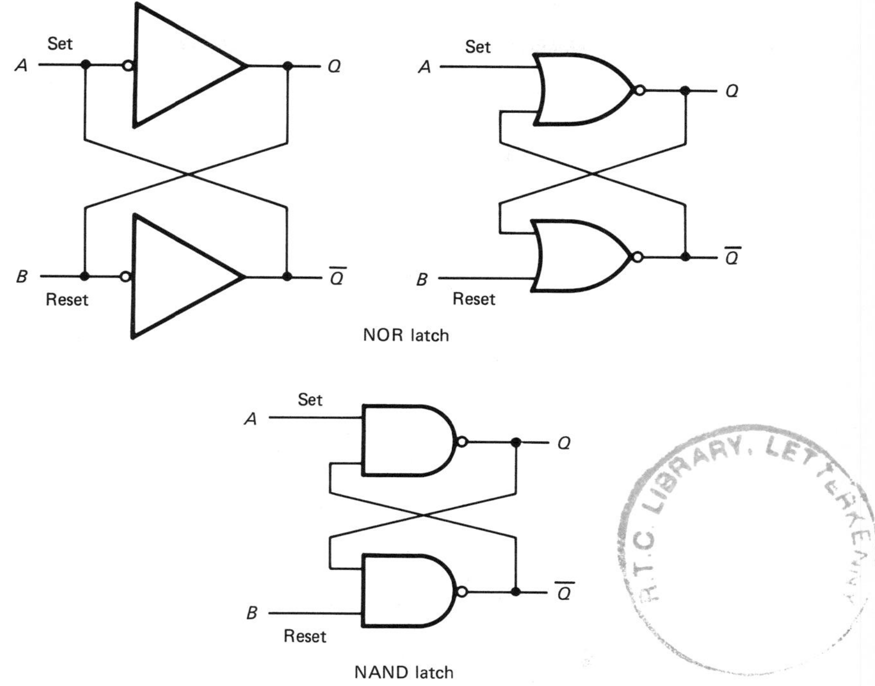

Fig. 9-18 Gates are combined so that they latch, or remember the last condition that existed at their input. These asynchronous RS latches do not require a clock pulse to trigger their timing.

and inputs at the beginning of the alphabet.) The Q output has its inversion designated as $\overline{Q}$. Input *A* is a set input, and input *B* is a reset input. The output Q always remembers that last state of the set or reset inputs; they will latch. RS latching circuits operate asynchronously; that is, they are not stimulated by an external pulse other than their inputs. Other latches (ac-RS, D, etc.) can be controlled by a clock to increase their stability. This is vital as the speed of operation increases. More data means a higher speed is necessary; thus the timing of sequential is more critical.

The flip-flops described have one input condition that results in an indeterminate output state. The *JK* flip-flop overcomes this disadvantage. All possible *J* and *K* input combinations represent useful states. With the clock and the *J* and *K* inputs both zero, the *JK* will not switch or change state. However, when both *J* and *K* are high (logic 1), then the flip-flop will switch after each clock pulse. Proper operation of the *JK* flip-flop depends on the pulse width and magnitude of the clock pulse. The ac *JK* flip-flop differentiates or narrows the clock pulse, overcoming this problem. Another flip-flop, the master-slave, consists of two RS flip-flops internally connected. The clock is fed into two AND gates and then to the master flip-flop through the inverter to the slave. Figure 9-19 shows that when the clock goes from high to low, the *J* and *K* data are transferred to the Q output of the master. The inverter ensures that the slave is off (low) when the master is on (high). Then, as the clock returns to zero (low), the master transfers its data to the slave flip-flop. A *JK* flip-flop made especially for very-high-frequency use is the positive- and negative-edge-triggered flip-flop. In Fig. 9-20, a different response from various types of *JK* flip-flops is observed as a result of the same data being fed to each *J* and *K* input. The BMET can always find out what type of flip-flop is being used by referring to an IC manual. This information is also often given in the medical instrument service manual.

THE COUNTER. One of the most common medical instrument logic circuits is the counter. The asynchronous DOWN counter in Fig. 9-21 starts with the binary number 1111 and counts down for each clock pulse. The inverted Q ($\overline{Q}$) output is used to drive the successive flip-flops. The flip-flops will switch when the clock pulse goes from a 1 to a 0. Waveforms associated with this type of counter are shown in Fig. 9-22. The preset asynchronous DOWN counter in Fig. 9-23 can be preset to any desired number before counting. Once this preset number

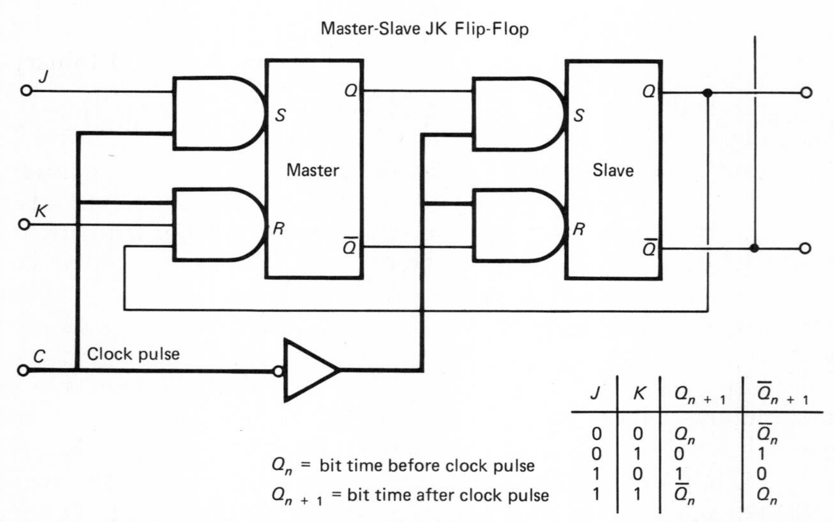

J	K	Q_{n+1}	$\overline{Q}_{n+1}$
0	0	Q_n	$\overline{Q}_n$
0	1	0	1
1	0	1	0
1	1	$\overline{Q}_n$	Q_n

Fig. 9-19 The master-slave *JK*-type flip-flop. The slave is always off when the master is on. The truth table explains the relationship between the outputs (Q_n) and the inputs (*J* and *K*).

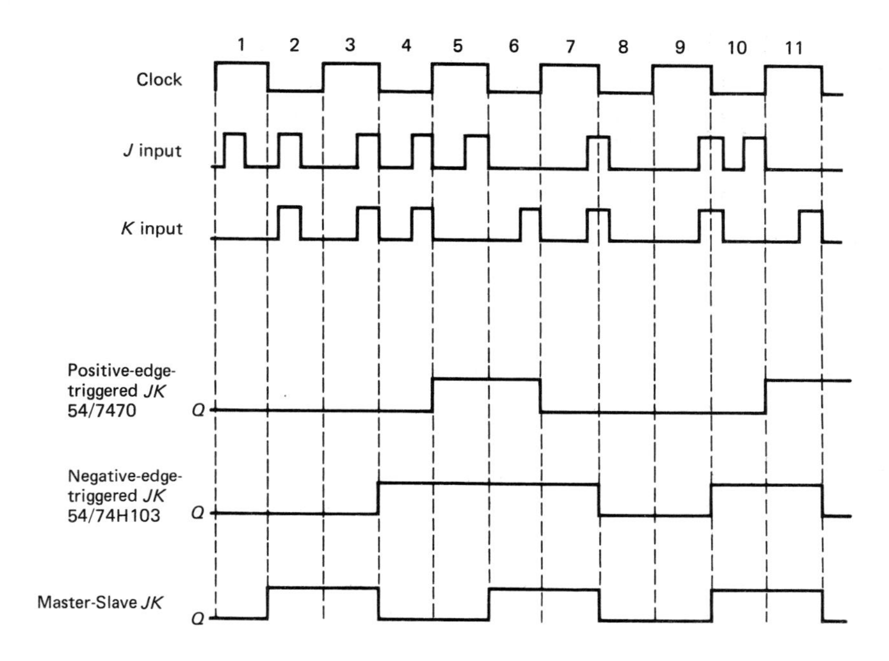

Fig. 9-20 Waveforms that indicate how positive-edge-triggered, negative-edge-triggered, and master-slave flip-flops react when the same input data are fed to each one.

has been programmed, the counter will count down to zero and then stop.

A modulo counter will count to a programmed number, then stop, reset, and recycle automatically. In the asynchronous BCD (binary-coded decimal) counter of Fig. 9-24, the clock pulse at flop-flop *D* must represent the least significant bit or number. Hence, this input repre-

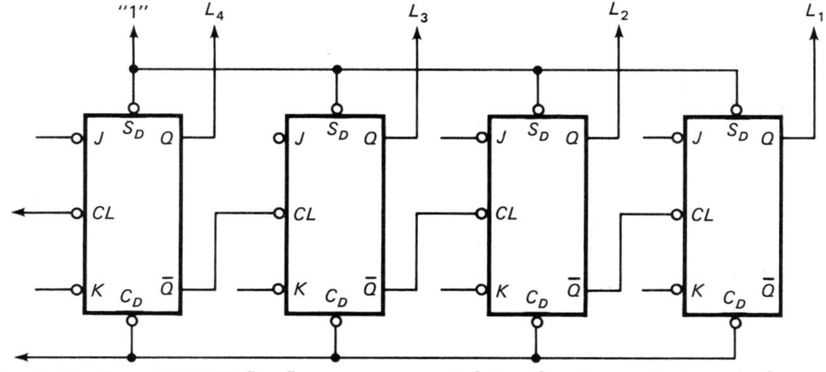

Fig. 9-21 Four 7476 IC flip-flops are connected together to create an asynchronous binary DOWN counter. All *J*, *K*, and C_D terminals should be connected to a logic 1.

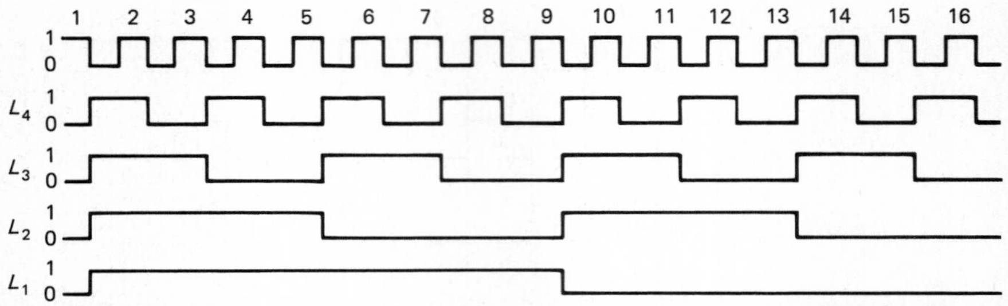

Fig. 9-22 Time relationships between the various waveforms found in the binary DOWN counter in Fig. 9-21. The numbered pulses at the top are the input pulses being counted. The least significant bit is counted at the L_4 output. The most significant bit is counted at the L_1 output, or the flip-flop at the extreme right in Fig. 9-21.

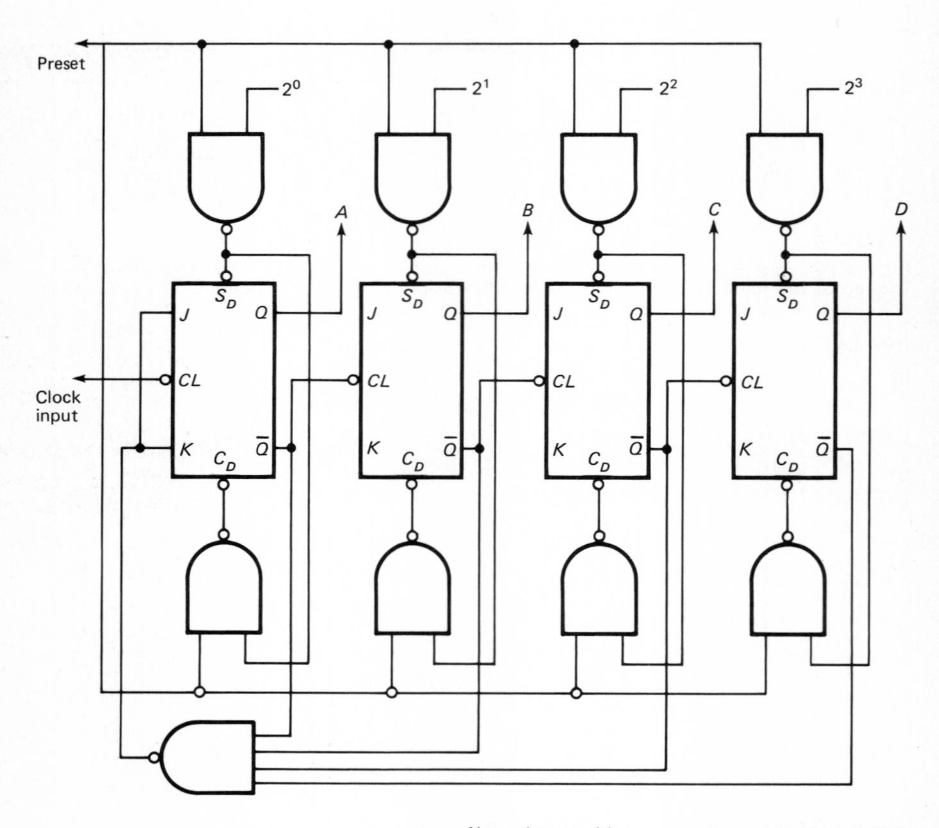

Fig. 9-23 A preset asynchronous DOWN counter. The preset pulse is fed to input 1 to start the count down to zero. Output D becomes the most significant bit, while output A becomes the least significant bit.

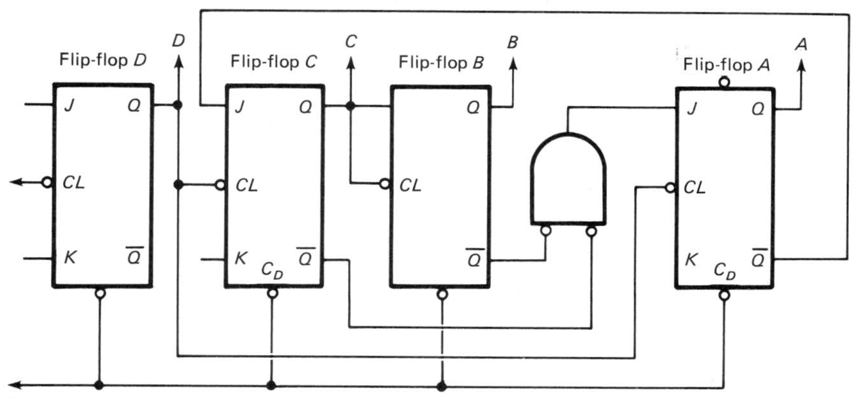

Fig. 9-24 The asynchronous binary-coded decimal (BCD) counter. The least significant digit is fed to flip-flop *D*, which is also the pulse divider for successive flip-flops.

sents a divide-by-two counter. When the counter is cleared, the *J* input of flip-flop *C* will be high (1) because this input is tied directly to the *A* output; the *J* input will be high (1) until the binary count of 1000. Flip-flop *C* is a divide-by-four counter until the count of 1000. The NOR gate output will be high at the binary count of 0111.

An up-down counter will count up when grounding the down pins and will count down when grounding the up pins.

PULSE RISETIME AND AMPLITUDE. When a logic circuit does not function, we can look for a defective IC by using the signal-substitution method described in Sec. 9-3. Often, logic curcuits may work in an erratic fashion, resulting in nonuniform and dubious readouts. In these cases, it may be necessary to examine the pulse itself. To guarantee reliable operation, input signals feeding a TTL device should have a risetime of no less than a microsecond. A longer risetime may cause oscillations on the output.

The Schmitt trigger is a circuit (or an IC) that "cleans up" a signal with a slow risetime or a degraded shape. TTL input level for low (0) should be below 0.4 V. The on (high or 1) input should be between 2.4 and 3.6 V. For good noise immunity, the clock pulse should have a risetime and falltime of less than 150 ms. If the low level or zero is higher than 0.4 V, trace that circuit backward, looking for defective ICs or transistors that will not saturate. If a high (1) is less than 2.4 V, check all collector pull-up resistors along that signal path. Look for resistors that have increased in value. When the oscilloscope shows ringing or overshoot, look for impedance mismatch, especially where interconnecting lines drive separate pieces of equipment.

A TTL MEDICAL APPLICATION

The ability of the human nerve to propagate electric signals is extremely important. This nerve conductivity allows us to move muscles and gives us sensual feelings. The time required for a pulse (stimulus) to travel along the nerve to a pickup electrode (response) located near the nerve is called the nerve's *conduction latency*. This time difference can be seen on an oscilloscope. The medical specialist must then interpret this reading into the actual conduction latency. Several manufacturers today make nerve-conduction analyzers with conduction latency read directly on an LED readout display.

In Fig. 9-25, the stimulus signal is fed into a Schmitt trigger, where it is shaped into a well-defined pulse. This pulse is amplified and sets the flip-flop (M203). The AND gate (M1103) goes high, and the binary-coded counter (M231) begins to count. After the stimulus has traveled along the nerve, it reaches the response or pickup electrode. The response is fed into signal-conditioning circuits which amplify and shape the response signal. The response then turns off flip-flop M203, thus changing the AND gate output to low or zero. At this instance, the BCD counter stops its count and the LEDs remain at the number corre-

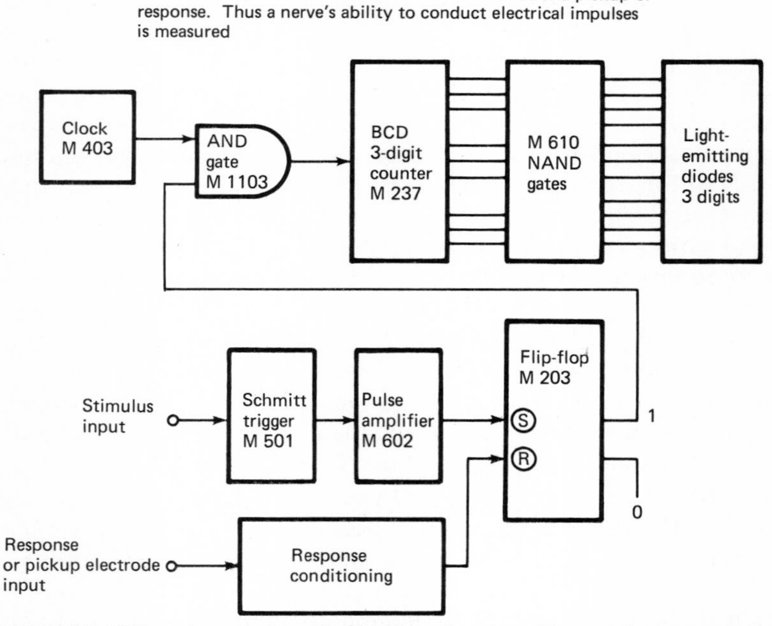

Fig. 9-25 This TTL system produces a digital readout in milliseconds corresponding to nerve-conduction latency or time delay. The modules are made by Digital Equipment Corp., Maynard, Mass.

sponding to the last pulse before the flip-flop was turned off. The digital readout displays the amount of time required for the stimulus signal to travel from the proximal point (area of stimulus pulse) to the distal or response pickup point. The clock frequency is set so that clock pulses will relate to time in milliseconds.

Most medical applications require more sophisticated logic circuitry than the nerve-conduction analyzer discussed here. However, the basic principles remain the same. As logic functions became more complex, TTL circuitry presented a problem. The total instrument or system became bulky and power-consuming. As a consequence, cost increased and portability suffered. It was for these reasons that TTL technology was slowly replaced by CMOS technology.

TROUBLESHOOTING CMOS

The previous chapters show that some computerization of biomedical data can be seen in almost any recently manufactured instrument. In addition, biomedical computerization applications are proliferating at so rapid a pace that one might call it a technological explosion. TTL techniques used in early equipment had severe handicaps. It was difficult to filter out TTL noise, and multiple logic functions were bulky and required heavy-duty power supplies. For these reasons several IC manufacturers made rapid breakthroughs in CMOS (complementary metal-oxide semiconductor) technology. Although CMOS has many inherent advantages over the old TTL circuitry, it presents an entirely new set of problems for the troubleshooter and designer. The following is presented so that the BMET may understand CMOS technology and be fully prepared for the pitfalls encountered when servicing biomedical equipment using it.

CMOS is not a full-fledged family of IC logic and medium-scale integration (MSI) functions. Most manufacturers have implemented or are implementing standard outputs and loading rules. While actual implementation of the functions is not consistent, variations encountered are almost always for improved operating parameters. Input-protection circuits, however, are not consistent from manufacturer to manufacturer, from device type to device type, and, unhappily, sometimes even between inputs of the same device. This last phenomenon is not a result of manufacturing parameter variation but is due to chip design. Admittedly, certain parts require various different schemes of input protection, such as some types of ac-coupled circuits do (astable and monostable multivibrators, for example).

INPUT PROTECTION. What about input protection? Probably the most notorious feature of CMOS logic is the susceptibility of the gate to damage by discharge of static electricity. Such static charges are of low energy but can have potentials in excess of 1000 V, while the breakdown voltage for the thin-gate oxide of CMOS circuits (1000 Å) is in the range of 50 to 90 V. In CMOS IC design there are three viable input-protection schemes now being used by manufacturers. The protection circuitry is included on the IC chip. Each of these protection methods is a compromise. Figure 9-26 shows the schematic differences of these protection circuits. The *single-diode protection scheme* (Fig. 9-26*a* to *c*) is simple and requires a minimum of chip area. However, the protection afforded by this method is also minimum. There are several circuits which require the use of this method, notably because of input swings which may greatly exceed the power-supply bias in one direction under normal operation. The *double-diode-plus-resistor scheme* of

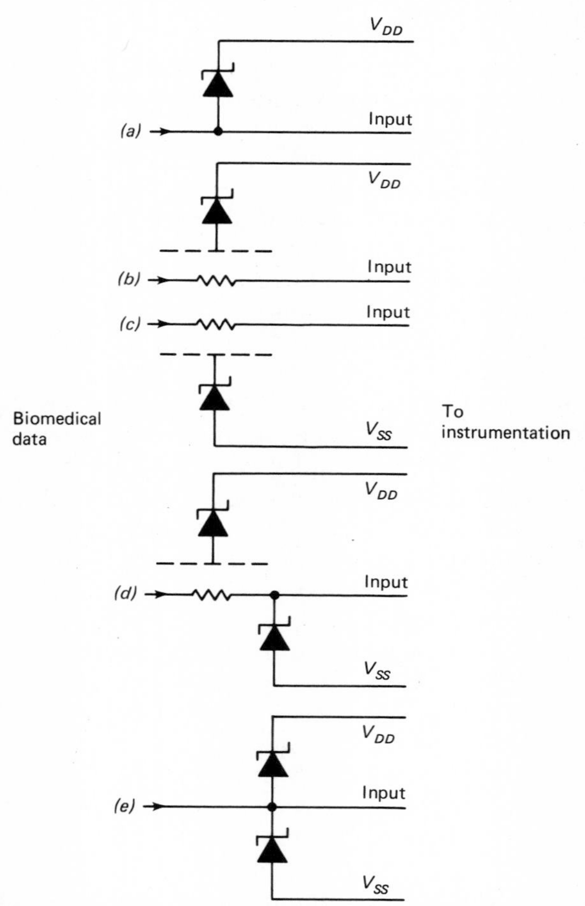

Fig. 9-26 Typical CMOS input-protection network in IC chips. The resistor-diode symbol represents a distributed diode structure. Typical breakdown voltages for diodes are between 35 and 100 V. Typical resistance values are from 200 to 2500 Ω.

Fig. 9-26*d* offers the best protection for CMOS inputs, but requires two to four times more chip area than the single-diode method. This scheme exhibits good clamping of transients to the power-supply terminals and also provides, in combination with the circuit capacitance, an *RC* delay characteristic before the zener diode avalanches to ground. This is the most widely used CMOS gate-protection scheme and has many variations in actual implementation. The third method of CMOS input protection, Fig. 9-26*e*, is called the *transmission-switch method* and uses the parasitic diodes of a CMOS transmission switch to obtain its clamping action. This scheme can use an effective area of zero on the chip but is susceptible to rupture of the transmission-switch control gates. As with the double-diode method, this protection scheme provides good clamping to the voltage-supply rails. The transmission-switch method is usually combined with the single-diode resistor protection characteristics to become, in effect, the double-diode method of Fig. 9-26*d*. The transmission-switch method is usually found at either the parallel-or serial-data inputs of shift registers, counters, and flip-flops.

At this time, Motorola Semiconductor is the only major manufacturer of CMOS ICs which does not consistently use double-diode (Fig. 9-26*d*) protection circuitry. In the light of this variation of input-protection circuitry, I suggest that if a Motorola part is specified in an ac-coupled circuit, you should use a Motorola part. On the other hand, if a part from, say, RCA, Solid State Scientific, or Siltek has been specified, you may use the same part from any other manufacturer except Motorola. Otherwise, different waveforms and possibly different operation may result. A Motorola part may be used provided that a silicon diode is added to the circuit in shunt with the input, as in Fig. 9-27. *Note:* Do not use a germanium, hot-carrier, or other type of diode which exhibits a forward voltage of 0.5 V or less. Also, there is no need to use a power diode. A good choice would be a 1N914 or similar device. You should

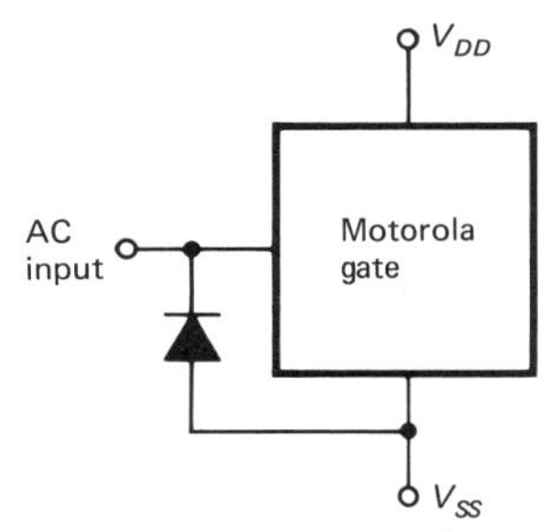

Fig. 9-27 Use of an internal diode as a V_{ss} clamp when using Motorola gates in ac circuits. CR_1 is a 1N914 or similar diode.

realize that this mechanism is not to afford extra input protection but only to make the circuit perform in a more predictable manner.

As mentioned earlier, input-protection networks have been designed into CMOS circuits for the primary purpose of protecting the fragile gate oxides from damage due to accumulated static charge. The gate circuit of MOS devices may be considered as a low-value capacitor, typically 0.5 pF, and does not provide a dc path for current flow as does a bipolar input circuit (see Fig. 9-28). Static charge which may accumulate on this gate capacitance through handling cannot be "bled off" without input-protection circuitry (Fig. 9-28*b*). Any charge of 25 to 50 picocoulombs (pC) impressed on a minimum-size unprotected CMOS input may destroy the gate dielectric. In contrast, normal operating bias usually covers the range from 1.5 to 7.5 pC for the same size devices. Consider for a moment now that you, as a human being, average about 300 pF of capacitance and by normal activities can store up to 15 kV. This works out to 4.5 μC. But, you also average around 50 to 100 kΩ of series resistance, which, together with the input-protection networks of CMOS circuits, reduces these charges to safe on-chip values.

If you have trouble visualizing this, consider the equation for charge, $Q = CV$. The gate oxides of CMOS devices exhibit a typical rupture potential of 50 to 90 V, while their normal operating range is 3 to 18 V. The obvious conclusion would be: *Handle with care.* This precaution was a strict requirement before the days of gate-protection circuitry. While this is not to say that you should be irresponsible in handling CMOS devices, it does mean that grounded working surfaces and static-free environments are not essential for their use. At the very least you should use a grounded soldering iron tip. Any other power tools to be used on the equipment should also have grounds attached. This is

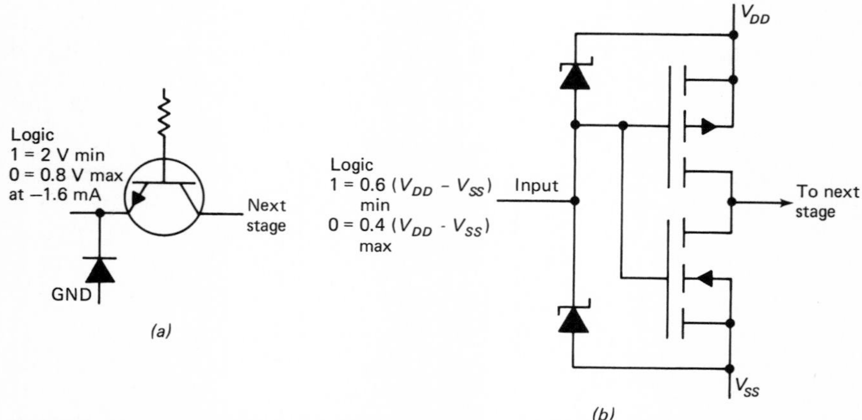

Fig. 9-28 (*a*) The typical TTL input with voltages specified for the two binary states. (*b*) the CMOS input shows that "turn-on" voltage requirements are much lower.

easily provided if you have a three-wire ac power system and conscientiously select and use the proper tools. A recommended soldering iron is the Ungar Imperial.

Don't throw away your old soldering irons, because with a little ingenuity you can make a workable arrangement by using an alligator clip or banana plug and a length of shield braid from RG-58U or RG-59U coaxial line. Secure one end of the braid to the tip of your soldering iron or gun and either plug the banana plug into a ground terminal of a three-wire ac system or slip it on to your cold-water pipes. The ground and power pins of your circuit board or chasis should be shorted temporarily and also attached to the same ground system in a similar manner. Aluminum foil is a good way to do this. Other power tools (drills, saber saws, etc.) should also be grounded in a like manner, especially if they will be used on this equipment after CMOS parts have been installed. You should also remove fabric rugs from workbench areas. Rubber mats are usable.

One final note on the protection devices is that CMOS circuits generally come packed in black conductive foam or black plastic and metal handler sticks. Try to leave the devices in these protective mediums until you are ready to use them.

TERMINATE ALL INPUTS. The unprotected CMOS gate, being a capacitor, provides a mechanism for charge storage instead of dissipation. Unlike bipolar circuits, where the logic levels are dependent on current flow, in CMOS circuits the logic levels are dependent on voltage levels. Figure 9-28 illustrates these differences. This characteristic alone sets CMOS apart from all other logic families, especially where energy-stingy applications are concerned, such as when battery and portable operation is intended. Because there is no dc flow, another caution in respect to CMOS must be mentioned. When designing and constructing CMOS circuits, all unused inputs must be biased. If this is not done, excessive power-supply current drain and/or malfunctioning of circuits may occur. Since there is no way for an accumulated charge to drain, there may be a static bias which can put the device in a high current-dissipation mode or, just as bad, might put it on the "wrong side of the truth table." This same consideration goes for inputs which might see an open or closed state of a switch. Either the switch should be a double-throw type with both terminals tied to a valid logic level or the normally open condition should be resistor-biased to either V_{dd} or V_{ss} as appropriate.

Input-protection networks and gates of CMOS devices may also be damaged if they are inserted or removed from sockets while power and signals are applied. Always turn off power and low-impedance sources before replacing CMOS ICs. Another caution along this line is that

CMOS devices may be damaged if low-impedance signal sources are on and driving these circuits without V_{dd}/V_{ss} power applied. Always turn power supplies on first and off last.

WHO MAKES CMOS? The list of CMOS manufacturers and their device codes should be very helpful in parts procurement if your favorite distributor does not stock the brand of ICs specified. There are three major subfamilies of CMOS. These are:

1. CD4000 series. This is the oldest and most firmly established CMOS family. It contains a good representation of gates, flip-flops, and MSI functions. This is the most widely "second-sourced" family of CMOS, but it suffers from some system compatibility faults. With the announcement by RCA, the family's innovator, of its β-series specification, the family will now take on standard output parameters.
2. MC14500 series. Motorola introduced early members of this series in 1971 to supplement several obvious holes in the CD4000 series of CMOS ICs. Since then the family has added systems-oriented MSI functions, including several functions patterned after some SN7400-series TTL functions.
3. MM74COO series. This family and its sister family (MM54COO) were the first CMOS families which could truly live up to the title of a logic family. National Semiconductor, which announced the family in early 1972, notes that its features are true TTL-level compatibility, pin-for-pin CMOS logic equivalents for the SN7400 series parts from which they take their numbers, and true family characteristics.

The CD4000 series is the most widely second-sourced CMOS family. National Semiconductor's MM74COO series has the next widest second-source capability. Many of the MC14500 series parts, as well as several of the MM74COO series parts, are now being second-sourced by RCA and several other manufacturers. RCA and the few suppliers who second-source the MC14500 series parts use the 4500 series numbers. RCA has begun using CD4000-series part numbers for those MM74COO parts which they second-source.

SUPER CMOS. Inselek, Fairchild Semiconductor, and Harris Semiconductor do not produce conventional bulk-substrate CMOS. These manufacturers use special substrates and/or special isolation techniques in the fabrication of their parts, which are most generally seen by the user as higher speed of operation and lower quiescent power dissipation. The parts from these vendors should not be mixed with those of the other suppliers unless careful consideration is given to the possibility of spike (glitch) hazards in the logic system.

BUFFERED GATES. Buffered gates, like buffered aspirin, offer some advantages. The buffered gate is contrasted to the simple gate structure in Fig. 9-29. The prime distinctive feature of buffered gates is the addition of two inverters after the logic block. These inverters contribute some delay to the signal but add beneficial features: loading on each stage is minimized, input capacitance is reduced because smaller devices are used in the logic stage, overall chip size is smaller, output characteristics are symmetric and independent of the number of active inputs, the transfer curve is sharper, noise immunity is better. Also, buffered gates exhibit less propagation delay in real systems. Inverting gates may be either simple or buffered depending on the supplier and/or part number. Noninverting gates are always buffered.

Because of the extra inverters in their circuits, buffered gates have unique properties. Buffered gates have higher propagation delay in lightly loaded systems, but they show lower propagation delay when heavily loaded by capacitance. This is due to their more symmetrical output characteristics, achieved by isolating the logic function from the output driving function. The most unique difference in buffered gates is that there is a significant phase shift through them. This may result in erratic performance in oscillator, one-shot, and linear circuits. Again, for ac circuits and for linear uses, it would be best to try to stick to the original manufacturer, but if you are careful in your choice or are willing to do a little "cut and try," parts from other manufacturers can be used.

CMOS is the most energy-conscious logic family. Its price per gate structure is the most attractive available. These considerations will

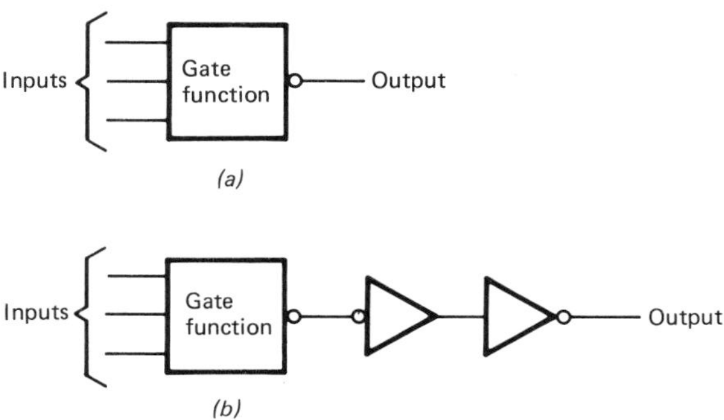

Fig. 9-29 The difference between (*a*) a simple (unbuffered) IC gate structure and (*b*) a buffered CMOS gate structure.

make CMOS the logic family for 85 to 95 percent of all biomedical data processing applications.

9-15 DIGITAL TROUBLESHOOTING

When troubleshooting analog circuits, the task is one of verifying characteristics such as resistance, capacitance, or turn-on voltages of components with two or three nodes. While the function of the total circuit may be complex, each component in that circuit performs a simple task, and proper operation is easily verified.

Each diode, resistor, capacitor, or transistor can be tested using a signal generator, voltmeter, ohmmeter, diode checker, or oscilloscope. When this circuit is built in IC form, these components are no longer accessible. It is necessary to test the complete circuit function.

It is now necessary to observe complex digital signals and decide if these signals are correct according to the function the IC was meant to perform. Verifying component operation requires stimulating and observing many inputs while simultaneously observing several outputs.

Figure 9-30 shows a typical TTL signal. This could just as well be any analog signal viewed on an oscilloscope. The oscilloscope displays absolute voltage with respect to time, but in the digital world absolute values are unimportant. A digital signal exists in one of two or three states—high, low, and undefined or in-between level—each determined by a threshold voltage. It is the relative value of the signal voltage with respect to these thresholds that determines the state of the digital signal, and this digital state determines the operation of the IC, not absolute levels. If the signal is greater than 2.4 V, it is a high state and it is unimportant whether the level is 2.8 or 3.0 V. Similarly, for a low state the voltage must be below 0.4 V. It is not important what the absolute level is as long as it is below this threshold.

Within a digital logic family, such as TTL, the timing characteristics of each component are well defined. Each gate in the TTL logic family

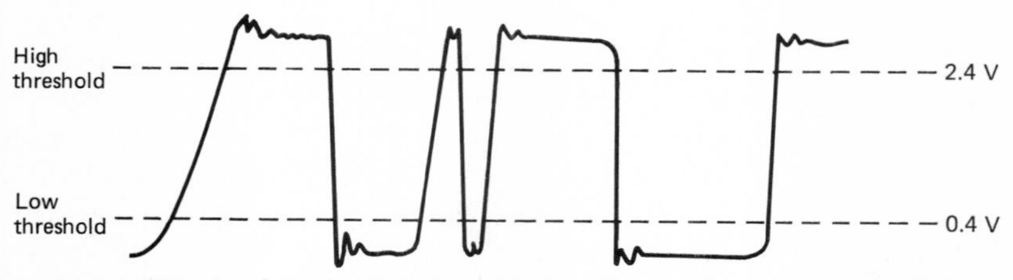

Fig. 9-30 A TTL signal. In the digital world, the relative value of a signal voltage with respect to the threshold voltages determines the operation of the circuit. A signal above the high threshold is in the high state, and whether it is 2.8 or 3.0 V is unimportant to the operation of the circuit.

displays a characteristic propagation delay time, risetime, and falltime. The effects of these timing parameters on circuit operation are taken into account by the designer. It is to be hoped that once a design has been developed beyond breadboard or prototype stage and is into production, problems due to design have been corrected.

An important characteristic of digital ICs is that when they fail, they fail catastrophically. This means that timing parameters rarely degrade or become marginal. Thus observing on an oscilloscope and making repeated decisions on the validity of timing parameters is time-consuming and contributes very little to the troubleshooting process. Once problems due to design are corrected, the fact that pulse activity exists is usually enough indication of proper IC operation without further observation of pulse width, repetition rate, risetime, or falltime.

FAILURE MODES OF DIGITAL ICs

It is important to understand the type of failures found in digital circuits. These can be categorized into two classes—those caused by a failure internal to an IC and those caused by a failure in the circuit external to the IC.

Four types of internal failure can occur to an IC. These are (1) an open bond on an input or an output, (2) a short between an input or output and V_{cc} or ground, (3) a short between two pins (neither of which is V_{cc} or ground), and (4) a failure in the internal circuitry (often called the steering circuitry) of the IC.

In addition to these four internal failures, four failures can occur in the circuit external to the IC. These are (1) a short between a node and V_{cc} or ground, (2) a short between two nodes (neither of which is V_{cc} or ground), (3) an open signal path, and (4) a failure of an analog component.

The first failure internal to an IC is an open bond on either an input or output. This failure has a different effect depending on whether it is an open output bond or an open input bond. In the case of an open output bond (Fig. 9-31), the inputs driven by that output are left to float. In TTL and DTL circuits a floating input rises to approximately 1.4 to 1.5 V and usually has the same effect on circuit operation as a high logic level. Thus an open output bond will cause all inputs driven by that output to float to a bad level, since 1.5 V is less than the high-threshold level of 2.0 V and greater than the low-threshold level of 0.4 V. In TTL and DTL, a floating input is interpreted as a high level. Thus the effect will be that these inputs will respond to this bad level as though it were a static high signal.

In the case of an open input bond (Fig. 9-32), the open circuit blocks the signal driving the input from entering the IC chip. The input on the

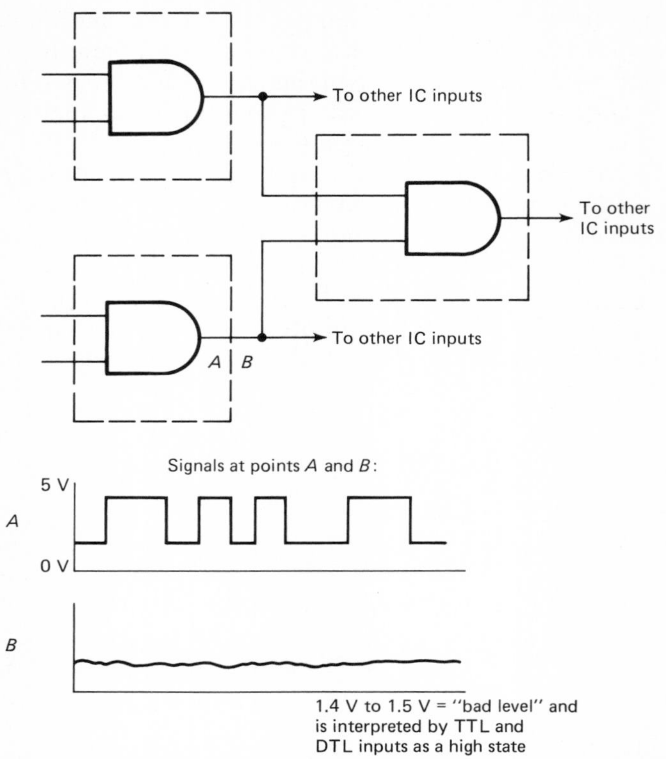

Fig. 9-31 The effect of an open output bond upon circuit operation. An open output bond allows all inputs driven by that output to float to a "bad level." This level is usually interpreted as a logic high state by the inputs. Thus the inputs driven by an open output bond will respond as though a static logic high signal was applied.

chip is thus allowed to float and will respond as though it were a static high signal. Since the open occurs on the input inside the IC, the digital signal driving this input will be unaffected by the open and will be detectable when looking at the input pin (such as at point *A* in Fig. 9-32). The effect will be to block this signal inside the IC, and the resulting IC operation will be as though the input were a static high.

A short between an input or output and V_{cc} or ground has the effect of holding all signal lines connected to that input or output either high (in the case of a short to V_{cc}) or low (if shorted to ground) (Fig. 9-33). In many cases, this will cause expected signal activity at points beyond the short to disappear, and thus this type of failure is catastrophic in terms of circuit operation.

A short between two pins is not as straightforward to analyze as the short to V_{cc} or ground. When two pins are shorted, the outputs driving those pins oppose each other when one attempts to pull the pins high

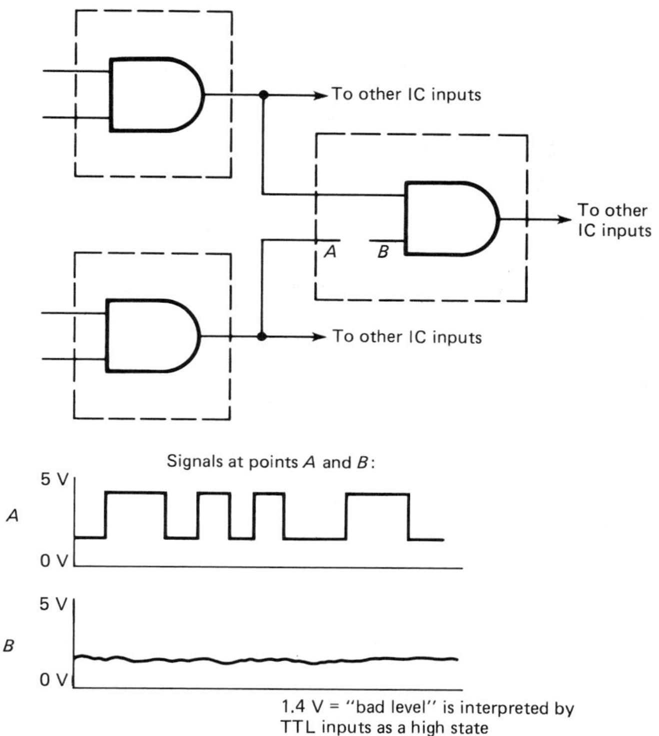

Fig. 9-32 The effect of an open input bond on circuit operation. This has the effect of blocking the input signal from reaching the chip and allows the input of the chip to float to a "bad level." Thus even though the signal can be viewed at an external point such as point *A*, the input of the chip responds to the bad level as though it were a static high level.

while the other attempts to pull them low. In this situation the output attempting to go high will supply current through the upper saturated transistor of its totem-pole (vertically stacked) output stage, while the output attempting to go low will sink this current through the saturated transistor to ground. Whenever both outputs attempt to go high simultaneously or to go low simultaneously, the shorted pins will respond properly. But whenever one output attempts to go low, the short will be constrained to be low.

The fourth failure internal to an IC is a failure of the internal steering circuitry of the IC. This has the effect of permanently turning on either of the upper transistors of the output totem pole, locking the output in the low state. Thus this failure blocks the signal flow and has a catastrophic effect upon circuit operation.

An open signal path in the circuit has an effect similar to that of an open output bond driving the node (Fig. 9-34). All inputs to the right of the open will be allowed to float to a bad level and will thus appear as a

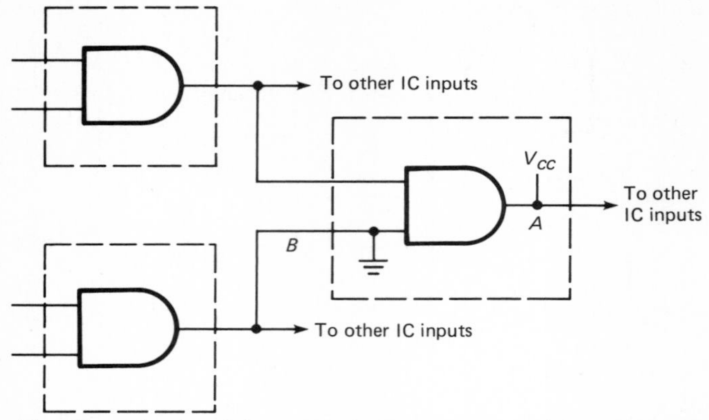

Fig. 9-33 The effect of a short between an input or output and V_{cc} or ground. All signal lines connected to point A are held in the high state. All signal lines connected to point B are held in the low state.

static high level in circuit operation. Those inputs to the left of the open will be unaffected by the open and will thus respond as expected.

DIGITAL TOOLS

We have seen how digital troubleshooting is an art of its own. It is possible to use the scope, voltmeter, and other instruments designed for analog applications in the specialized digital area. However, digital tools have been especially designed for these applications. The most valuable of these new tools are the logic probe, the logic pulser, and the logic clip.

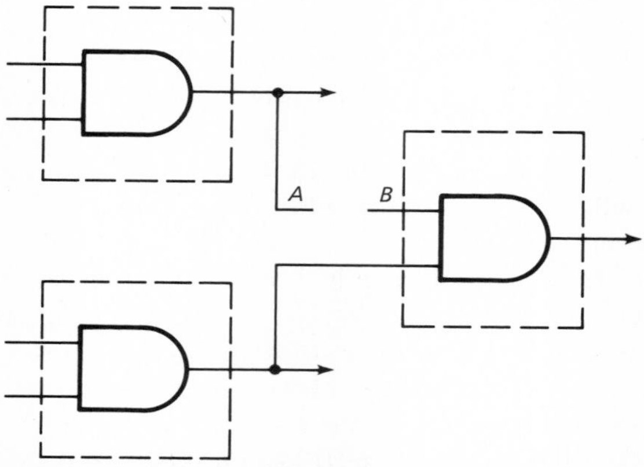

Fig. 9-34 The effect of an open in the circuit external to an IC. All inputs attached to the node at point A will be driven properly. All inputs to the right of the open (point B) will be left to float to a "bad level" and will therefore look like a static high state.

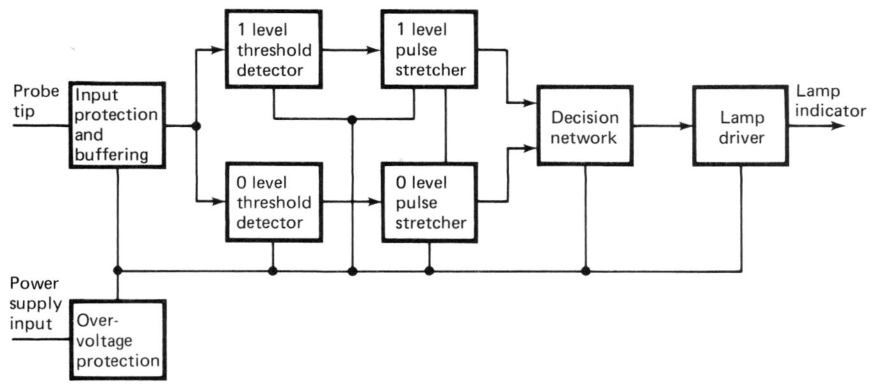

Fig. 9-35 Block diagram of HP Model 10525 logic probe. Threshold detectors advise the decision network whether the probe is receiving a 0 or a 1 bit. A lamp is the indicator.

LOGIC PROBES. The logic probe (Figs. 9-35 and 9-36) greatly simplifies tracing logic levels and pulses through IC circuitry to find nodes stuck HIGH/LOW, intermittent pulses, and normal pulse activity. It instantly tells whether the node probed is high, low, a bad level, open-circuited, or pulsing.

Probes have two preset logic thresholds which correspond to the high and low states of conventional logic families. When touched to a high level, a bright band of light appears around the entire probe tip; when touched to a low level, the light goes out. Open circuits or voltages in the bad-level region between the preset thresholds cause lamp illumination at half brilliance. Single pulses are easily viewed by stretching to 0.05 s. The lamp flashes on or blinks off depending upon the pulse's polarity. Pulse streams to 50 MHz cause the lamp to blink off and on at a 10-Hz rate.

Since most IC failures show up as a node stuck either HIGH or LOW, the logic probe provides an inexpensive yet remarkably easy way of detecting the fault. With a logic probe, these single-shot, short pulses that

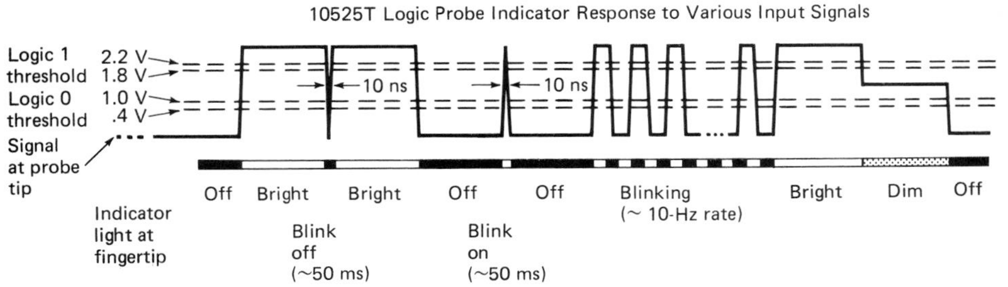

Fig. 9-36 The HP logic probe light can be seen responding to the various input levels. At the extreme right, the 1.4-V logic level does not represent a true 1; thus the light is only dim.

are nearly impossible to see with even the fastest of scopes are readily displayed.

Logic probes such as the HP Model 10525T also function quite well with logic families other than TTL and DTL, such as 5-V CMOS, as long as the logic levels are TTL-compatible.

LOGIC PULSER. The HP Model 10526T logic pulser solves the old problem of pulsing ICs on digital logic boards for troubleshooters using TTL-DTL circuits. Merely touch the pulser to the circuit under test, press the pulse button, and all circuits connected to the node (outputs as well as inputs) are briefly driven to their opposite state. No unsoldering of IC outputs is required. Pulse injection is automatic, so the user need not be concerned with whether the test node is in the high or low state: high nodes are pulsed low and low nodes high each time the button is pressed.

The pulser is essentially a single-shot pulse generator with high output-current capability packed in a convenient probe. The ability to source or sink up to 0.65 A ensures sufficient current to override IC outputs in either the high or low state. Output pulse width of 0.3 μs limits the amount of energy delivered to the device under test, thereby eliminating the possibility of destruction. Additionally, the pulser output is tristate, so that circuit operation is unaffected by probing until the pulse button is pressed.

Combining in-circuit pulse injection with the detection capabilities of the HP 10525T logic probe and 10528A logic clip focuses new power on solving the problems of fault isolation. Pulser-probe and pulser-clip combinations let digital troubleshooters have complete stimulus-response capability at their fingertips. Questions such as: "Is a gate functioning?"; "Is a pin shorted to ground or V_{cc}?"; "Is a counter counting?"; are quickly and easily answered without unsoldering pins or cutting PC traces.

Gate operation is tested with the pulser driving the input and the probe monitoring transmitted pulses at the output. When pulses are not received, the pulser and probe on the same pin can detect if the failure is due to a short to ground or V_{cc}.

LOGIC CLIP. The HP Model 10528A logic clip is a handy service tool. This unit clips onto TTL or DTL Dip ICs and instantly displays the logic states of all 14 or 16 pins. Each of the clip's 16 LEDs independently follows level changes at its associated pin; a lighted diode corresponds to a high logic state. The logic clip has no controls to be set, needs no power connections, and requires practically no explanation as to how it is used.

The logic clip is much easier to use than either an oscilloscope or a voltmeter when the question is whether a lead is in the high or low state (1 or 0 state), rather than its actual voltage. The clip, in effect, is 16 binary voltmeters, and users do not have to shift their eyes away from the circuit to make the readings.

The intuitive relationship of the input to the output—lighted diodes corresponding to high logic states—greatly simplifies the troubleshooting procedure. Users are free to concentrate their attention on the circuits, rather than on measurement techniques. Timing relationships become especially apparent when clock rates can be slowed to about one pulse per second. The misbehavior of gates, flip-flops, counters, and adders then becomes readily visible as all the inputs and outputs are seen in perspective.

QUESTIONS

1. A medical instrument is inoperative. What is the very first test that should be made?
2. Describe the signal-substitution method of troubleshooting.
3. In evaluating the amplifying ability of a transistor, would you be more interested in the ac current gain or the dc beta?
4. True or false: A proportionally large change in transistor base current causes a small change in collector current.
5. In the circuit of Fig. 9-1, $R_1 = 1150\ \Omega$, $R_2 = 50\ \Omega$, $R_3 = 2\ \Omega$. The collector current is 100 mA. What is the base-emitter bias voltage? Assume that there is no base loading.
6. If you measured 2 V from emitter to ground in Fig. 9-1, what has occurred?
7. In TTL logic, when an IC input or output is shorted to ground, how will all connected lines read?
8. Current flow in the reverse direction between collector and emitter is called __________.
9. Why is the collector-base leakage current the most critical kind of leakage current?
10. Describe the consequences of a failure in the internal steering circuitry of an IC.
11. What is the result of failing to bias any unused CMOS input?
12. CMOS ICs can be replaced with the power source and drive circuits on, so that these devices are under actual load conditions. Would you follow this advice? Give your reasons.
13. True or false: Digital troubleshooting can be satisfactorily performed by merely verifying the operation of specific components. Explain your answer.
14. What are the two proper digital states and the third possible condition?
15. We have a series of digital signals. Their signal levels occur in the following sequence: 2.8 V, 0.03 V, 0.35 V, 2 V, and 5 V. List the corresponding digital states in the correct sequential order.
16. What are the two primary causes of digital IC failure?

17. Pick out the failure in the following list that does not belong with the others. Explain your answer. (*a*) Short between IC input and output. (*b*) Short between V_{cc} and ground of an IC. (*c*) An open signal path to an IC. (*d*) A failure in the steering circuit of an IC.
18. When there is an open output bond in the IC, what will the consequent result be?
19. When an IC input or output is shorted to V_{cc} (power source), all connected signal lines will be in what state?
20. If the input of an input line driving an IC is open, what condition or state will exist at the IC output?

chapter 10

Troubleshooting the System

INTRODUCTION

In the last chapter we learned how to test semiconductors and integrated circuits. Various methods of signal tracing were used to identify a particular faulty section of a biomedical system. This was followed up by locating the offending component.

In this chapter, a source of trouble will be covered not so much as it relates to a single component (even though a single component may be faulty), but more in terms of the total system concept. To start with, further exploration of the use of the dipper will be covered. Having learned to use this tool earlier, we should have some familiarity with it. However, in this chapter, more sophisticated dipper applications will be covered.

The entire system concept as it relates to overall frequency response will be covered. This will include the dangers of deteriorated lower and upper frequency response and the advantages of extending lower and upper frequency response. Instances where a reduction of frequency response might be useful will be explored. An effective technique for determining frequency response using inexpensive test instrumentation will be discussed.

The BMET often finds that the hospital or research budget imposes severe limitations on the test equipment that can be made available. As the capability of any worker depends on the tools used, the BMET must see to it that the tools (even though inexpensive) are highly reliable. Because of this, the calibration of these tools becomes a key factor in determining the standard of excellence of the BMET. Simple, straightforward, yet reliable calibration techniques are discussed so that the BMET will be able to get the most out of inexpensive equipment.

When biomedical instruments are built into a system, by far the biggest headache is the ground loop problem. This is explored in detail. Specific types of sources used with certain amplifiers can severely aggravate this problem. In matching amplifiers to both additional systems and the originating-source device, care must be taken to minimize the ground loop problem. Ground loop currents will create troublesome interference. Worse than that, they will kill the patient.

10-1 DIPPER SERVICING TECHNIQUES

In Sec. 4-9, it was shown that high-frequency interference could be eliminated by placing parallel or series traps or filters in the patient leads. The resonant frequency of such traps is determined by tuning the dipper using various plug-in coils until the dipper meter shows a sharp dip. The dipper-calibrated frequency dial then indicates the resonant frequency of the filter circuit. Using the dipper as a filter-design aid is only one of its many applications. The Millen No. 90652 solid-state dipper has a wide variety of biomedical applications. Starting with its use in tuning resonant traps, here is a listing of possible dipper applications.

PARALLEL RESONANT TRAPS

The dipper may be used as a dip oscillator. Traps may be tuned or checked either before or after connection in the desired circuit. If they are tuned before installation, the adjustment will remain correct upon installation if the inductance is physically removed from other conductive components which may alter the inductance value. This is not usually the case, so further minor adjustment will probably be required after installation. When in the circuit, it is possible that a trap's resonant frequency may be quite a bit off, as indicated by the solid-state dipper. Actually, the trap itself will still be tuned to approximately the correct frequency, but the dip oscillator reading may be found at some other frequency (usually lower) due to circuit "strays" across the trap. Final precise adjustment may be made by tuning the trap under actual operation for the desired effect.

SERIES RESONANT TRAPS

Follow the same general procedure as with the parallel resonant trap. To check or tune prior to installation, the trap may be first connected as a parallel trap. At high frequencies or where the trap inductance is low, the lead completing the parallel circuit should be of large wire or wide copper ribbon to keep its inductance low, and care should be taken not to permit this lead to be positioned so as to add stray capacitance. Leads to be used upon final installation must also be included when external measurements are being made.

RF CHOKES

To determine self-resonance of RF chokes, use the solid-state dipper as a dip oscillator. Put the coil of the RF choke close to the dipper coil for best sensitivity.

CIRCUIT Q OR COIL Q

Use the solid-state dipper as a signal generator. Connect a VTVM (vacuum-tube voltmeter) across the circuit to be measured. Couple the dipper to the circuit (Fig. 4-30*a*) and resonate for maximum, or peak reading, on a VTVM and diode placed across the test circuit. Note the frequency at which this occurs. Then shift the instrument each side of resonance to the frequency where the voltmeter reading drops to approximately 70.7 percent of that at resonance. Note the frequency of these two points and calculate the circuit Q from

$$Q = \frac{F_r}{\Delta F}$$

where F_r = resonant frequency
ΔF = difference between the "off-resonance" frequencies just found

The original coupling should be adjusted for a convenient maximum reading of the VTVM and then should be left fixed at this position for the remainder of the procedure.

RELATIVE CIRCUIT Q AT A GIVEN FREQUENCY

Use a dip oscillator and observe the character of the dip, whether broad or sharp, for a fixed setting of sensitivity control. The sharper the dip, the higher the Q.

MEASUREMENT OF CAPACITANCE

Several methods may be employed. All involve the use of the solid-state dipper as an oscillator. A small jig (Fig. 10-1*a*) must be made, into which may be plugged any one of the solid-state dipper coils.

To check an unknown capacitor, it is only necessary to clip the jig, with a coil inserted, across the unknown capacitance. Find the resonant frequency and refer to the calibration chart (Fig. 10-2) for the value of the capacitor with the coil employed. For overall accuracy, it is best to use one of the coils from the medium-frequency range.

Because of the distributed capacitance of the coils, there will be a slight error at very-low-capacitance measurements. Likewise, because of the self-inductance of large capacitors, there will be a small error

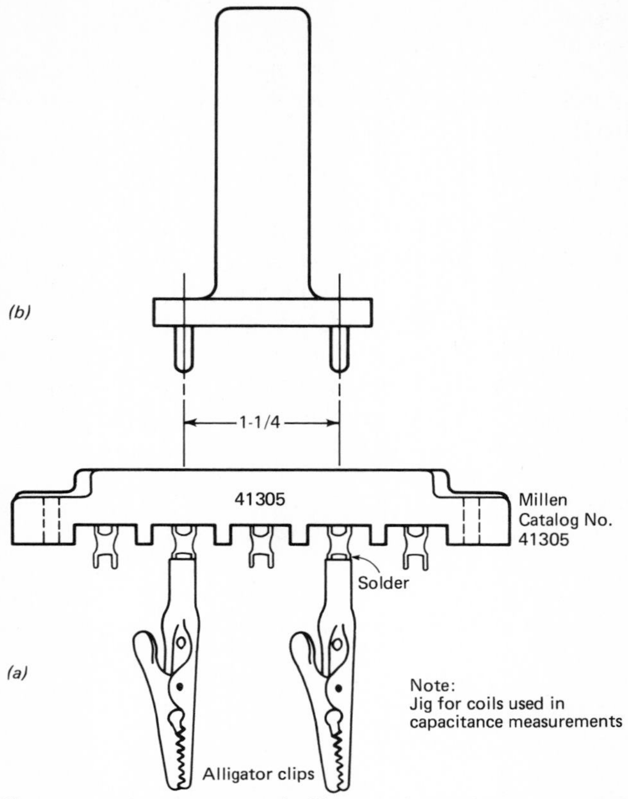

Fig. 10-1 When a capacitor is suspected of having changed value, or when its value is unknown, use this jig to determine capacitance. The alligator clips will hold the capacitor. The Millen socket allows coils to be changed. Thus capacitances from 7 pF all the way up to 4000 pF might be measured.

when these are measured. These errors will be negligible for most practical purposes.

Measurements of capacitance of below 50 pF are generally not obtainable because resonance at these values usually falls out of range of the coils left available for frequency checking. For measurements below 50 pF an additional calibrated coil is required.

For these measurements, in a great number of cases, the capacitor need not be removed from the circuit in which it is wired unless the capacitor is heavily loaded.

Another method, similar to that above, is to employ a known inductance and find the resonant frequency with the unknown connected across it. With the resonant frequency known and the inductance known, we may calculate the value of the capacitance C_x (in farads) by

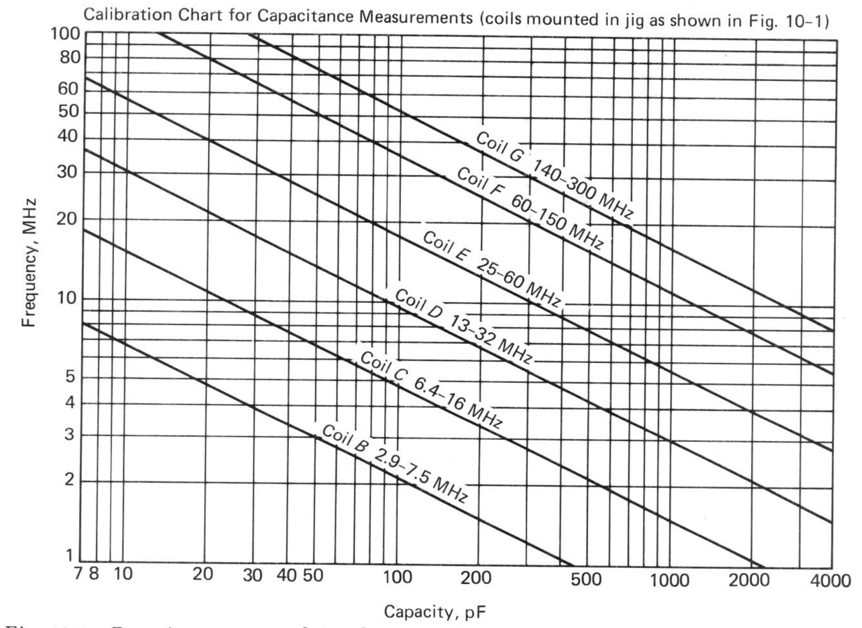

Fig. 10-2 By using any one of six plug-in coils with this chart, unknown capacitor values are found. Capacitors and resistors change value as equipment ages. In neurography, electromyography, and intracellular measurements, small time increments are vital to correct medical diagnosis. Changes in capacitor values in critical time-base and marker circuits can create false instrument readings.

$$C_x = \frac{1}{4\pi^2 F^2 L}$$

where F = resonant frequency, Hz
L = inductance, henrys (H)

A third method, for capacitors up to about 1000 pF, requires an inductance which is shunted by a calibrated variable capacitor. The capacitor is set at maximum, and the resonant frequency of the circuit is found. The unknown capacitor is then connected across the variable capacitor and the capacitance of the latter decreased to a point where the circuit resonates at the original frequency. The difference between the first and last setting of the calibrated variable capacitor is the value of the unknown capacitor.

MEASUREMENT OF INDUCTANCE OF RF COILS

Connect a capacitor of known value across the coil and use the dipper as a dip oscillator to find the resonant frequency of the resulting *L*/*C* combination. The inductance L_x (in henrys) of the coil may be calculated from

$$L_x = \frac{1}{4\pi^2 F^2 C}$$

where C = known capacitance, F

or reference may be made to an L/C resonance chart.

In measuring small values of inductance, be sure to employ a low-inductance standard condenser, connected to the unknown coil by a wide ribbon, to obtain the most accurate results. Due to the distributed capacitance, especially in large coils, some slight error will result; however, if the value of the low-inductance known capacitor is fairly high, the error will be negligible. Relative Q of capacitors or inductances at a given frequency may be noted by observing the character of the dip, as previously described.

FINDING INTERNALLY GENERATED SIGNALS

The dipper has still another valuable application, possibly its most valuable one. As biomedical equipment ages, it may generate unwanted signals. If the instrument has an oscilloscope output, erratic activity in the form of wandering spikes, noise, hash, etc., may be seen. If the instrument's paper recording system displays erratic and unaccountable activity, connect an oscilloscope and watch for the spurious activity previously described.

To rule out interference coming from the instrument's data input terminals, short them together and connect the short to ground. If the unexplainable activity persists, then it is apparent that impulses are coming from the power line or the instrument itself. Plug the Millen line-noise detector (refer to Chap. 4) into the same ac receptacle as the medical instrument and observe the activity on the power line. Should there indeed be activity on the power line, then go through the procedure as described in Sec. 4-8 under the subsection entitled Using a Line-Noise Detector. However, if the line-noise indicator shows a quiet power line, then the medical instrument itself is at fault. The instrument is radiating spurious or parasitic signals. How does this happen? There are three sources: the power supply, oscillators, and amplifiers.

When switching devices, rectifiers, and diodes in the power supply age, their internal inductance and stray capacitance form resonant circuits. These resonant circuits form a high impedance at specific frequencies, and erratic oscillations result. This spurious activity is then picked up by sensitive circuits and fed through the instrument system in the form of interference. When you find this condition, short circuit the offending component or components with a capacitance whose reactance is extremely low in the portion of the spectrum where the interference is being generated. Also, ground the path coming from the offending component into the instrument circuitry.

A biomedical instrument usually has one or more internal oscillators designed to generate either a time base, a calibration marker, or a delay signal. As the resonant components in the oscillator age, their Q, or quality factor, deteriorates. The net result here is that the oscillator signal, which was clean when the instrument was new, now has additional unwanted components. These can be classified as parasitics or spurious activity. They may have a mathematical relationship to the oscillator frequency ($2F$, $4F$, $\frac{1}{2}F$, etc.) or they may have no mathematical connection whatsoever. The offending coils or capacitors can be air-cleaned thoroughly with a high-pressure air gun. If that technique fails to cure the interference, the offending components must be replaced. If the power supply is clean and all the oscillators have been discounted as a source of internally generated interference, then the last remaining possibility is amplifiers.

Remember that every amplifier produces gain. Wherever there is gain, all that is required to sustain oscillation is an in-phase feedback path. In most biomedical instrument systems, stabilization is a prime virtue. Stabilization or self-balancing (as in pen recorders) is achieved by a feedback loop. This loop, when its components deteriorate, is a notorious troublemaker. Stray capacitance, inductance in leads, and impedance changes in solid-state devices all create situations where amplifiers become low-grade oscillators when shock-excited. Coupling capacitors between various stages and decoupling capacitors that isolate different stages increase in impedance as they age. This also contributes to spurious and parasitic activity. Transistor base-bias resistors change value, and bypass capacitors no longer bypass unwanted activity. These changes add to the problem of interference from internally generated signals. Under any of these conditions, every wire in the circuit becomes a high-frequency inductor and a potential source of trouble.

The fact that this type of interference is often erratic makes it even more ominous, for the physician may mistake this for occasional physiological data. Thus there is a possibility that a serious diagnostic error can take place as a result of the undetected presence of instrument-generated spurious signals.

10-2 THE AM RADIO PROBE

When you observe the spurious activity on an oscilloscope, set the oscilloscope course-frequency control to various positions. If individual cycles of this activity can be seen in the higher millisecond positions, then the activity is low in frequency. However, if individual cycles cannot be seen at these horizontal sweep positions but become more discernible in the low-microsecond course-frequency control setting, then the unwanted signals are of a much higher frequency. It is most likely that they will turn out to be in the medium- to higher-frequency parts of the spectrum.

Use an ordinary AM pocket radio as a probe; move it back and forth under the chassis or printed circuit board. Bring the pocket radio especially close to the components listed previously as the most common sources of this type of interference. The radio volume control should be at maximum, and it should be tuned to the extreme low end of the dial (540 kHz). Listen carefully for noise coming from the medical instrument. If noise is heard, tune the radio dial to the extreme high end (1600 kHz). If the noise decreases at this end of the dial, then its major component is probably below the AM broadcast band or at the low end. Once the exact component has been located, and using the *LCXf nomograph* (pp. 356–358), bypass capacitors can be inserted at the places previously described, or the offending component can be replaced.

This test will usually locate offending solid-state switches, diodes, rectifiers, motors, flashers, and other relatively low-frequency sources. But if the noise is higher at 1600 kHz, or if no noise is ever heard on the AM radio probe, then another technique must be used.

10-3 THE DIPPER PROBE

Plug a pair of medium- to high-impedance earphones into the dipper phone jack. Turn the oscillator-detector control to the detector position. The dipper is now a weakly oscillating detector. Starting with the lowest-frequency coil at 1.6 MHz, tune the dipper dial back and forth over its frequency range. At the same time, move it back and forth under the instrument chassis or printed circuit board. Listen in the earphones for whistling or buzzing noises during this procedure.

These noises are called *heterodynes.* When the dipper is tuned near the wavelength of the offending signal, a heterodyne will be heard. If no results are obtained, try the next higher-frequency coil in the dipper and repeat the process. Continue using higher-frequency coils until auditory activity is heard. If the heterodynes are strongest near a particular component and drop off sharply away from this component, then replace the troublesome component. But if the heterodyne is heard near several components and does not peak in one place, then a number of components may be contributing to the problem. If this is the case, it may become difficult to replace components. Using the reactance table, build a bandpass or tuned filter and insert it in the circuit so that it will block or bypass the unwanted frequency or the unwanted part of the spectrum.

10-4 ULTRASONIC TRANSDUCERS

As discussed earlier, use of ultrasonic techniques in the medical field is increasing rapidly. Ultrasonic arteriography does not present the hazards of x-rays and can define the interface between flowing blood and the arterial wall. Other ultrasonic techniques measure blood-flow velocity with many advantages over electromagnetic flowmeters. Ultrasonics is used to sample quantities of body fluids in intact subjects, for example, enterohepatic circulation of bile. Ultrasonics is widely used in the detection of tumors, foreign bodies, and obstructions.

The heart of the ultrasonic system is the piezoelectric transducer. As discussed in Chap. 3, these devices present a high Q and a high impedance at a given frequency. As their resonant frequency increases, they are more fragile, and hence they become more vulnerable to damage. As the resolution (or detail capability) of an ultrasonic system increases with higher frequency, ultrasonic frequencies are constantly increasing. At the present state of this art, ultrasonic frequencies as high as 5 MHz are being used for arteriography. The dipper offers an excellent way to test ultrasonic transducers.

Obtain a hollow cardboard or plastic tubing 2 in long and 1 in in

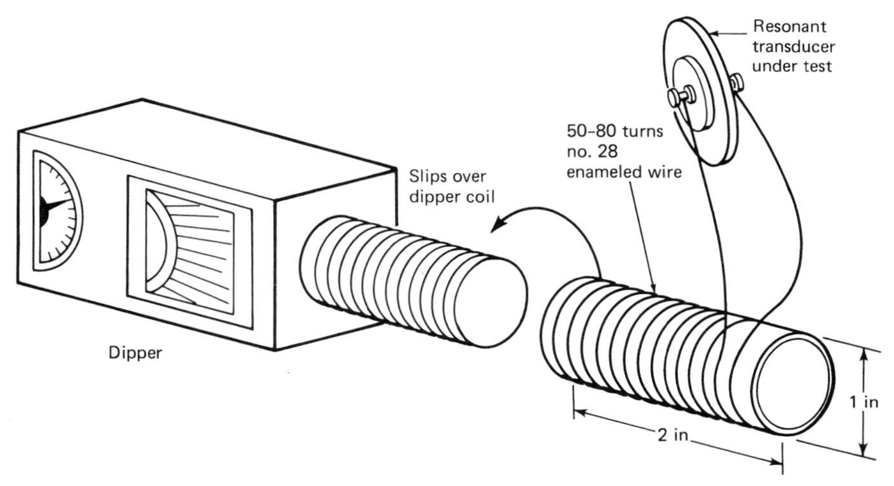

Fig. 10-3 The coupling coil is wound on any plastic or cardboard cylinder that will fit over the dipper coil. This test is valuable for resonant transducers. The medical instrument instruction manual will specify the transducer operating frequency. Look for the meter dip at this frequency.

diameter. Wind 50 to 80 turns of No. 28 enameled wire on this tubing. As shown in Fig. 10-3, this coil will fit easily over the dipper coil. Referring to the ultrasonic instrument operating manual, find the transducer operating frequency. Using the proper dipper coil covering this frequency, tune the dipper to the specified frequency. With the transducer connected as shown (Fig. 10-3), the dipper should dip sharply at the transducer's operating frequency. If no dip is observed, then the transducer is defective. And quartz crystal found in a crystal oscillator may be tested using this same technique.

10-5 FREQUENCY RESPONSE

After working with several medical specialists, you will discover that many of them have developed "pet theories" over the years. These theories may have to do with highly specific types of data in their field of interest. For example, Dr. Smith, a neurologist, feels strongly that to determine whether an end-plate spike (nerve potential) or a fibrillation potential is being observed, the nerve-response pulse duration and shape must be critically measured and analyzed. Dr. Jones, an electromyographer, feels strongly that the risetime of short-duration spikes in myotonia is the key parameter to the prognosis of this disease. Dr. Williams, another muscle specialist, feels that pulse falltime in myotonic dystrophy and very active polymyositis is the only distinguishing feature between the two diseases. An electroencephalographer feels that the close examination of EEG "spindles" can reveal crucial information. And Dr. Stone, a cardiologist, believes that a careful study of the depressed U segment of the electrocardiogram is called for.

In all these examples, the specialists are very concerned about data appearing in either the upper or lower limit of the frequency spectrum they are working with. Consequently, they will be most anxious to know what the frequency response of the instrumentation is.

MEASURING FREQUENCY RESPONSE

There are three ways to measure frequency response. One is to feed a signal generator into your instrument, with a multimeter measuring the instrument voltage output. Obtain the multimeter reading at approximately the center-frequency range of the medical instrument. Then tune the signal generator higher in frequency until the multimeter output falls to 50 percent of its original or midfrequency value. This is the upper frequency response of the instrument. Now tune the signal generator lower in frequency until the multimeter output falls to 50 percent of its original or midfrequency value. This is the lower frequency response of the instrument. This method is simple but presents a serious problem. The sine/square-wave signal generator at its very best will generate a signal down to 20 Hz, so it is only possible to measure low-frequency response down to approximately 10 Hz. The problem is that for most medical applications it is imperative to know the low-frequency response far below 10 Hz. This method leaves much to be desired.

A second method is to use a low-frequency spectrum analyzer displaying frequency down to 0 Hz and feed a sweep-frequency generator into the medical instrument. The spectrum analyzer will then display amplitude vs. frequency, or precisely how the medical instrument handles that portion of the spectrum fed to it by the sweep generator. This is the ideal method. The only problem is that the cost of a good low-frequency spectrum analyzer–sweeper combination is prohibitive.

There is a third method of frequency-response measurement which permits determination of low-frequency response down to 0.01 Hz and makes use of the test equipment we already have.

LOSS OF FREQUENCY RESPONSE

Whether or not the physician has a pet theory that makes the very-low frequency response, or the high-frequency response, of the instrument important, data obtained through these band limits are sometimes critical to correct diagnosis. Long time constants (low-frequency response) are vital to the analysis of slowly changing medical data, whereas the preservation of high-frequency response is the key to the analysis of spikes, transients, and other fast data.

By feeding our sine/square-wave generator into the instrument under test and picking up the instrument output with a dc oscilloscope, it is possible to calculate both low- and high-frequency response. In Fig. 10-4*a* the original square wave injected into the instrument has been retrieved at the instrument's output without distortion. In Fig. 10-4*b*, there is poor low-frequency response, and in Fig. 10-4*c*, low-frequency response has deteriorated even further.

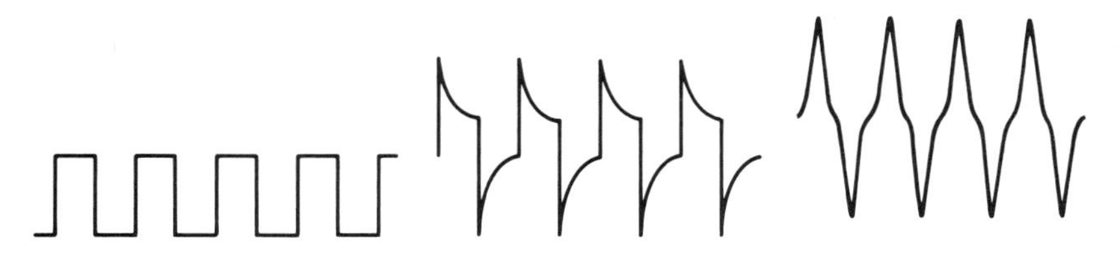

Fig. 10-4 (*a*) The square wave has been perfectly reproduced. (*b*) The leading edge of the square wave (positive and negative) is not distorted, but the flat top is not reproduced. Here low-frequency response is poor. (*c*) The lack of both upper and lower frequency response has caused the leading and trailing edges of the square wave to be badly distorted.

SQUARE-WAVE FREQUENCY-RESPONSE TEST

To obtain a perfect square wave from the instrument under test, the square-wave frequency (pulse repetition rate) must be at least 50 times higher than the instrument's low-frequency response (F_{cL}). Also, the square-wave frequency must be at least 50 times lower than the instrument's upper-frequency response (F_{cU}). For example, a 20-Hz square wave is fed into the instrument; the oscilloscope display shows a perfect square wave. It is then known that at the very least the instrument's frequency response is

$$F_{cL} = \frac{20\ \text{Hz}}{50} = 0.4\ \text{Hz}$$

and

$$F_{cU} = 20\ \text{Hz} \times 50 = 1000\ \text{Hz}$$

For a particular ratio of square wave to F_{cL} or F_{cU}, a particular pattern will be displayed on the oscilloscope. In Fig. 10-5, the percentage of tilt (slant) is measured in relation to the perfectly horizontal top.

Another indicator of the ratio is the percentage increase in peak amplitude over the perfect square wave. Using the 20-Hz square wave, if the F_{cL} were 2 Hz, then $F = 10F_{cL}$. In this case, the imperfect pulse top would show a 27 percent slant or tilt. In addition, the peak value of the response would increase over the height of the perfect square wave (V_0) by 16 percent (a ratio of 1.16 to V_0). The phase angle in relation to the perfect square wave would be 5.8°. As the square-wave frequency approaches the F_{cL}, the tilt becomes more severe, the peak amplitude increases, and the phase angle increases. If F_{cL} were 200 Hz, using the 20-Hz square-wave frequency ($F = 0.1F_{cL}$) the peak amplitude would be $V_0 \times 2$, or twice that which would normally be seen if the instrument's frequency response permitted the perfect square wave to be observed.

F_{cL} TEST PROCEDURE

Increase the square-wave-generator frequency until the pulse top is perfectly horizontal. Then, using the equation of square-wave frequency in hertz divided by 50, calculate F_{cL}. If it is impossible to obtain a perfectly horizontal top, increase the square-wave frequency until the tilt = 47 percent, then, using square-wave frequency in hertz divided by 5, calculate F_{cL}. For example, a 47 percent tilt is observed at 20 Hz. Then $F_{cL} = 5$ Hz.

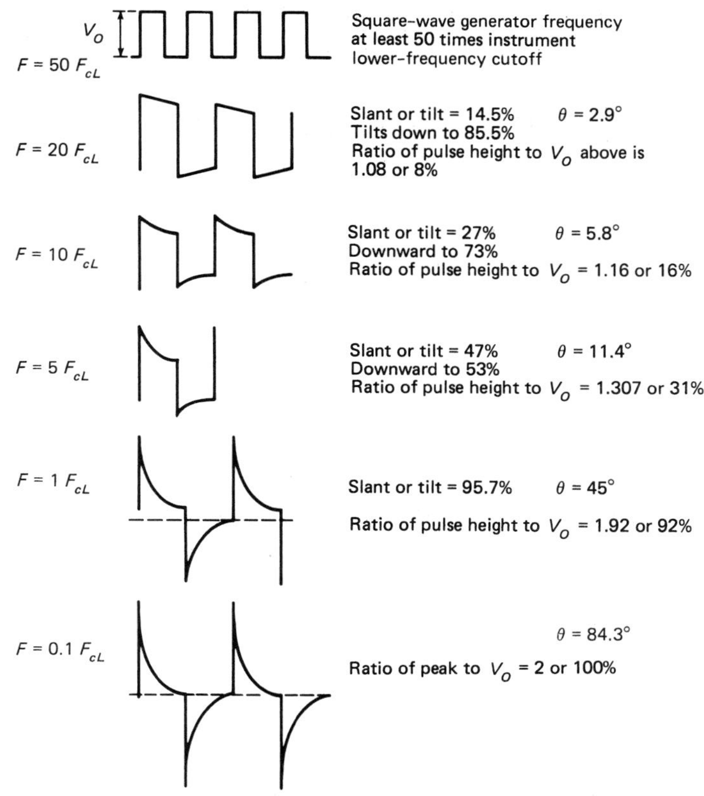

Fig. 10-5 The ratio of a square wave to the medical instrument's low-frequency response. The perfect square wave shows that the medical instrument's low-frequency response is at least one-fiftieth of the square-wave test frequency. As the test frequency moves closer to the medical instrument's low-frequency response, the square wave shows greater distortion. When the square wave is equal to the medical instrument's low-frequency response ($F = F_{cL}$), the square-wave trailing edge has disappeared.

PULSE-TILT LINEARITY. A quick method of estimating the ratio of the square-wave-generator frequency to F_{cL} is by observation of the linearity of the slant. Down to $F = 10F_{cL}$, the slant will be linear. At a ratio of 5, the slant will appear curved (Fig. 10-6), and when the square-wave generator frequency is equal to F_{cL} (ratio = 1), the curve will be severe.

DECREASING F_{cL}. Where the low-frequency response is above the manufacturer's specification, in tube instruments measure all grid-leak resistors and cathode-bypass capacitors to detect changes from the original value. In solid-state equipment measure the base-bias resistors and emitter-bypass capacitors. In all equipment, changes or deterioration in coupling capacitors and frequency-governing components in feedback loops will affect low-frequency response. When the low-

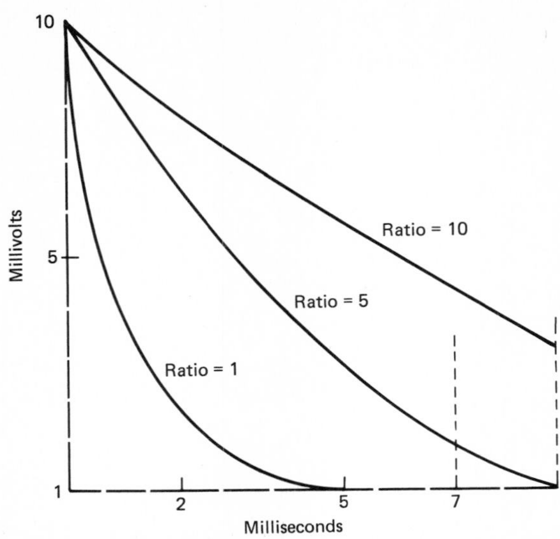

Fig. 10-6 A quick method of determining the low-frequency response of the medical instrument makes use of the linearity and angle of descent of the distorted wave reproduced by the medical instrument. At 10 times F_{cL}, the flat top only drops to 50 percent of the leading-edge voltage. At $F = F_{cL}$ there is a sharp sag, and the trailing edge is gone.

frequency response of an instrument must be decreased, then increase the capacitance of critical coupling capacitors and bypass capacitors. Also decrease the *RC* time constant of all feedback circuits.

UPPER-FREQUENCY RESPONSE: F_{cU}

Referring to Fig. 10-7, as the high-frequency limit of the instrument is approached, the top of the leading edge of the square-wave pulse becomes rounded or nonlinear, and the bottom of the trailing edge also becomes nonlinear. In addition, when the square-wave frequency is at or above F_{cU}, the pulse height falls off sharply.

To determine the instrument's upper-frequency response, increase the square-wave-generator frequency until the horizontal pulse top disappears. This occurs when the pulse edge is so nonlinear that it actually joins the pulse trailing edge. At this frequency, 50 percent of the pulse height will appear 32 percent away from the beginning of the leading edge. The phase angle compared to the perfect square wave will be 45°, and the pulse height will be 0.935 in relation to the perfect square wave. The square-wave generator is now at F_{cU}, the instrument's upper-frequency limit.

REDUCED F_{cU}. Where F_{cU} is found to be below the instrument manufacturer's specification, check for changes in the load resistance of output amplifier stages and check for increased values of filter resistors in

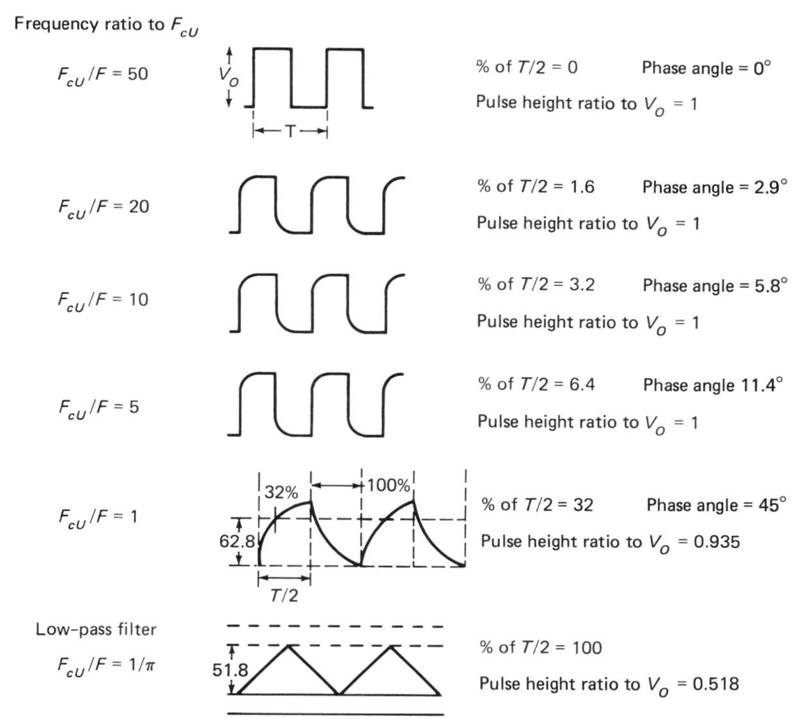

Fig. 10-7 The ratio of the square wave to the medical instrument's upper frequency response. When the test wave is 20 times the instrument's F_{cU}, the top of the test wave's leading edge is rounded. When the square wave equals the medical instrument's upper frequency cutoff, ($F_{cU}/F = 1$), a series of "sharkfins" are seen. At the ratio of $1/\pi$ the square wave has now become a perfect triangular wave.

high-frequency filter circuits. Also check for *RC* filter changes in feedback networks and an increase in the internal resistance of transistors or tubes. An increase in the flux leakage of output or coupling transformers will also reduce upper-frequency response.

Where it is necessary to increase F_{cU}, feedback-network time constants can be increased, and low-leakage (low-capacitance) coupling and output transformers may be installed.

DECREASING F_{cU}. Where the physician finds noise to be a problem, check for noise in tubes, transistors, or resistors. When the noise is not due to a particular component but is due to a combination of instrument age and low signal-source input (high instrument sensitivity), the possibility of decreasing the F_{cU} might be considered.

Before any thought is given to this, it is absolutely essential to determine whether decreasing the F_{cU} will cause any fast medical data to be lost. If it is found that no pertinent medical data will be lost, then two

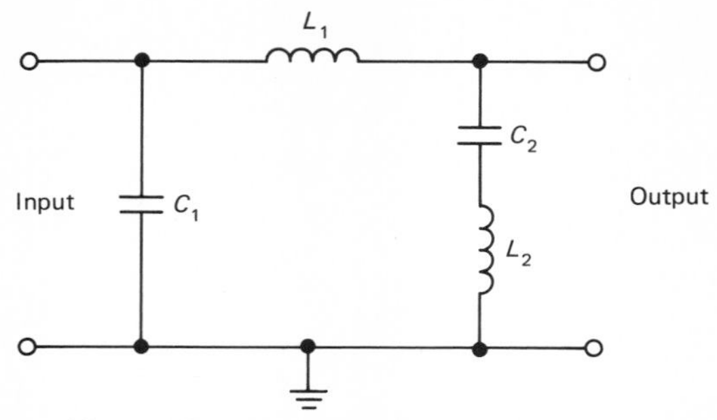

Fig. 10-8 Low-pass filter to decrease instrument noise. It should be inserted between the first and second amplifier stages where some attenuation can be tolerated. L_2 and C_2 should resonate 10 percent higher than the highest frequency carrying medical data. The value for C should be low in high-impedance circuits and high in low-impedance circuits.

approaches can be used. A commercial low-pass filter may be purchased to pass only the part of the spectrum containing useful medical data, or a low-pass filter can be designed according to Fig. 10-8 by using the *LCXf* nomograph (pp. 356–358).

A MASTER PATTERN FOR FREQUENCY-RESPONSE DETERMINATION

To accelerate the determination of lower and upper frequency limits, a transparent master pattern can be placed over your dc oscilloscope (Fig. 10-9). This handy device determines the ratio of the square-wave-generator frequency to that of the instrument by displaying the

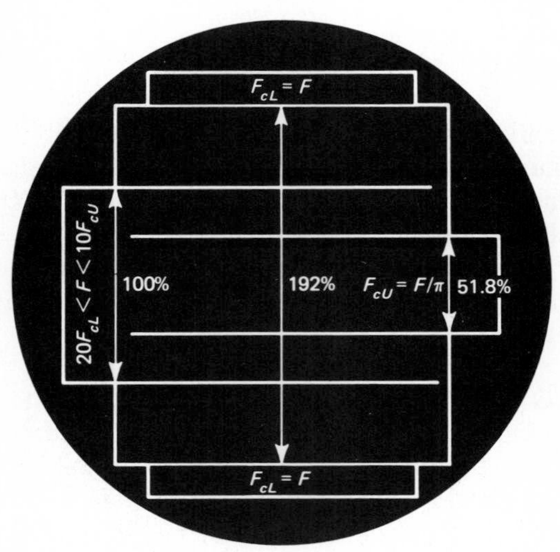

Fig. 10-9 A master pattern for rapid upper and lower frequency-response determination. Photograph this pattern, then enlarge the negative to the size of your oscilloscope display. Exact size is unimportant, as only the percentages are meaningful. Attach the negative to the oscilloscope screen with Scotch brand tape.

amplitude variation. Variation of the frequency ratio produces marked variations in the amplitude of the output voltage, particularly toward the ends of the range. The Y gain of the oscilloscope is continuously variable, and the 100 percent level can readily be adjusted at the frequency $20F_{cL} < F < 10F_{cU}$. Then, the square-wave frequency is increased until the amplitude falls to 51.8 percent or the two horizontal lines closest to the center. F_{cU} is then calculated from $F_{cU} = F/\pi$. To find F_{cL}, decrease the square-wave frequency until the amplitude is 192 percent of the square-wave F and the lower cutoff frequency is then the generator's frequency. The corresponding Y amplitude markings also appear on the pattern.

Photograph the master pattern as shown and enlarge the negative to fit over your oscilloscope screen. This allows any inexpensive oscilloscope and square-wave generator to test the bandpass characteristics of medical instruments. The costly sweep generator and spectrum analyzer method is avoided, and the same results are obtained with the master pattern of Fig. 10-9. Some of the most significant medical data are often obtained near the upper and lower frequency limits of the medical instrument or system. One of the more common effects of instrument aging is the loss of either F_{cU} or F_{cL}, or both. Thus, instrument frequency response becomes a very important parameter in troubleshooting biomedical systems.

10-6 THE GROUND LOOP PROBLEM*

The system ground loop is the largest source of electric noise between electronic modules. More than one ground on a signal circuit or signal cable shield produces a common impedance coupling or ground loop between these two points. This generates large 60-Hz electric noise currents which are in series and combined with the useful signal. The magnitude of ground loop current is directly proportional to the difference in absolute potential between the two grounds. In most cases a ground loop through either a cable shield or signal circuit will produce so much 60-Hz noise that it will obscure millivolt-level signals.

Two separate grounds are seldom, if ever, at the same absolute voltage. This potential difference creates unwanted current in series with one of the signal leads. In Fig. 10-10 the potential difference between earth ground 1 and earth ground 2 produces ground loop current in the lower signal lead from the signal source to the input of the amplifier, causing ground loop noise to be combined with the useful

* Parts of this section have been condensed from the booklet "Signal Conditioning" by D. Nalle, Gould Instrument Systems Div., Cleveland, Ohio.

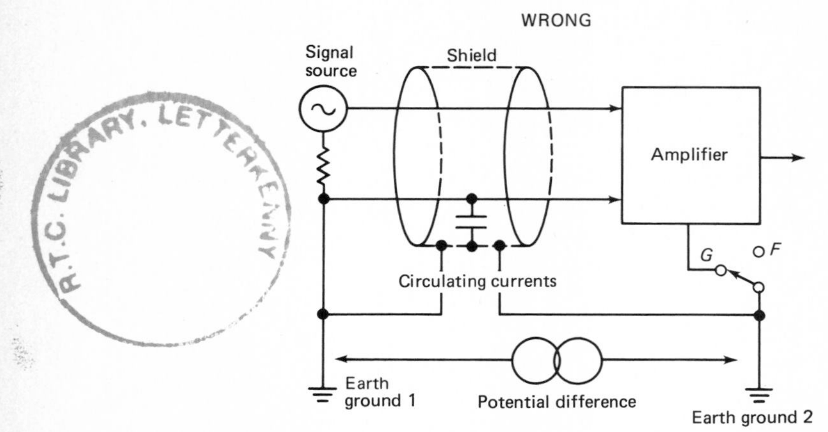

Fig. 10-10 A ground loop created by more than one ground.

signal. There is a second ground loop in Fig. 10-10 through the signal cable shield from the signal source to the amplifier. The ground loop current in the shield is coupled to the signal pair through the distributed capacity in the signal cable. This current is returned through the output impedance of the signal source and back to earth ground 1, adding a second source of noise to the useful signal. Either one of these ground loops is capable of generating a noise signal that is at least 100 times larger than a typical millivolt-level signal.

The amplifier shown in Fig. 10-11 is capable of being floated a few volts off ground. The ground loop through the signal lead can be broken by simply lifting the amplifier grounding strap. The amplifier enclosure is still solidly grounded to earth ground 2, but this will not create a ground loop, since the amplifier enclosure is insulated from the signal circuit. The ground loop through the signal cable shield is eliminated by removing the jumper from the cable shield to earth

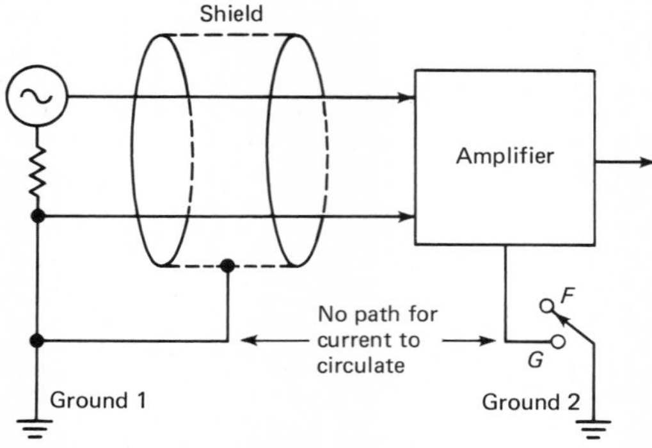

Fig. 10-11 Loop is eliminated by floating the amplifier off ground and removing the jumper from ground 2 to the signal cable shield.

ground 2. Now the signal source and the signal cable shield are grounded only at the signal source, which is the proper configuration for minimum noise pickup.

In off-ground measurements, the signal cable shield should *not* be grounded. Effective shielding is secured by stabilizing the signal cable shield with respect to the useful signal. The signal cable should be connected to either the center tap or the low side of the signal source. Since the signal cable shield is being driven by an off-ground common-mode voltage, it is necessary that the cable have appropriate insulation between the shield and the outside of the cable. *This is very important.*

GROUNDING THE INPUT

The single-ended grounded amplifier has two input terminals, one of which is common with the output. This direct connection from input to output is normally grounded through the third conductor in the ac power cord. The amplifier enclosure is usually internally connected to this common point. This type of amplifier works well with balanced floating signal sources or single-ended floating signal sources, but it will not operate properly with any type of grounded signal source unless it is connected to the same ground as the amplifier, or unless one of the grounds is disconnected. Any difference in potential between the signal-source ground and the amplifier ground will add to or subtract from the true value of the signal being measured. This erroneous noise signal is generally referred to as a *ground loop* and must be avoided.

The balanced-to-ground amplifier has two active input terminals which have equal resistance to a common ground terminal. This common input terminal is firmly grounded through the third wire in the ac power cord. Both the enclosure and the low side of the output are normally grounded to this same point inside the amplifier case. This type of amplifier can be operated as a balanced-to-common amplifier by removing the ground connection in the ac power cord. In this case, the amplifier would normally be connected to one ground at the signal source. It can also be operated as a single-ended grounded amplifier by simply installing a ground strap from one active input terminal to ground. The major limitation of a balanced-to-ground amplifier is its restricted off-ground voltage capability, which decreases as the input attenuator is advanced to a more sensitive position. This type of amplifier will work well with a single-ended floating signal source, with a balanced floating signal source, and in most cases with a balanced grounded signal source.

The single-ended floating amplifier has two input terminals that are electrically isolated from the output terminals. It is normally provided with an internal floating shield which is internally connected to the low side of the input. Both input terminals are free to float up or down in compliance with any common-mode voltage that may appear at the signal source but the capacity to ground of its "hot" input terminal. It is, therefore, important to connect this amplifier so that any common-mode voltage at the signal source is used to drive the low side of the input. The amplifier enclosure and the low side of the output are normally grounded through the third wire in the ac power cord. This type of amplifier works well with single-ended grounded signal sources, single-ended floating sources, or single-ended driven off-ground sources and can be used down to millivolt levels with balanced floating signal sources.

The balanced, floating, and guarded amplifier is the most sophisticated for all dc amplifier types and can be used with all types of self-generating signal sources. Both input terminals are isolated from the amplifier chassis and isolated from the output. The input terminals also have equal impedance to a third terminal called the *guard shield* or simply *guard*, which is a full-floating internal shield. The guard is used to minimize internal capacity from signal input terminals to chassis ground and to improve the ac common-mode rejection of the amplifier.

Both amplifier input terminals are free to float up or down in compliance with any common-mode voltage that may appear at the signal source. Since both input terminals are floating and have very low capacity to chassis ground, the incoming signals may be grounded, floating, or driven off-ground without affecting accuracy or system noise. When the guard shield is properly connected, the ac noise-rejection characteristics are quite good, so this amplifier can be used over a wide range of signal amplitudes, down to and including the microvolt level. The guard shield is *not* internally connected, but it is brought out to separate terminals in the amplifier input connector so that it may be properly connected for all types of signal sources.

SINGLE-ENDED GROUNDED AMPLIFIER

When a single-ended grounded amplifier is used with a single-ended floating signal source, the low side of the source and the signal cable shield are connected to the grounded amplifier input terminal, as shown in Fig. 10-12. The other side of the source is connected to the active amplifier input terminal. When a single-ended grounded amplifier is used with a balanced floating signal source, the grounded amplifier input terminal may be connected to either side of the signal source. The other side of the source is connected to the active amplifier input terminal. The signal cable shield is connected to the grounded amplifier terminal, as shown in Fig. 10-13.

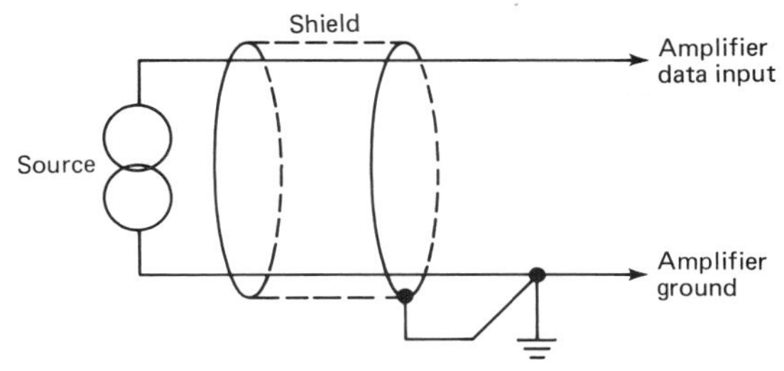

Fig. 10-12 Single-ended grounded amplifier operating with a floating signal source.

A single-ended grounded amplifier can be operated at millivolt levels with a single-ended grounded signal source provided one of the grounds is disconnected. Where possible, remove the ground at the source and connect the cable shield to the amplifier ground as shown in Fig. 10-12. If this is not practical, the amplifier ground must be disconnected so that the amplifier can float a few volts away from power-line ground. This is done by using a ground-isolation adapter on the ac power plug. In this configuration, the grounded side of the signal source is connected to the amplifier ground terminal and the signal source is connected to the amplifier, as shown in Fig. 10-14. The amplifier enclosure is still grounded, but to the signal-source ground instead of the power-line ground. When the source ground is used, all channels in a multichannel system must be connected to a common signal-source ground.

The single-ended grounded amplifier is *not* appropriate for low-level applications because it has no common-mode rejection and would, therefore, be quite noisy. It should not be used with a balanced grounded signal source because the amplifier ground would disturb or unbalance the source. It should *never* be used with a driven off-ground source because the single-ended grounded amplifier input would destroy the source or burn off the amplifier grounding connection, or both.

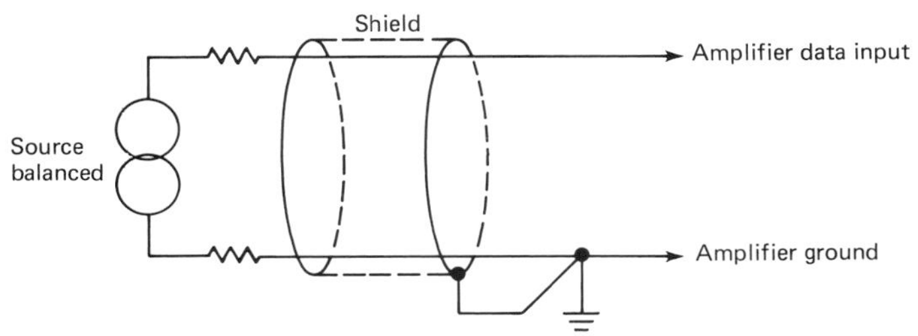

Fig. 10-13 Single-ended grounded amplifier operating grounded with floating signal source.

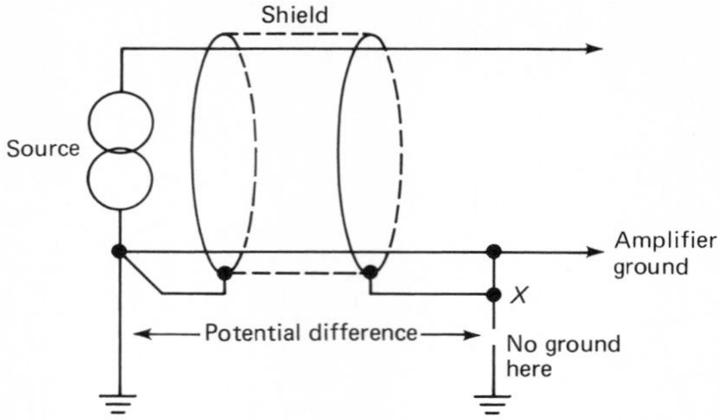

Fig. 10-14 Single-ended grounded amplifier operating floating from grounded signal source.

BALANCED-TO-GROUND AMPLIFIER

When a balanced-to-ground amplifier is used with single-ended floating or balanced floating signal sources, the two active amplifier input terminals are connected to both sides of the signal source. The connections can be reversed if a change in polarity is desired. The signal cable shield is connected to the grounded input terminal on the amplifier, as shown in Fig. 10-15. The optional ground strap may be installed or omitted depending on which condition provides minimum electric noise.

The balanced grounded signal source can be used with a balanced-to-ground amplifier and operated at full sensitivity if the potential difference between the signal-source ground and the amplifier ground is quite small. In this case the difference in absolute potential between the signal-source ground and the amplifier ground would show up as a common-mode voltage, as shown in Fig. 10-16. For example, if the two grounds differed in absolute potential by 2.8 V p-p and the amplifier has a common-mode rejection of 1000 to 1 (60 dB) at 60 Hz, then 2.8 mV would show up as an error or noise signal at the amplifier input.

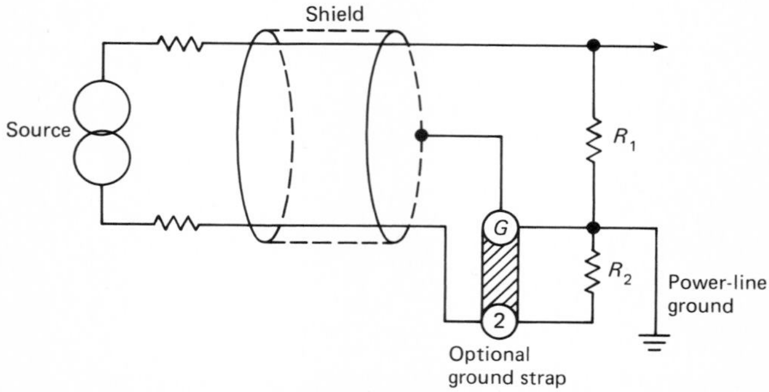

Fig. 10-15 Balanced-to-ground amplifier operating grounded with single-ended floating source.

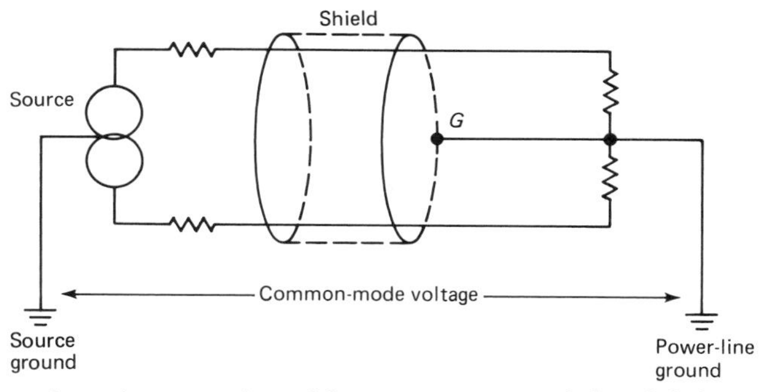

Fig. 10-16 Balanced-to-ground amplifier operating grounded with balanced grounded signal source.

For this balanced-to-ground application the active amplifier input terminals are connected to both sides of the signal source. These connections can be reversed if a change in signal polarity is desired. The signal cable shield is connected to the grounded input terminal on the amplifier and to the grounded center tap on the signal source, as shown in Fig. 10-16. The common-mode problem could be eliminated by lifting the ground at the amplifier and operating it as a balanced-to-common amplifier, as shown in Fig. 10-17. When the signal-source ground is used, all channels in a multichannel system must be connected to a common-source ground.

The balanced-to-ground amplifier can *not* be used with a single-ended grounded signal source. The best solution would be to remove the ground at the signal source and operate the amplifier single-ended grounded. If this is impractical, then the amplifier will have to be operated single-ended floating. This can be done by installing the ground strap from input terminal 2 to the ground terminal and then lifting the ground in the ac power cord as shown in Fig. 10-18. When the signal-source ground is used, all channels in a multichannel system must be connected to a common-source ground.

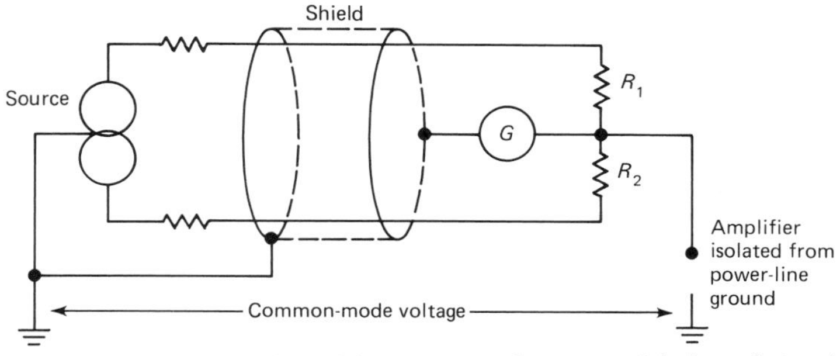

Fig. 10-17 Balanced-to-ground amplifier operating floating with balanced signal source.

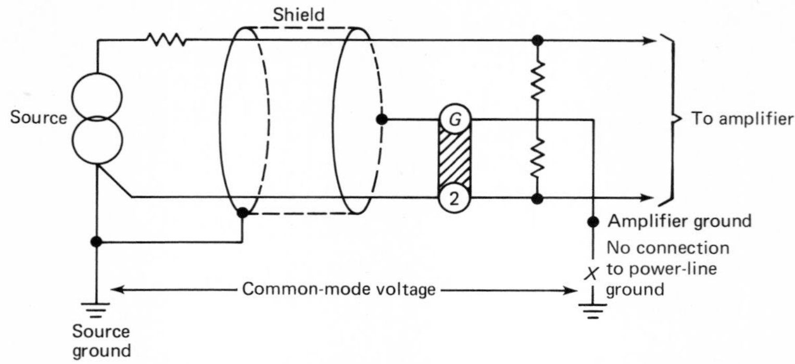

Fig. 10-18 Balanced-to-ground amplifier operating floating with single-ended grounded source.

The balanced-to-ground amplifier can be used in some low-gain applications where the signal source is driven off ground by a common-mode voltage, as shown in Fig. 10-19. The magnitude of the off-ground voltage is limited by the maximum common-mode voltage that is permitted on the amplifier at various sensitivity settings and by the amount of common voltage error that can be tolerated. For example, a typical amplifier has a common-mode rejection of 60 dB (1000 to 1) at 60 Hz, which means that a 20-V p-p common-mode voltage would produce a 60-Hz error voltage of 20 mV. If the recorder sensitivity was 1.0 V full scale (20 mV per chart division), this would represent a common error of 2 percent of full scale, which would probably be all right for most applications.

If the amplifier common-mode rejection is 40 dB, 100 to 1, the error would be 20 percent, which can *not* be tolerated for any application. This problem could be resolved by operating the amplifier balanced to

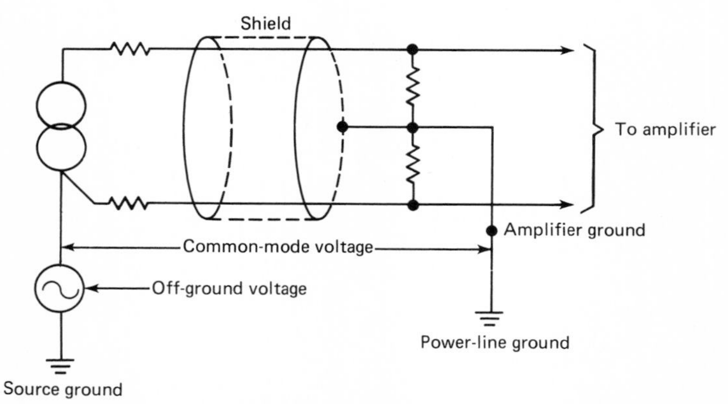

Fig. 10-19 Balanced-to-ground amplifier operating grounded with balanced driven off-ground source.

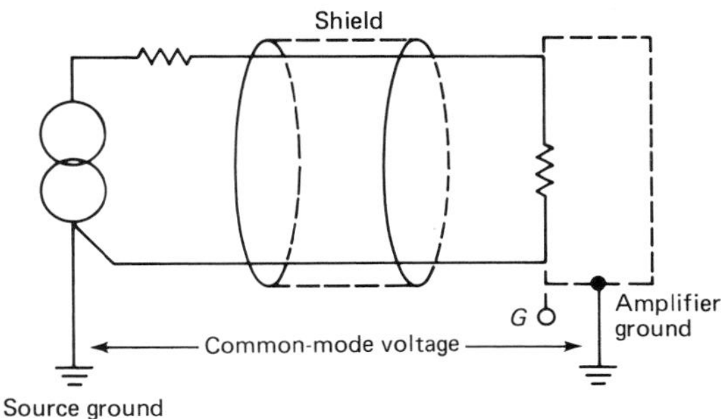

Fig. 10-20 Single-ended floating amplifier operating from single-ended grounded signal source.

common as shown in Fig. 10-17 providing the user is willing to assume the responsibility of operating the amplifier enclosure and output circuit 20 V off ground. Otherwise, an isolation amplifier would be required.

SINGLE-ENDED FLOATING AMPLIFIER

For single-ended grounded signal sources, the low side of the single-ended floating amplifier input is connected to the grounded side of the source. The cable shield is connected to the grounded side of the signal source, as shown in Fig. 10-20. In those cases where a single-ended floating amplifier is operated at maximum sensitivity from a high-impedance single-ended grounded signal source or where the common-mode rejection of the amplifier is quite low, it may be necessary to operate the amplifier free-floating to improve its common-mode rejection. This requires the following additional connections, as shown in Fig. 10-21. Connect the signal cable shield to both the amplifier ground terminal and the low-input terminal. Then be sure to install a

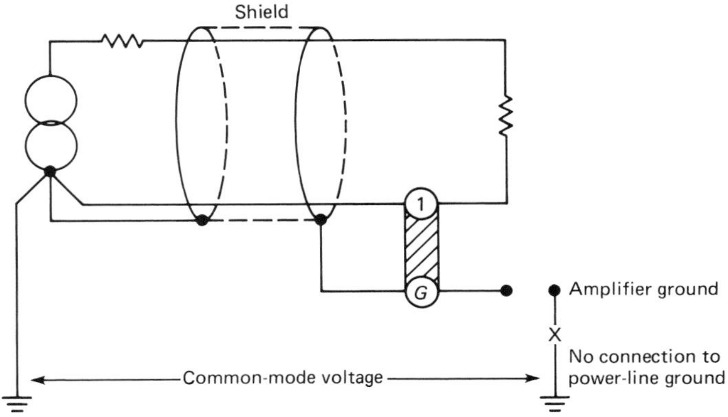

Fig. 10-21 Single-ended floating amplifier operating free-floating from grounded signal source.

ground-isolation adapter in the power cord. When the signal-source ground is used, all channels in a multichannel system must be connected to a common source ground.

For single-ended floating signal sources, the low side of the amplifier is connected to the low side of the signal source. The signal cable shield is attached to the low side of the amplifier input and grounded at the amplifier, as shown in Fig. 10-22. In cases where input leads are quite long, where the signal level is very low, or where the source impedance is high, it will be better to ground the low side of the source and the cable shield at the signal source and operate the amplifier free-floating, as shown in Fig. 10-21. If this is done, the power-line ground must be disconnected by installing the ground-isolation adapter in the ac power cord.

The single-ended floating amplifier was never intended for use with high-impedance balanced grounded signal sources, but it can be used down to millivolt levels if the source impedance is quite small and the amplifier common-mode rejection is quite high. The active-amplifier input terminals are connected to both sides of the signal source. The connections can be reversed if a change in polarity is desired. The signal cable shield is connected to both the signal-source ground and the amplifier ground terminal. A ground-isolation adapter is installed in the ac power cord, so the amplifier enclosure is driven through the cable shield by the signal-source ground, as shown in Fig. 10-23. When the signal-source ground is used, all channels in a multichannel system must be connected to a common source ground.

The single-ended floating amplifier can be operated grounded from a balanced floating signal source if the cable length is short and the source impedance is quite small. The active amplifier input terminals are connected to both sides of the signal source. The connections can be reversed if a change in polarity is desired. The signal cable shield is grounded at the amplifier to the power-line ground and connected to

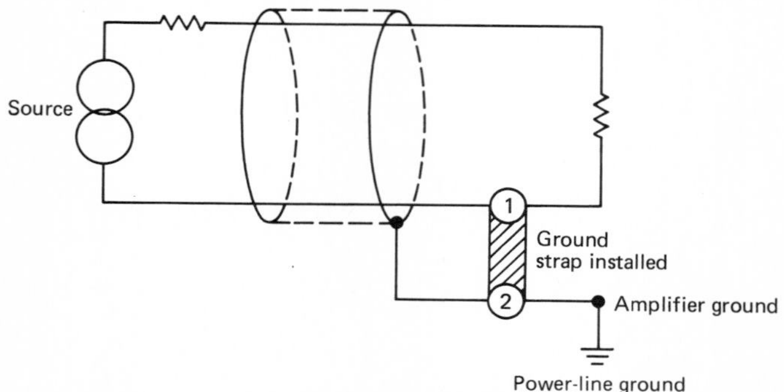

Fig. 10-22 Single-ended floating amplifier operating grounded from floating single-ended source.

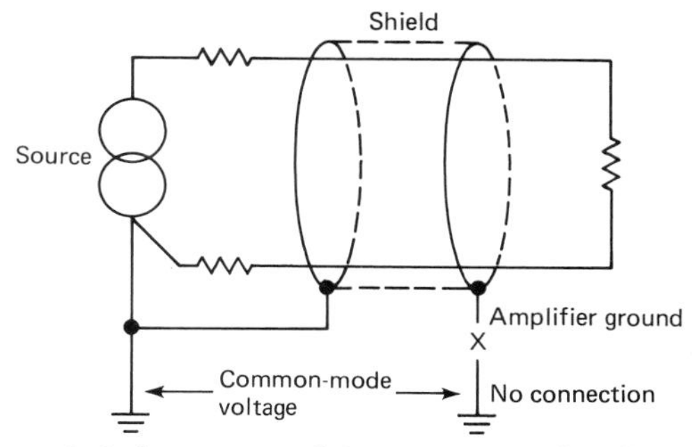

Fig. 10-23 Single-ended floating amplifier operating free-floating from balanced grounded signal.

the low side of the amplifier input by using a ground strap, as shown in Fig. 10-24.

Where a single-ended floating amplifier is used with a long cable length to a high-impedance balanced floating signal source, the signal cable shield and one side of the source should be connected to a low-impedance ground at the signal source. The low side of the amplifier is connected to the grounded side of the signal source. The common-mode rejection of the system can be further improved by also connecting the cable shield to the amplifier ground terminal and to the low side of the amplifier input.

Then the ground-isolation adapter is installed in the power cord, as illustrated in Fig. 10-25, so that the amplifier enclosure is driven by the signal-source ground. When the signal-source ground is used, all channels in a multichannel system must be connected to a common-source ground.

In applications where there is a large potential difference between the signal-source ground and the amplifier ground or where the

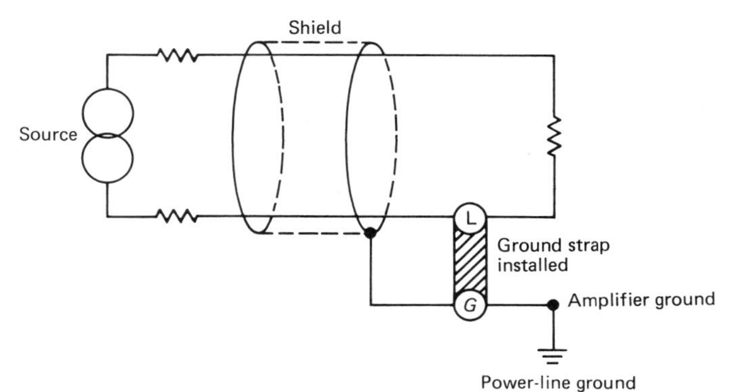

Fig. 10-24 Single-ended floating amplifier operating grounded from balanced floating source.

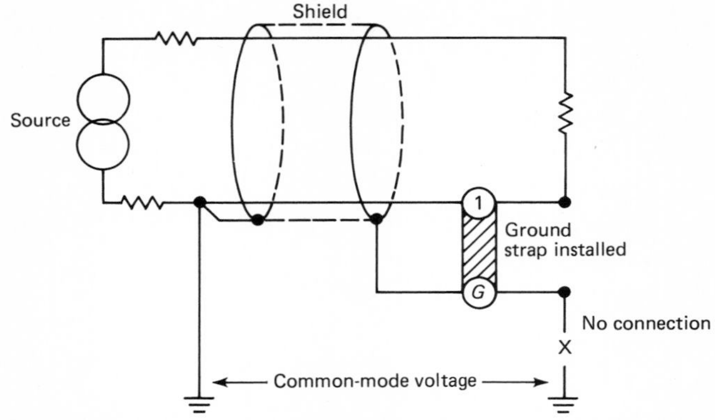

Fig. 10-25 Single ended floating amplifier operating free-floating from balanced signal source.

common-mode rejection of the amplifier is inadequate, it will be beneficial to operate the amplifier free-floating. This is done by connecting together the signal cable shield, the low side of the amplifier input, and the amplifier enclosure and lifting the power-line ground at the amplifier as shown in Figs. 10-21 and 10-25. In this case the amplifier enclosure is grounded to the signal-source ground through both the signal cable shield and the low side of the signal cable. The common-mode rejection of the amplifier is improved, since the amplifier enclosure is now acting as a guard shield and is driven by the low side of the signal source.

The single-ended floating amplifier operates best with single-ended signal sources because the capacity to ground of its low input terminal is greater than the capacity to ground of its "hot" input terminal. It was never intended for use with high-impedance balanced grounded or balanced driven off-ground signal sources.

The source and amplifier combinations described here should cover all situations of coupling a source to an amplifier. By carefully following the grounding techniques suggested, the ground loop problem can be minimized or eliminated completely.

10-7 CALIBRATION

Biomedical instrumentation technique has advanced to the point where small differences in measured voltage amplitudes or time increments can cause a completely different medical diagnosis. The biomedical engineers or technicians must be able at all times to certify that their calibration of biomedical measuring instrumentation is accurate. To do this it is absolutely mandatory that all test equipment used to calibrate and check medical instruments is itself calibrated against a trusty standard.

The better oscilloscopes have built-in circuits to calibrate the vertical amplitude. A 1-V p-p test signal or a calibrated step attenuator may be used for this purpose. Likewise, the horizontal sweep (time base) may have a step-type sweep attenuator which will calibrate the sweep from 2 s/cm up to 200 ms/cm. However, in the less expensive oscilloscopes there is no reliable built-in calibration circuitry; if a less expensive oscilloscope must be used, it may be necessary to build your own calibrator. To calibrate voltage or amplitude, an ac and dc amplitude calibrator can be made with very little effort. A fresh, size D, $1\frac{1}{2}$-V flashlight battery makes an excellent amplitude calibrator for scopes that have a dc input (Fig. 10-26). The horizontal sweep is turned off, and the CRT electron spot is focused to its smallest size or smallest dot. With the vertical-sensitivity switch at 0.1 V/cm (make certain this switch is on the dc side), the spot should sit on the lowest or bottom horizontal graticule. The voltage-divider output is connected to the red or + vertical input terminal and the negative battery terminal to the black vertical input. The spot appears as a vertical line. Adjust the vertical-gain control until this line rises $7\frac{1}{2}$ graticules. This is 0.75 V, and the scope's vertical circuit is now calibrated for direct current. For ac calibration, connect the voltage divider of Fig. 10-26 to the secondary of a 6.3-V filament transformer, as shown in Fig. 10-27.

Now connect the divider output to the scope vertical input (red). This time turn the coarse-frequency sweep control to 50 ms/cm, set the sync selector to line, and adjust the horizontal fine-frequency control so that the 60-Hz sine wave from the filament transformer is perfectly still—no left to right or right to left movement. The voltage divider has

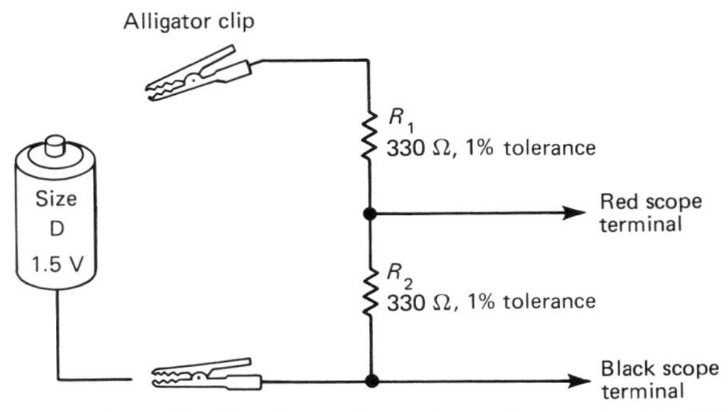

Fig. 10-26 Simple voltage divider that reduces the battery output to 0.75 V across R_2. The oscilloscope vertical axis is then calibrated at 750 mV. The output across R_2 might be connected to additional voltage dividers. Thus vertical calibration could be accomplished at lower levels. A second divider with a dropping resistor, 90 Ω, and voltage taken across 10 Ω would allow calibration at 75 mV. A third divider with the same resistance values would allow calibration at 7.5 mV.

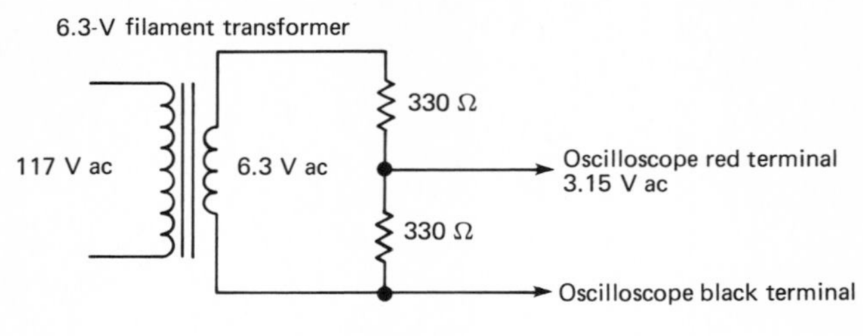

Fig. 10-27 Time base and ac voltage calibrator. AC voltage can be calibrated at 3.15 V. Additional voltage dividers will allow voltage calibration at lower levels. The 60-Hz power-source frequency allows successive ac peaks of 16.66 ms to be seen. These peaks are maintained at an accuracy of better than 0.1 percent.

reduced the 6.3-V rms transformer output to 3.15 V rms; and 3.15 V rms × 1.414 (to obtain peak value) × 2 = 8.9082 V peak value. Now set the vertical-sensitivity control to 10 V/cm (make certain it is on the ac side) and center the sine wave with the vertical-centering control. Adjust the vertical-gain control until the distance from the bottom peak to the top peak is almost 9 graticules, or 8.9082 to be exact. The ac vertical amplifier is now calibrated. More accurate calibration can be achieved using an IC Voltage Standard.

To calibrate the sweep or time base, the same standard (Fig. 10-27) for ac vertical amplitude calibration is used. Set the coarse-frequency control to the 2-ms/cm position. Adjust the horizontal-gain control until the horizontal distance between two positive sine-wave peaks is slightly less than 8½ graticules, or 16.6 ms. If the oscilloscope does not have a 2 ms/cm position, then set the coarse-frequency control to 1 ms/cm. This time, adjust the horizontal-gain control until the horizontal distance between a positive peak and the next negative peak is slightly under 8½ graticules, or 8.3 ms. In the last method only half or 180° of the complete sine wave was the total sine wave.

Our time standard was the 60-Hz frequency regulation provided by the electric power company. Although there is some variation throughout the United States, we can be safe in assuming that our time calibration standard (16.6 ms) is always precise to within a small fraction of 1 ms. This accuracy might cause concern if it were our standard when sending a space probe to the planet Mars, but for biomedical applications it is more than sufficient. To verify the accuracy of the time base for shorter time periods, a high-quality signal generator should be used.

The B&K precision solid-state RF signal generator, Model E200D, is pictured in Fig. 10-28. With its internal crystal calibrator, this instrument will furnish frequency accuracy of better than ±0.05 percent at 100 kHz and 1 MHz. At 100 kHz, the time duration per cycle is 10 μs,

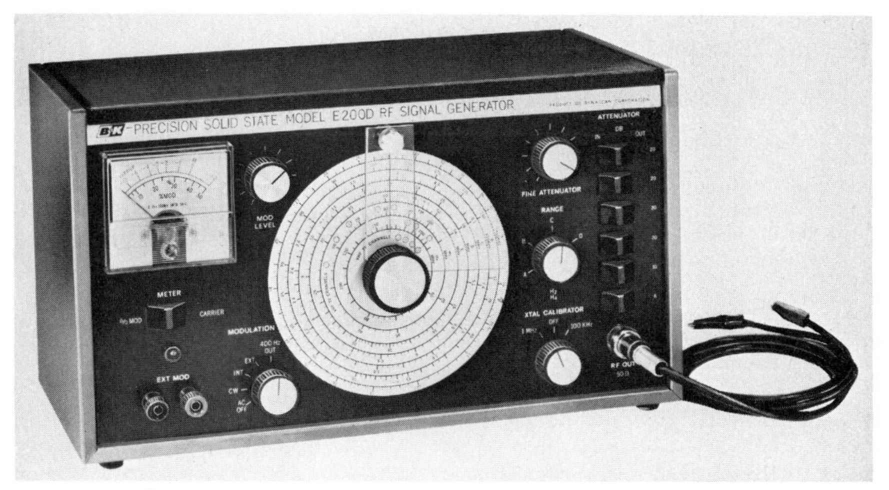

Fig. 10-28 The B & K solid-state signal generator. Stable output is obtained from 100 kHz up to 250 MHz. The attenuator can produce 96 dB of attenuation. Thus this instrument can be fed into medical circuits to determine either gain or loss of an amplifier. The 100-kHz and the 1-MHz crystal calibrators are useful for calibrating a medical instrument or an oscilloscope to an accuracy of 1 μs.

and at 1 MHz, the time duration per cycle is 1 μs. If medical instruments are constantly in use where frequent time calibration is necessary in the 100-μs to 1-ms range, the audio-frequency sine/square-wave generator can be used as a time-base calibrator. Its 1-kHz output will calibrate 1 ms, and its 10 kHz output will calibrate 100 μs.

10-8 NOISE IN TRANSISTORS

It is common to find that noise in biomedical instruments is not being generated externally but rather comes from a noisy transistor in the instrument itself. Starting with the first transistor at the input of the instrument, continue the following test all the way up to the last transistor before the readout. Place a 10-μF capacitor between the base and emitter of the transistor under test. Connect the scope vertical input probe to the collector of the transistor under test, making sure the scope is grounded to the medical instrument ground. A noisy transistor will show up as the very wide pattern of close spikes in Fig. 10-29.

To simplify this procedure, connect the oscilloscope probe across the instrument's output stage (collector to emitter) which drives the readout device. The noisy pattern of Fig. 10-29 should be seen with the instrument's input terminals shorted. Now connect the 10-μF capacitor at the input of that stage (base to emitter). The noisy pattern should disappear, indicating that the noisy transistor (or other component) is

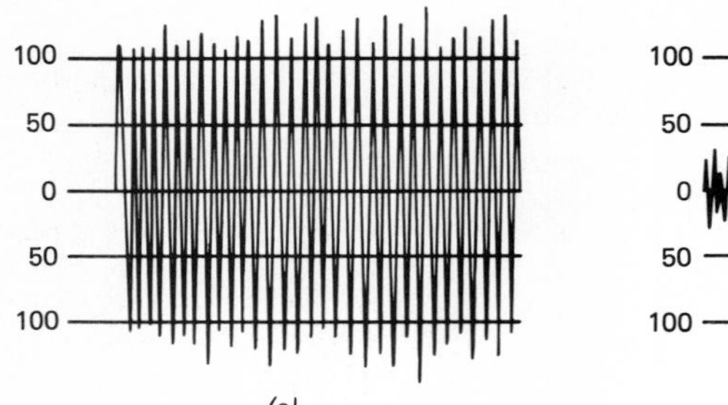

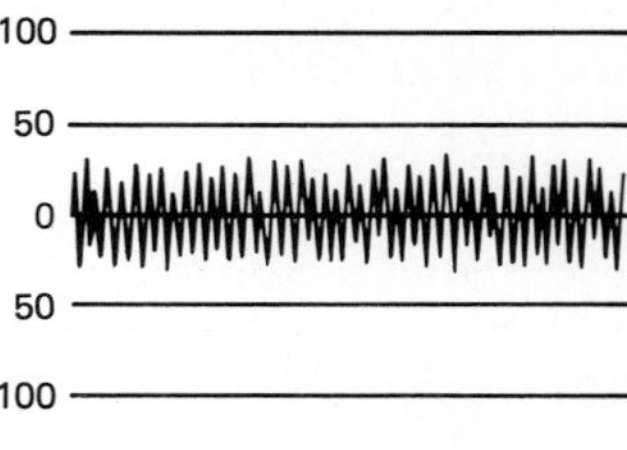

Fig. 10-29 (*a*) Oscilloscope display showing noisy transistor; (*b*) same oscilloscope display after noisy transistor has been replaced. Both oscilloscope vertical scales are calibrated in microvolts.

located prior to our capacitor short. Reconnect the shorting capacitor between the emitter and base of preceding stages, working your way back to the input.

The stage will be reached where the capacitor short does *not* remove the noisy pattern. The capacitor is now connected between base and emitter of the noisy transistor.

QUESTIONS

1. Draw the circuits for both the parallel and the series resonant filter (trap).
2. When using a dipper to measure circuit or coil Q, do you first tune the dipper for maximum or minimum VTVM reading?
3. Using Fig. 10-2, calculate the unknown capacity in picofarads for the following examples. (*a*) Coil *C* is used, and the dipper dips at 5 MHz on its dial. (*b*) Coil *D* is used, and the dipper dips at 7.2 MHz on the dial.
4. If the instrument input is shorted and the interference disappears, would a line-noise detector be used? Explain.
5. How are unwanted oscillations generated in a medical instrument?
6. List at least three functions of oscillators in common medical circuits.
7. What is a parasitic? How are they generated?
8. Describe one method of eliminating parasitics.
9. How would an AM pocket radio be used as a probe for circuit-noise detection?
10. Describe the procedure to be used to test an ultrasonic transducer with the dipper.
11. What are three methods for measuring the frequency response of an instrument?
12. When you are using the square-wave frequency-response method, a 30-Hz square wave appears on the scope without distortion. Calculate the lower- and upper-frequency response of the medical instrument.
13. The magnitude of ground loop current is directly proportional to the voltage difference __________.
14. What is the first test to determine the presence of ground loop currents in an instrument system?
15. What type of dc amplifier could be used with all types of signal sources?

16. When the single-ended grounded amplifier is operated with a single-ended grounded signal source, what precaution should be taken?
17. Can a single-ended grounded amplifier be used for low-level medical applications? Explain your answer.
18. If you had a balanced grounded signal source, what type of amplifier would you use?
19. Once the correct amplifier has been installed in Question 18, what possible problem could develop?
20. What is the time interval between two positive sine-wave peaks of the ac power source as seen on an oscilloscope? Why is this time interval a reliable tool for calibration of an oscilloscope time base?

LCXf NOMOGRAPH

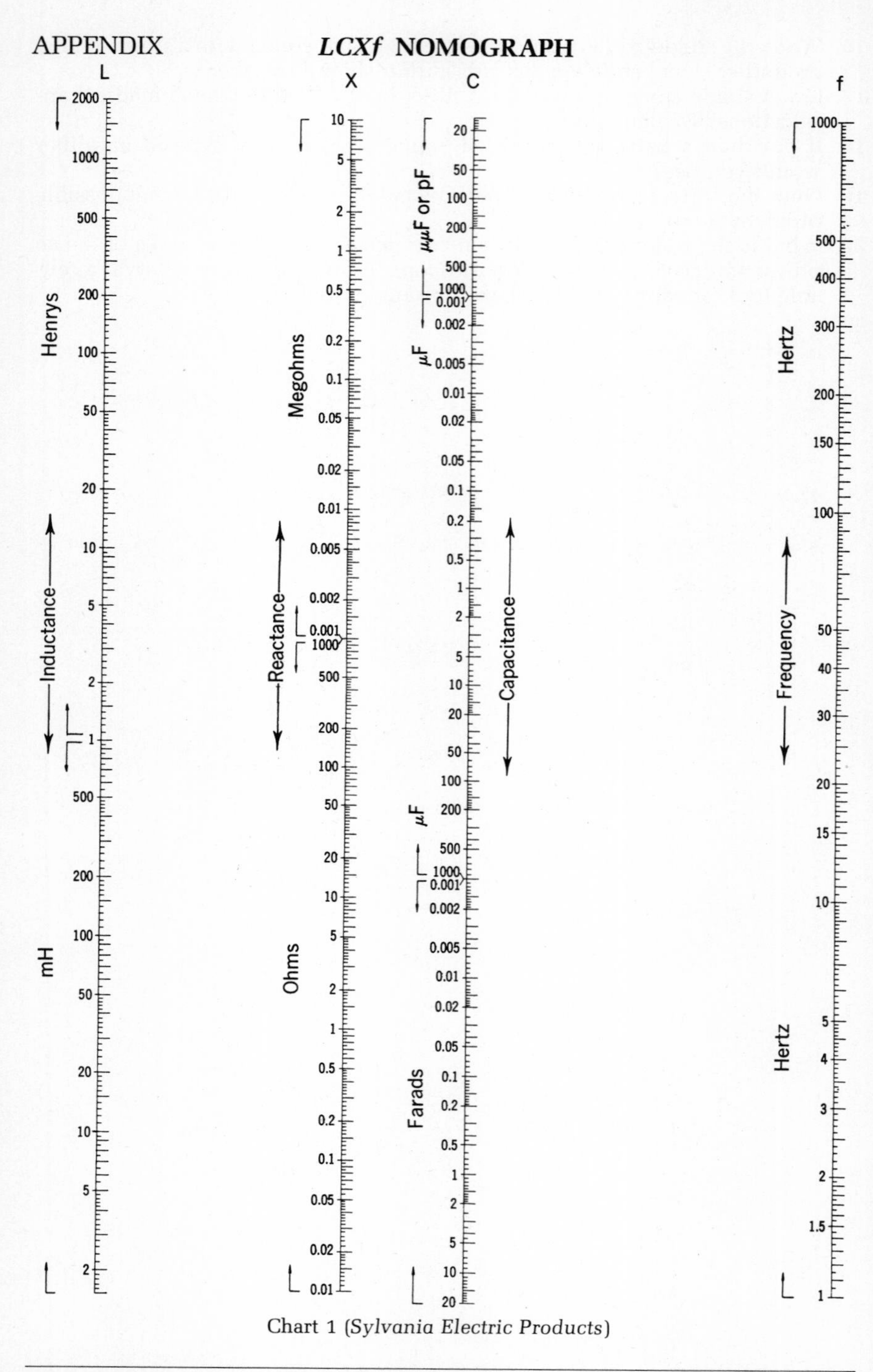

Chart 1 (*Sylvania Electric Products*)

LCXf NOMOGRAPH (continued)

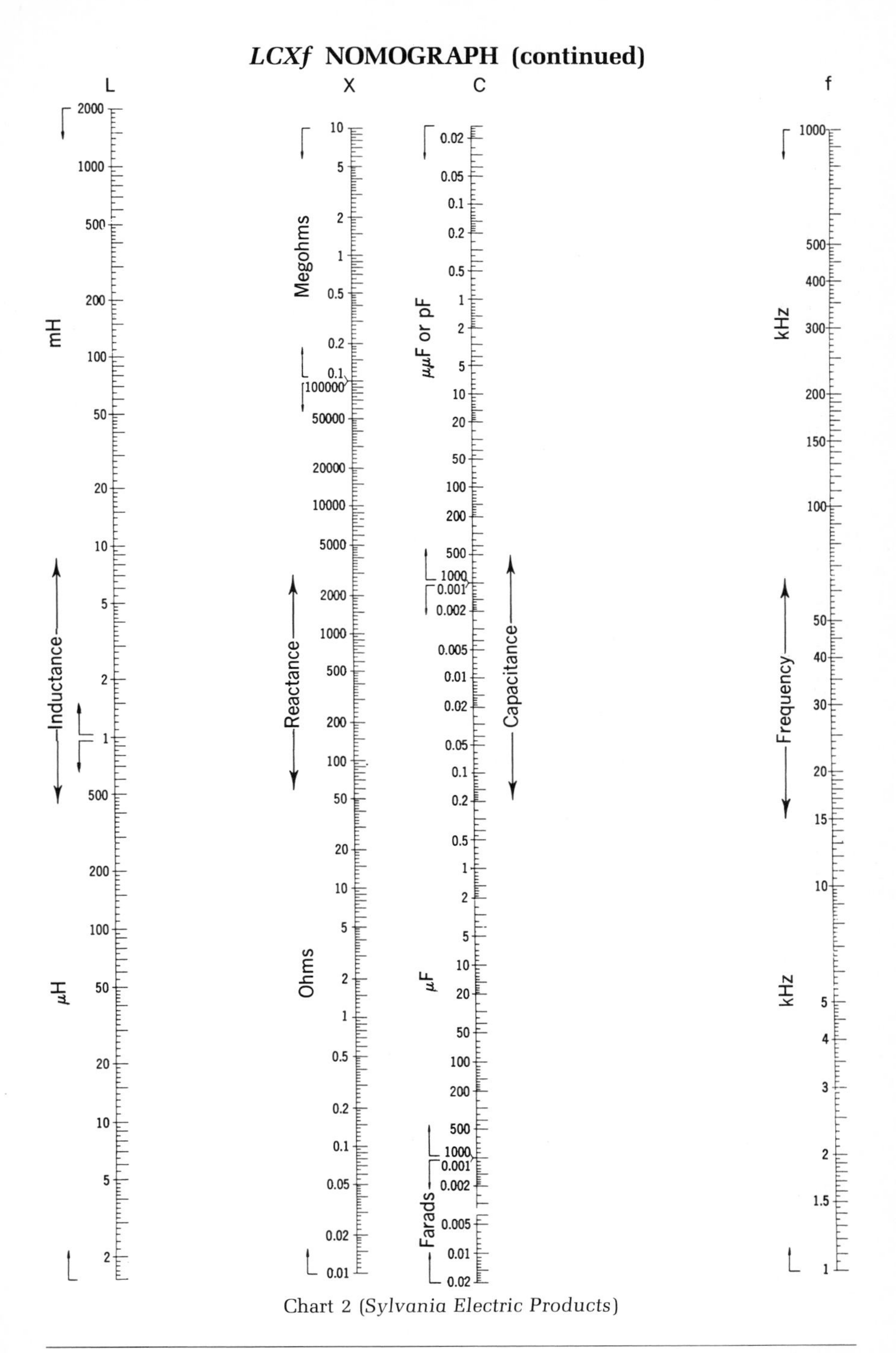

Chart 2 (*Sylvania Electric Products*)

LCXf NOMOGRAPH (continued)

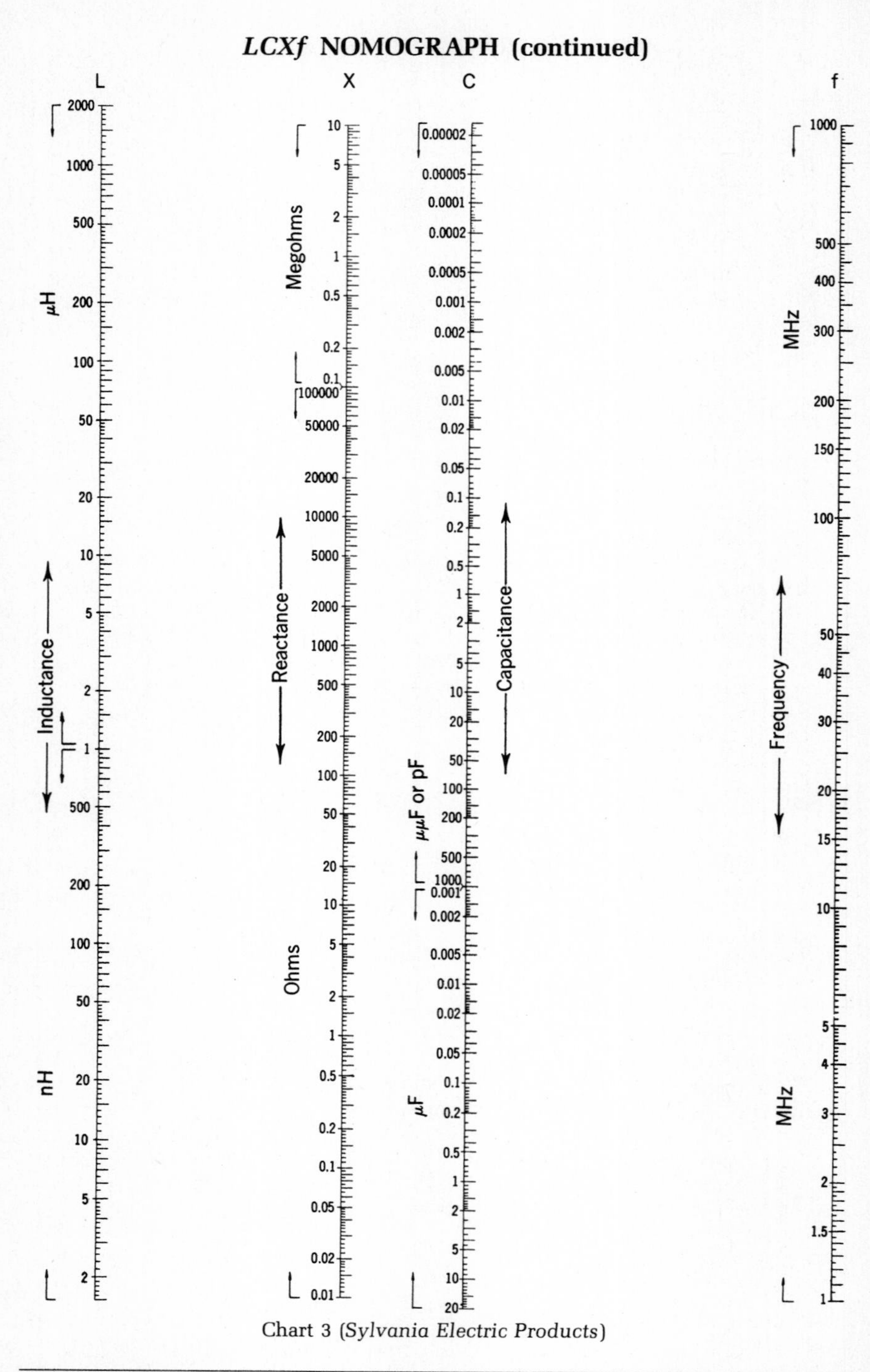

Chart 3 (*Sylvania Electric Products*)

Answers

CHAPTER 1

1. Molecule.
2. False.
3. Oxygen.
4. Ionized.
5. They are charge carriers, conducting electric charges through both majority and minority carriers. Majority carriers may be sodium, chlorine, or potassium ions in large concentrations. These carriers are extremely mobile. Nature seeks to balance the concentration gradient this way.
6. Only hydrogen.
7. Ion concentration in the calibrated-buffer solution becomes the reference. The test solution outside (unknown ion concentration) is then compared to this buffer reference.
8. The cell.
9. Osmosis.
10. Osmoreceptors.
11. CO_2 and O_2.
12. The voltage difference is 65 mV.
13. Potassium. Sodium. Chloride.
14. Mitochondria is the cell's energy plant.
15. Positive. Negative.
16. These tissues oxidize oxygen.
17. Both higher temperature and the larger diameter will cause the electric signals to speed up.
18. At the nerve's critical level, the fiber is triggered into total response. Prior to reaching this level, (submaximal) fibers are not excited.
19. Ganglion cells.
20. These fibrillation potentials would indicate that the muscle cell membrane is unstable. It might reveal denervation, where the muscle's nerve is not supplying the muscle properly. Then the muscle would become abnormally active electrically. Spinal shock, electrolyte unbalance, or an inflammatory process might also be the cause of this activity.

CHAPTER 2

1. Violent muscle contraction upon electrical stimulation or the natural reaction to painful stimuli.

2. Ground.
3. A tingling sensation.
4. Ventricular fibrillation.
5. Ventricular fibrillation.
6. The fibrillation threshold for direct current is higher than for alternating current.
7. Hemorrhagic lesions of the mitral valve and ventricular fibrillation.
8. The magnetic field of an electric motor, auto ignition system, cautery, diathermy, microwave ovens.
9. Over 10 s can cause a fatality.
10. When there is a ground fault.
11. An ac voltage could exist on the bed frame because of capacitive coupling between the bed frame and the primary wiring in the bed.
12. Using the lowest-resistance scale (0 to 1 Ω) of a VTVM, FET-VOM, etc., measure the resistance between the instrument case and the power-cord ground pin.
13. False. A reading above 0.1 Ω indicates a hot case; excessive leakage currents exist between the hot case and the ground.
14. On the contrary, voltages between different grounds are common. They are caused by leakage currents, noise, inductive pickup, etc.
15. Before the circuit breaker opened, $\frac{1}{10,000}$ of the fault current of 15 A would flow, or 1.5 mA.
16. Common ground point connects all grounds together with heavy-gage (6 to 8) wire. The subground point should be as close as possible to the patient.

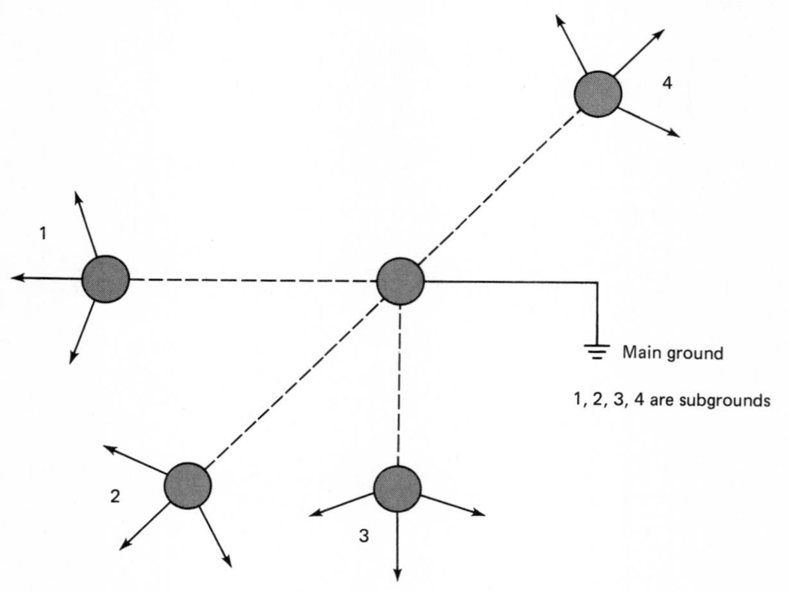

17. Yes.
18. Solder the connection, secure with heavy copper lugs, and use only noncorrosive hardware.
19. A 12 by 12 ft copper screen centered under the operating table will reduce ac interference considerably.

20. A line isolation monitor is connected to an impedence threshold detector which continuously observes the impedance between power line and ground. When this impedence drops below a set figure (60,000 Ω), an alarm sounds. At the same time, the circuit will trip.

CHAPTER 3

1. Gauze soaked in saline solution will cause an electrode-tissue resistance change due to evaporation.
2. pH of 7. This is ideal to ensure stability.
3. No. The problem should be solved in another way, as the shielded leads will attenuate and degrade fast pulses.
4. No. Surface electrodes will totalize the activity of many millions of cells. Use needle electrodes.
5. Zinc, stainless steel, tungsten, or platinum alloy.
6. Copper and silver.
7. False. The high capacitance degrades fast pulses.
8. No. The ohmmeter voltage may damage the fragile transducer crystal.
9. It has a wider dynamic range than other transducers.
10. Strain-gage transducer.
11. Strain-gage transducer.
12. R_4 must be 125 Ω for V to be zero and the bridge to be balanced.
13. Strain-gage resistance changes are translated into a variable-voltage output (or zero-voltage output) because the bridge is excited by a known, highly regulated voltage.
14. Quartz and other crystalline materials convert mechanical strain into an electric output (voltage). Thus physiological pressure is changed to a voltage and then amplified.
15. In manufacturing a crystal, the frequency-determining factors are how the crystal is cut, the dimension of the plate, and the kind of crystal material.
16. False. The resonant crystal has a high Q; thus it is far more efficient at a particular frequency.
17. The arterial blood-flow pattern will be changed by constriction. A reduction of the mean flow may result.
18. The length of the exposed vessel, the space around the vessel, proximity of adjacent organs, the depth of the vessel.
19. $E = (MLV) \times 10^{-8} = (1100) \times 10^{-8} = 0.000011 \text{ V} = 11\ \mu\text{V}$.
20. Total darkness resistance should be very high, over 1 MΩ. Resistance under strong light should be approximately 10 to 20 Ω.

CHAPTER 4

1. Most ECG amplifiers have a high-frequency response up to approximately 30 Hz. The 60-Hz interference is above the instrument's frequency response. Thus what does appear on the display is so badly attenuated and distorted that it appears as noise (high frequency) would on an audio amplifier.
2. 5 μV, 20 μV, 2 μV, 0.3 μV.
3. Perpendicular to, or at right angles to.
4. $F = NI = 87 \text{ turns} \times 5.2 \text{ A} = 452.4 \text{ maxwells}$

5. Spreading the loop should increase magnetic interference. Also, changing the loop's plane would change the amplitude of magnetic interference.
6. By twisting the wires together.
7. Shielded patient leads. Also capacitance between shield and conductor.
8. Impedance from both leads to ground is seldom equal, as least-resistance currents from one lead to ground will be greater than the other. This imbalance then creates a differential voltage (interference) between the two inputs.
9. $Z = (20 \times 10^{-9}\ \text{A}) \times 5000\ \Omega$
   $= 0.02 \times 5000 = 100\ \mu\text{V}$
10. Ground the object or person located between the instrument and the source; increase the size of the electrode area.
11. An unbalanced ground might result.
12. Look for a ground fault in one of the instruments in the system.
13. These devices convert a high input Z into a low Z, thus making any lead imbalance negligible.
14. False.
15. Active filter.
16. Active filters need a power supply. Also they might introduce noise into the circuit.
17. Low-pass, high-pass, bandpass, band-reject, and notch filter.
18. No. As can be seen in Fig. 4-17, this would create excessive phase and magnitude distortion.
19. With a high-Q filter, the rate of decay of the ringing increases (see Fig. 4-19). High Q also makes the filter extremely sensitive to parameter variations such as drift.
20. The TV interference disappears when the input terminals are shorted. Thus, the interference is picked up through the patient leads. We would determine the wavelength of the interfering signal. Then construct or purchase RF filters (wavetraps) to be inserted in each patient lead to tune out the TV signal. See X and Y in Fig. 4-28.

CHAPTER 5

1. A linear displacement voltage to develop position and a voltage from a velocity transducer which corresponds to velocity.
2. Frequency compensation automatically adjusts recorder frequency response to be flat up to 30 Hz for 100-mm pen deflection and up to 50 Hz for 50-mm pen deflection. This circuit also changes amplifier gain according to the pen motor used.
3. The position-feedback signal is obtained from a Wien-bridge oscillator. A demodulator attenuates this carrier and provides the position-feedback signal, which is then fed to the servocontrol amplifier.
4. High speed and high resolution permit a high sampling rate.
5. The commutator sequentially scans all selected input channels, connecting them to a common signal line (see Fig. 5-3).
6. Mode selector.
7. True.
8. An output (pen deflection) which is directly proportional to the input and to the pen-motor current. Equal increments of input signal should cause equal increments of changes in the trace.
9. Full-scale deflection.

10. Slope-based nonlinearity.
11. Using a variable-voltage source and an accurate digital voltmeter to calibrate this source, test to determine how closely equal input-voltage increments cause equal increments of pen motion. This should be done at all points along the channel.
12. Pen-motor coil.
13. The feedback loop compensates for nonlinearities in various circuits and can maintain system linearities of $\pm\frac{1}{4}$ percent down to ± 0.1 percent of full scale.
14. A feedback loop can be extended to the input side of the drive amplifier and also to the pen-motor circuit to cancel magnetic field nonlinearities.
15. The time base and the amplitude are fixed.
16. Data can be squeezed, stretched, elongated, and shortened; it is alive. A higher-frequency response than that achieved with a chart recording is possible.
17. No. The fast pulse would be gone before it could be studied.
18. Advantage: It will "freeze" the nonrecurring fast pulse so that it can be studied. Disadvantage: To successfully "freeze" data, the storage scope must be activated at the very instant the elusive transient appears. This is difficult to accomplish.
19. This feature allows the capture of a transient pulse after it has passed, even though the recorder has not been programmed to capture that particular type of pulse. When a trigger is not available to signal the approach of the desired data, pretrigger recording still permits the elusive transient to be captured.
20. The minimum sampling rate would be 240 Hz. Too low a sampling rate would eliminate much of the detail, possibly to the extent that the signal obtained would bear little or no resemblance to the input signal.

CHAPTER 6

1. This theory states that the acoustic impedance mismatch of a physical junction between two homogeneous media determines the reflection coefficient of ultrasonic radiation.
2. Most dense: muscle, blood, kidney; least dense: liver, brain, fat.
3. The higher the absorption coefficient, the more ultrasonic energy is converted into heat; thus, according to declining absorption coefficient, muscle, kidney, liver, brain, fat, blood.
4. The angle of incidence should be oblique or as small as possible.
5. The reflected wave is higher in frequency. As there are now more cycles per second, the wave has been compressed. Wave compression occurs when the reflector is moving toward the source.
6. $$F_c = \frac{\text{velocity} \times \text{frequency}}{\text{speed of sound}}$$
$$= \frac{0.1\ (800{,}000)}{1088\ \text{ft/s}}$$
$$= \frac{80{,}000}{1088\ \text{ft/s}} \approx 73\ \text{Hz}$$
7. Although its reflectance is low, the high velocity of blood will produce sufficient Doppler shift to make it a good reflecting medium.

8. $F_d = \frac{2 \times \text{blood-flow speed}}{1088 \text{ ft/s}} (1 \text{ MHz})(\sin 41.3°)$

$= \frac{0.02 \text{ s}}{1088 \text{ ft/s}} (660{,}000)$

$= 0.000\,018(660{,}000)$

$= 11.88 \text{ Hz}$

9. We would specify that the operational system focus on only highly selected, critical data as compared to an experimental system, which must provide a broad spectrum of data. In the operational system, the computation and collection of massive amounts of data is secondary in importance as compared to the method of data presentation. Data in the operational system must be presented in a manner that facilitates fast, correct decisions.
10. (*a*) Yes; (*b*) yes; (*c*) no.
11. P_C or $P_S = \frac{1}{2} C^2 = \frac{1}{2} (64) = 32$ W
12. In pulse modulation, either the duration, amplitude, or time position of pulses may be varied to provide data.
13. In a frequency-division system, if frequency components of one channel fall within a second channel, crosstalk will result. Subcarrier 2 was the second harmonic of subcarrier 1, and subcarrier 3 was the second harmonic of subcarrier 2. Operation of transistors in their nonlinear region further strengthens harmonic activity. The receiver with its limited selectivity could not discriminate against the already serious crosstalk situation; thus channels 2 and 3 contained many data from other channels and the three-channel system could only be used on one channel.
14. This circuit in a telemetry transmitter discriminates against the large-amplitude, short-duration pulses of a pacemaker while leaving cardiac input data unaffected.
15. $\frac{200 \text{ mA}}{0.675 \text{ mA}} = 296$ h or $12\frac{1}{3}$ days
16. (*a*) False; (*b*) false; (*c*) false; (*d*) true; (*e*) false.
17. Converts the high-frequency or intermediate-frequency receiver signal into the original biomedical modulating voltage.
18. Eight demodulators and eight subcarriers would be required.
19. High cost, low modulation sensitivity, crosstalk between channels, filter circuitry required to reduce crosstalk.
20. (*a*) False; (*b*) false; (*c*) false; (*d*) false; (*e*) false.

CHAPTER 7

1. The clock.
2. Establishes the computer's pulse rate and keeps the computer's operation on schedule.
3. In this case we would use a sequential or serial data format.
4. The parity bit would verify that the number of pulses is correct.
5. Execution time is the length of time required to address a particular location in the memory.
6. Sequential; high.
7. Source.
8. A set of instructions which performs a part of the main program.

9. A 16-bit MP. An MP with a shorter bit length would require additional instruction sets.
10. Define the problem to be solved, describe the input parameters to be processed, decide what processing is required, decide the details of the output to be produced.
11. A decision table.
12. To evaluate both the advantages and the value of the various instruction formats and to choose the best instruction for a particular task.
13. Governs the sequence of the program and holds the address of the next instruction to be taken from the program's memory space.
14. The operating code.
15. (*b*), (*a*), (*c*).
16. A 16-bit (word) MP.
17. Several independent data and address buses.
18. Low power consumption; isolation between different elements within the same gate; many more gates for the same size; greater density; and smaller chip size.
19. LSI is faster and more flexible than MOS technology.
20. Consideration of a new purchase should take into account gate complexity, power consumption, propagation delay (speed), type of programming available, availability of PROM, type of readout, second sourcing, and number of power supplies required.

CHAPTER 8

1. 12.12 V.
2. 82.4 V.
3. Output; reference.
4. No. Oscillators that deliver such large voltages directly cannot be made to produce high stability against load or line variations. We would have to design an oscillator (5000 V or under) and use diode-capacitor multiplier sections to build up the output voltage to 400,000 V.
5. CMRR equals 480.
6. With a CMRR of 10,000, a 1-μV signal will give the same output as the 10-mV interfering signal. Thus a 2-μV signal at minimum is needed to make our system function.
7. As large as possible. If this resistance were close to infinity, common-mode gain would ideally be zero.
8. The constant-current source artificially creates an infinitely high common-emitter resistance, looking into the constant-current source output or the collector circuit.
9. Cascading (adding additional stages) increases both the gain and the CMRR.
10. Equal; 180° out of phase.
11. It is true that a low impedance does not pick up stray interference. However, to eliminate current flow from the input terminals through the patient and to increase sensitivity, the highest input impedance possible is required.
12. (*b*).
13. (*c*).
14. (*c*).
15. (*c*).

16. Feedback returning to the transistor base is determined by the charging rate of C_1. Also, R_1 determines the oscillator base bias. Together, they form an RC circuit with a given time constant; $RC = T$.
17. 1 MΩ.
18. 120 pulses per minute.
19. The capacitance of both C_1 and C_2 will change according to the voltage (biological signal) impressed across them. C_1 is connected from the top of the oscillator tank coil to the neutral center tap, while C_2 is connected from the bottom of the tank coil to the neutral center tap. Thus both varactors are series-connected across the entire tank coil. A voltage that raises the capacity of C_1 also raises the capacity of C_2, increasing the voltage-capacitance coefficient. C_1 and C_2 now constitute the variable C in the LC resonant circuit that tunes the oscillator.
20. Figure 8-10*c*: A differential voltage between the base and the varactor is amplified at the collector, changing Q_1 current and changing capacity across the entire tank. As changing varactor C is in series with C_2, it tunes the tank from the center tap to ground. Figure 8-10*d*: The crystal frequency is "rubberized" by the varactor. C_1 changes the resonant frequency of C_1 and L_2. This effectively detunes the crystal's natural frequency, creating phase or frequency modulation.
21. (*b*) A discriminator.

CHAPTER 9

1. Test all power-supply voltages to determine if they correspond to those listed in the maintenance manual.
2. Replace the signal source with a sine/square-wave generator. Starting with the last stage before the readout device, connect the generator and check the readout device for an indication of output from the generator. If generator output is observed, go to the previous stage and repeat this test. In the process of moving the generator (signal replacement) back toward the input of the instrument, the defective stage will be located.
3. AC current gain.
4. False. It is the reverse.
5. The voltage divider R_1, R_2 places the base 0.5 V above ground. With 100-mA collector current (emitter current-collector-base current), R_3 has a 0.2-V drop. Thus the total base-emitter bias is 0.7 V.
6. Normal collector current (100 mA) should have created a 0.2-V drop across R_3. However, the 2-V drop indicates 1 A is flowing in the collector circuit. This 10-fold increase would reveal a collector-emitter short in Q_1.
7. All connected lines would read low.
8. I_{ceo} or leakage current.
9. The collector-base junction has the highest impedance; thus the same leakage becomes more critical here than at a lower-impedance junction. Also the transistor's gain is most dependent on this junction. I_{CBO} amplification is most affected, and the operating or Q point changes drastically.
10. This will have the same effect as locking the IC output in the low state, or blocking the signal flow.
11. Power-supply current drain or malfunction may occur, as there is no way for an accumulated charge to drain. A static bias could create a "bad" signal level.

12. This is bad advice. Both the power source and the drive circuits must be turned off when CMOS ICs are replaced. If these precautions are not taken, the input-protection networks and gates of CMOS devices could be damaged.
13. False. Digital circuits use integrated circuits. Individual components are no longer accessible. The complete circuit function must be tested.
14. High, low, and the undefined or in-between level.
15. High, low, low, undefined, high.
16. Failures caused by internal breakdown within the IC and failures caused by breakdown external to the IC.
17. (*c*) An open signal path to an IC is external to the IC itself. All the other failures occur inside the IC.
18. All inputs driven by that output will float to a static high level.
19. In the high state.
20. A high state will exist at the IC output.

CHAPTER 10

1.

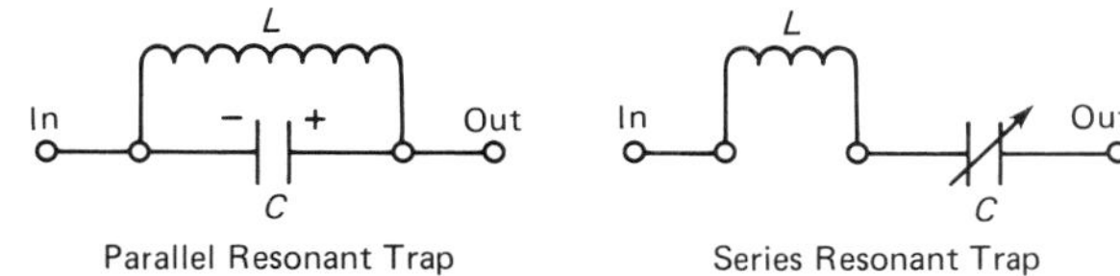

Parallel Resonant Trap   Series Resonant Trap

2. First tune the dipper for a maximum VTVM reading.
3. (*a*) 90 pF; (*b*) 170 pF.
4. No, a line-noise detector would not be used, as the interference is coming through the instrument's input terminals.
5. Unwanted oscillations are generated through the internal inductance and stray capacitance of switching devices, such as rectifiers and diodes. Resonant circuits form as these components age. High impedances create feedback paths and generate oscillations.
6. Oscillators are used as calibration markers, time-base generators, delay signals, pulse generators, etc.
7. As the Q of resonant components deteriorates, as bypass capacitors age, as new *LC* circuits are formed, parasitics develop. These unwanted oscillations are sometimes frequency-related to desired oscillations.
8. Clean coils and capacitors with an air gun. Test for leaky bypass and coupling capacitors, and for resistors which have changed value.
9. Move a pocket radio along different parts of the circuit. With volume at maximum, listen for "hash" (noise) at the bottom and then at the top end of the broadcast dial.
10. Connect a coupling coil to the transducer under test. This coil fits over the dipper coil. Rotate the dipper dial near the transducer frequency until a sharp dip indicates that the transducer is functioning properly.
11. (1) Variable-frequency generator feeds the instrument and a VTVM measures frequency response. (2) Low-frequency sweep generator used with spectrum analyzer. (3) Square-wave generator feeds the instrument; output is seen on oscilloscope.
12. Low-frequency response: 30 Hz/50 = 0.6 Hz
    Upper- (high-) frequency response: 30 Hz × 50 = 1500 Hz

13. Between two different grounds.
14. First check for excessive ac interference in any instrument in the system.
15. The balanced, or floating, or guarded amplifier.
16. Remove one of the signal-source grounds.
17. No. A single-ended grounded amplifier has no common-mode rejection. Noise and interference would become a serious problem.
18. A balanced-to-ground amplifier should be used.
19. Even though the balanced-to-ground amplifier has been installed, a voltage difference between the signal-source ground and the amplifier ground might exist. This would create a common-mode voltage and cause ac interference (see Fig. 10-16).
20. The peak-to-peak time interval for one cycle of 60 Hz has a period of 0.0166 s. This is equivalent to 16.6 ms. The electric power utilities maintain control of this frequency to a tolerance of 0.1 percent. The 16.6-ms power-source sine wave could then be trusted to be better than 16.6 μs in accuracy.

Index